Men's Health and Wellness for the New Millennium

Men's Health and Wellness for the New Millennium

Valiere Alcena M.D., F.A.C.P.

iUniverse, Inc.
New York Lincoln Shanghai

Men's Health and Wellness for the New Millennium

iUniverse books may be ordered through booksellers or by contacting:

iUniverse
2021 Pine Lake Road, Suite 100
Lincoln, NE 68512
www.iuniverse.com
1-800-Authors (1-800-288-4677)

Because of the dynamic nature of the Internet, any Web addresses or links contained in this book may have changed since publication and may no longer be valid.

The information, ideas, and suggestions in this book are not intended as a substitute for professional medical advice. Before following any suggestions contained in this book, you should consult your personal physician. Neither the author nor the publisher shall be liable or responsible for any loss or damage allegedly arising as a consequence of your use or application of any information or suggestions in this book.

ISBN: 978-0-595-45782-3 (pbk)
ISBN: 978-0-595-69676-5 (cloth)
ISBN: 978-0-595-90084-8 (ebk)

Printed in the United States of America

Contents

Acknowledgments

I would like to thank Sabina Ivanova for providing me with technical computer help during the writing of the book.

I would like to thank my children and grandchildren for their love and supports during the writing of this book.

Preface

This book is written to catalog some of the many medical conditions that some men suffer from. Many men suffer from diseases such as Diabetes Mellitus type I&II, Hypertension, Heart diseases, Cancer, High cholesterol, Obesity, Stroke, Enlarged prostate, Erectile dysfunction, COPD/Emphysema, Asthma, Peripheral Vascular Disease, Glaucoma, Osteoarthritis, Osteoporosis/Osteopenia, and Anemia etc and some of these men wait too late to seek medical attention.

This book explains some of the reasons why these diseases occur, how to evaluate them and how to best treat them.

The book is written in an easily readable and understandable manner so that anyone can understand the materials it contain.

Introduction

The health care industry in the United State of America is in crisis. The US health care industry is among the biggest industries in the US. It is a two trillion dollar annual industry and yet it is the most inefficient when compared to other health care industry in several other industrial countries in the world. There are 47 million uninsured people in the US. The life span in the US is 76 years and ranked 45th in the world. Infant mortality in the US is higher than some developing countries. The Health Maintenance Organizations (HMO) controlled the health Care delivery system in the US. They have kidnapped it under false pretense and they are not about to release their grip from its financial throat. Over 93% of employed people in the US are forced to be part of an HMO and they are given no alternatives. The HMO'S have a parasitic relationship with working men and women in the US and with physicians and all other health care providers Most HMO's executives have a cozy relationship with the head of many Industries in the US. HMOs are in it strictly for the money plain and simple. They have **Zero interest in quality care. It is a" managed cost" financial philosophy and not manage care philosophy.** There are many recent examples of how greed drives some health providers. Some doctor do unnecessary tests and give medications to patients for their own financial benefit. In 2004, some for profit dialysis centers is said to have billed the government 1.8 billion dollars for providing Epogen/Procrit injections to dialysis patients unnecessarily which raised their hematocrit above 36% causing some of these patients to have stroke and heart attack. Source: JAMA, April 18, 2007-Vol 297, No 15 The fact the hematocrit of these patients was raised above 36% causing some to have strokes and heart attacks apparently did not matter to these doctors (some nephrologists). Another example is the one that shows that some doctors (some Cardiologists) placed (PCI) Stents in the coronary arteries of some patients with stable angina. The report shows that treating these patients conservatively with medications would have been just as efficacious and less costly. Source: Circulation. 2005; 111:2906–2912.

The health care system is burdened with punitive regulations and yet 100.000 patients die because of medication errors every year in the US ...

The Brand drug business is about 325 billion dollars per year in the US and the Generic Drug business is somewhere in the neighborhood of 25 billion dollars per year. Generic drugs have many potential pitfalls; the most glaring is the fact that it is totally uncontrolled and people have no idea where these medications are made, how they are made and in what countries they are made. The pharmacists are pushing doctors to prescribe the Generic drugs because they made huge profits selling them. The pharmacists buy the generic medications from countries where there is no control as to what are in these medications and no one knows how safe they are. Now both the HMOs and the government have gotten involved in the mess by forcing doctors to prescribe these medications to patients for the sake of saving money that goes into the bank account of the HMO's ... Many state governments in the US are in bed with the HMOs as partners because they have contracted out their Medicaid programs to the HMOs to manage at the expense of the poor in their states. The lobbies for the HMO's control many politicians at all levels of governments in the US and because of that, the health care system in the US is likely to remain under the control of the HMO's for years to come.

The only real solution to this problem is to establish Universal Health Care in the US. Universal Health Care will do away with the "Status Syndrome" in the health care delivery system in the US.

21.5 million men smoke tobacco in the US and tobacco smoking contributes to over 400,000 deaths in the US every year. Obesity is an epidemic in the US. Sixty eight per cent of adults and adolescents are obese/overweight and obesity is associated with diseases such as certain cancers, diabetes, high cholesterol, stroke, hypertension to name a few. Over 440, 000 deaths every year are associated with obesity and its many complications in the US every year. Depression, drug addiction and alcoholism are quite common in men in the US and are discussed in details in the book.

Because of the" **Status Syndrome**", poor men have less access to quality of health care in the US than do men who are rich. Poverty plays a major role in the diseases that poor people are afflicted with. Malnutrition predisposes people to diseases. Poor education predisposes people to diseases. Poor housing predisposes people to diseases. Poor working environment exposes poor people to the development of many diseases that work related. The poorer a .be the victim of disparity in health care which is so prevalent in the US. "An estimated 800,000 lives have been lost due to racial or ethnic health disparities in the past 10 years." Source: **US Department of Health and Human Services. Data 2010. Accessed at www. Healthypeople.gov/ on 17 May 2007.**

Universal Health Care will do away with "The Status Syndrome" in the health care delivery system in the US.

CHAPTER 1

HYPERTENSION IN MEN

HYPERTENSION IS ONE OF THE most common diseases that afflicts men and is a disease that is associated with other diseases such as obesity, diabetes mellitus, and high lipid in the blood.

Worldwide about 1 billion people have hypertension and by 2025 it is said that half a billion more will develop hypertension.

In the US, 72 million individuals have hypertension. Hypertension is more common in blacks than whites, in fact 40 per cent of blacks in the US have hypertension. There are 13.8% blacks in the US, which, translates into 40.2 million blacks, and 16 million of them have hypertension.

The overall prevalence of hypertension in the U.S. population is 72millions or 24%. The prevalence of hypertension in men in the US is 29.4 00,000 or 31.5% of men in the US are hypertensive. 30.6% of white males are hypertensive, 41.8% of black males are hypertensive and 27.8% Mexican American males are hypertensive. The prevalence of hypertension in Hispanics or Latinos is 18.2%. The prevalence of hypertension in Asians is 16.7% and the prevalence of hypertension in American Indians or Alaskan Natives is 21.2%. The total number of deaths attributed to hypertension in the year 2002, was 261,000. The total yearly mortality due to hypertension in the US is 49.700-20.500 of the yearly mortality due to hypertension in the US is in men and 14.700 is in white males and 5.300 is in black males. In 2002, the over death rate from hypertension in the US was 17.1 per 100,000. The actual death rates for white males who died because of hypertension were 14.4 per 100,00 and the death rates for black males who died because of hypertension were 49,6 per 100,00. In 2005, it is estimated that the direct and indirect costs of the treatments of hypertension in the US was be $59.7 billion.

Metabolic Syndrome is frequently associated with essential hypertension in men. In the US an estimated 47 million individuals have Metabolic Syndrome. Metabolic syndrome in men is Obesity (waist circumference greater than 40 inches)
Fasting blood sugar of 110mg/dl or higher
High density lipoprotein (HDL) cholesterol less than 40mg/dl
Blood pressure of 130/85 mm Hg or higher
Serum triglycerides level of 150mg/dl or higher
Mexican Americans have the highest prevalence of Metabolic Syndrome 31.9%. Whites have a prevalence of metabolic syndrome of 23.85, blacks have a Metabolic Syndrome of 21.6%, and those who refer to themselves as others in the US have a prevalence of Metabolic Syndrome of 20.3%. Complications associated with these diseases commonly caused suffering and death of men.

What is hypertension?

Hypertension is when the systolic part of the blood pressure is higher than normal and when the diastolic part of the blood pressure is higher than normal.

What is the systolic part of blood pressure?

The systolic part of the blood pressure is the upper part of the number in the blood pressure reading machine.

What is a normal systolic blood pressure?

A normal systolic blood pressure ranges from 100 to an upper limit of 139.

What is normal diastolic blood pressure?

A normal diastolic blood pressure ranges from 60 to an upper limit of 89.

CLASSIFICATION OF BLOOD PRESSURE IN ADULTS AGE 18 YEARS AND OLDER

Category	Systolic mm/Hg	Diastolic mm/Hg
Normal	100–130	60–85
High Normal	130–139	85–89
Hypertension		
Stage I	140–159	90–99
Stage II	160–170	100–109
Stage III	180–209	110–119
Stage IV	210	120 or greater

(Archives of Internal Medicine, Volume 153, January 1993)

New blood pressure Classifications

Classification	Systolic		Diastolic
Normal	<120	and	<80
Pre-hypertension	120–139	or	80–89
Stage 1	140–159	or	90–99
Stage 2	160+		100+

Source JAMA Volume 289, No 19 May 21, 2003 The JNC-7 Report

What instruments are needed to take the blood pressure?

The instruments that are needed to take the blood pressure are:

1. A blood pressure cuff, which is attached to a manometer on which is listed different numbers—from 20 mm/Hg to 300 mm/Hg.
2. A stethoscope, which is placed on a pulsating artery, most often at the bend of the arm, on the inside part of the arm.

What are some of the pitfalls in taking the blood pressure?

If the cuff is too small, the blood pressure can be falsely high, as much as 10 to 20 mm/Hg systolic or diastolic. If the cuff is too large, the reverse can happen, namely the blood pressure can be too low by as much as 10 to 20 mm/Hg. Make sure the blood pressure cuff is neither too large nor too small.

Both errors can have serious negative impact in the care of a man being treated for hypertension, in that either he can receive too much or too little medication, which in either case can be harmful.

Make sure that the blood pressure cuff is functioning properly, before using it. In particular, check to be sure that the blood pressure cuff is not leaking, because, if it is leaking air, then, it is sure to give a false reading.

Use a small cuff for a man with a small arm, medium-size cuff for a man with a medium-sized arm and a large cuff for a man with a large arm. There are very large cuffs made to suit the needs of very obese men, and as just stated above, using an undersized cuff to take the blood pressure of a man with a very large arm can cause a false reading in the blood pressure of that man.

An example of such a situation is a man with a large arm whose blood pressure reading is 140/90 with an undersized cuff, when in fact the blood pressure is 130/80 when a large blood pressure cuff is used to take him blood pressure. That type of error must be avoided because the man's psyche can be quite seriously affected because he has been told that him pressure is high when in fact the pressure is perfectly normal when it is taken with the proper cuff. When the person applies for life insurance, that particular error can adversely affect him ability to be insured. If insurance is obtained, higher premiums are likely to be charged because of the falsely taken blood pressure.

One should make sure that the stethoscope being used to take the blood pressure is in good working order, because if it is not, that can also cause improper blood pressure readings. Be certain there are no holes in the diaphragm of the stethoscope, which is the bottom part, and check the rubber tubing for holes and cracks. If these problems are found in the stethoscope or the blood pressure machine, do not use them, because air will escape while the doctor is trying to listen to the blood pressure, resulting in false blood pressure readings.

Automatic blood pressure machines are okay, if you know how to use them.

Always take the blood pressure in three positions:

1. When the man is lying down.
2. When the man is sitting down.
3. When the man is standing up for at least 3 to 5 minutes.

Why is it important to take blood pressure in this way?

It is important to take the blood pressure in that way because most active men are either sitting up or standing up most of the time, and they lie down only to sleep at night or to take a nap during the day. Several antihypertensive medications work best when the man is standing up. It is, therefore, important to know what these men's blood pressure readings are when they are standing up, sitting down or lying down. If a man is bleeding or dehydrated, him blood pressure will drop when he is sitting up or standing up as compared to when he is lying down. The pulse rate when the person is sitting up or standing up who has lost a lot of blood or fluid is likely to go up. That is the cause of orthostatic hypotension. That is, the pulse goes up and the blood pressure goes down. The pulse rate going up is a much more sensitive sign of orthostatic hypotension than the blood pressure dropping by itself. Of course, that maneuver depends on the age of the person because the older the individual, the less proper will be the tone within the wall of their vessels. When one stands them up, that can in itself cause the blood pressure to drop. These individuals tend to have what is called a wide pulse pressure and all that has to be taken into consideration when one is talking about volume loss that is either blood or fluid from the body. It takes a minimum of 1200 to 1800 cc of either fluid or blood loss for orthostatic hypotension to occur. Again, it depends on the age and the size of the man, because an older man who has lost between 800 and 1000 cc of either blood or fluid may have him blood pressure drop significantly. That is because a man's intravascular volume becomes contracted as the man ages. Therefore, that statement has to be made in light of knowing the man's size and age. A younger man is more likely to tolerate the loss of 1800 cc of either blood or fluid with only slight evidence of orthostasis, as opposed to an older man who might in fact develop cardiovascular collapse just on the basis of 1800 cc of either blood loss or fluid loss.

Other conditions that can cause an acute drop in blood pressure include:

1. Too much antihypertension medications
2. Acute heart attack
3. Certain abnormal rhythms of the heart, either too fast or too slow a heart rate
4. Severe infection in the blood, such as sepsis
5. Oversensitivity of the carotid bodies, which are located in both sides of the neck, can frequently cause orthostatic hypotension to occur.

Vasovagal reaction can also cause a man's blood pressure to drop. In fact, it can also cause the person to collapse based on certain emotional factors, and so on, as when someone receives bad news such as the loss of a loved one or some other major crisis. These things can cause a person to collapse suddenly because of vasovagal reaction. Also, a vasovagal reaction in an older person with underlying cardiac disease can actually cause him blood pressure to drop when having a bowel movement, by the fact of straining that activates the vaso-vagal reaction mechanism. In addition, acute and severe vomiting with retch-ing can also cause an older individual to collapse because of the activation of the vasovagal reaction mechanism of the human body.

that system just outlined is closely associated with the control of posture in the human body, namely in terms of its proper function, speaking specifically of the carotid body sensitivity. There are many other factors or conditions that can cause a man's blood pressure to drop, which can result in collapse.

It is mandatory and necessary to take blood pressure in the elderly in both arms, and when feasible, lying down, sitting down and standing up as outlined above.

As a man gets older he loses muscle elasticity within the blood vessels, resulting in what is called wide pulse pressure (the term for a large difference between the systolic and diastolic blood pressure), and a drop in blood pressure can occur in the standing position as a natural physical phenomenon in elderly men.

That situation is partly responsible for the higher systolic blood pressure seen frequently in the elderly. Although it is important to treat hypertension in the elderly, it is prudent to make all efforts not to be too aggressive with antihy-pertensive medications in the elderly so as not to cause too great a drop in the systolic blood pressure.

The elderly need the systolic blood pressure to remain in the range of 130 to 140 for proper perfusion to take place in the brain.

As the blood vessels of the veins are stiffened and narrowed due to plaques that occur because of aging, a higher systolic pressure head is needed to push blood to the brain circulation to deliver the necessary oxygen for proper brain functions.

Dropping the systolic blood pressure too low in the elderly can lead to a stroke and that is something that must be avoided. On the other hand if the systolic blood pressure is allowed to remain too high—170 to 180 range, for example—for too long a period of time, the result can be a stroke, a heart attack or congestive heart failure, and possibly death can result.

The root causes of hypertension in men are many, and chief among the causes of hypertension in men are the following:

1.   Salt sensitivity
2.   Salt-rich diet

3. Obesity
4. Stress
5. Genetic component of the salt sensitivity being transferred from the forebears of men in Africa to them who are now living in the New World and also those who are still living in Africa.

Of these causes, salt sensitivity is the most important as the genesis of hypertension in men. Salt sensitivity in men of color is a genetic problem, as just mentioned. The gene responsible for causing salt sensitivity in Blacks originated in Africa. Salt retention in the body of Blacks living under the severest conditions that existed in Africa thousands of years ago, and to some degree still exists today, was necessary for survival, though, hundreds of years ago. Working in the hot sun in the fields of Africa was associated with massive salt loss due to sweating through the skin that existed then and that exists today for those who still have to toil the land under these circumstances in Africa and also in other tropical countries of the world. That massive salt loss leads to water loss, resulting in dehydration. To prevent deaths, which would have been the result of that severe water loss, the body developed a gene, which is located in the kidneys of black people to retain salt in their body, thereby retaining water to preserve life.

Since it is undeniable, that the human race began in Africa, the concept of salt retention in the human body and salt sensitivity being responsible for the genesis of essential hypertension applies to all human beings no matter what ethnicity an individual belongs to. **This most important concept has been confirmed in 2002 by a multi institutional study which was published in the Proceedings of the National Academy of Sciences. It took 18 years to do the study and it shows that the kidneys of American Caucasians, Japanese and Ghanaians contain G protein coupled receptor kinase type 4 in the same amount in all three racial groups and it causes salt retention by the kidney in all of them, hence the basis of essential hypertension was discovered, and it is the same in every human beings.**
source: **Proceedings of the National Academy of Sciences (2002; 99: 3872–3877).**

This lifesaving gene was a necessity in the old world in Africa but is a detriment to health in the New World and results in the disease of hypertension in men. The salt-sensitive gene is extremely strong and highly penetrating. The diet that people like to eat contributes largely to several of the most common diseases that afflict men and women in this country. The interplay of hypertension, diabetes mellitus, obesity and high cholesterol, referred to as metabolic hypertension, or Syndrome X, is quite common in men. All four components of the disease are genetically transmitted. Presently 48.6% of African men are obese in this country. When a black baby starts out in life with that abnormal genetic package, by the time that infant boy grows up into manhood and has to go through all the psychosocial, social and economic stresses to survive in the present world, he is certain to suffer from the adverse effects of the metabolic hypertension. The history of salt sensitivity and secondary fluid retention resulting in elevation of blood pressure did not start thousands of years ago as a disease but rather as a God-given measure, to maintain life and prevent death, as outlined above. Living conditions in ancient Africa thousands of years ago where the human race began, and to a significant extent in present-day Africa, are quite harsh with people working in extremely high temperatures. Under these conditions, the human body loses a lot of salt through the skin and in so doing loses water along with salt through the skin as sweat. Wherever salt goes in the human body, water goes with it. When a person loses salt and too much water with it, the body can become dehydrated quickly. Once the intravascular system is depleted of fluid the body risks being collapsed. It takes between 1800 cc to 2500 cc of fluid lost ordinarily to cause the blood pressure to fall in a 70 kg man or a normal-sized man. Once the kidneys sense that the blood pressure is falling, their normal tendency is to prevent salt from going out of the body in the urine, thereby attempting to maintain the blood pressure in the normal range. Through that mechanism, salt remains in the body and keeps water with it to maintain blood pressure and to prevent the body from collapsing. The kidneys are able to do this because there are special genes that are located in the kidneys that enable them to hold on to salt. All the billions of men who live across the world have to face the fact that they suffer the same fate of salt sensitivity when it comes to the problem of hypertension as do those who are clearly African in appearance. Those who choose not to acknowledge any connection with their African ancestry do so strictly for psychosocial, social and economic reasons only. However, when it comes to the scientific facts, they are clear and obvious, because the African gene is quite penetrating, regardless of the percentage, degree and extent to which one is associated with it from a genetic (DNA) standpoint. It clearly will show up when it comes to certain disease entities that are of a hereditary nature. Men in the New World have largely had the syndrome of salt sensitivity to thank for their existence. That is so because when the original human beings left Africa, they traveled on wooden wharfs on the open sea to come to what is now the new world and one can imagine the adversities they had to overcome, including dealing with the hot sun and storms of different intensities as well as hunger and thirst. Those who survived did so in part because their kidneys were able to hold on to enough salt, which kept some water in their bodies, preventing those who survived from dying because of dehydration. They went on to become the forebears of the human race in the new world, as it exists today. The kidneys of these people contained a gene (known today as G protein coupled receptor kinase-4) which enabled them to hold enough salt in their bodies to hold on to water, which kept them alive. We thank this gene to a great degree for our existence. The immediate forebears of blacks in the new world never would have survived the voyage, the horrible voyage of torture and brutality across the Oceans, to arrive in the Americas and elsewhere. The fact that their kidneys were able to hold on to enough salt and water kept them alive. Those of us who are alive today and refer to ourselves as Blacks and other races or what ever we wish to call ourselves and carry the salt sensitivity gene in our kidneys (and all humans do so to one degree or an other), owe our African ancestors a debt of gratitude for our existence..

Along with all the good qualities that the forebears of men have passed on to them, they also passed on the gene for hypertension. Hypertension and its associated complications have caused and are causing more deaths than any other diseases in men in the United States and worldwide

Blacks and Asians have hereditary low renin hypertension. This form of hypertension is called low renin or high volume hypertension.

Blacks have low renin because the high salt content in their bodies suppresses renin production there by causing the level renin to become low, and Asians have low renin because the high salt diet they eat suppresses renin production there by causing the level of renin to become low.

This is very important clinically because they are certain medications such as beta-blockers and simple angiotensin converting enzyme inhibitors that work to lower blood pressure only when the renin level is high, so prescribing these types of medications to individuals in these two racial groups to lower blood pressure may not work Hypertension causes problems for men because it affects their hearts, their brains, their kidneys and their eyes. These four organs are called end organs. The damage done to men's by hypertension causes atherosclerotic plaques to be deposited within their coronary arteries, resulting frequently in heart attacks and death. Hypertension also causes the heart of men who suffer from it to become enlarged because the heart has to pump against a high load and that high load is the high blood pressure and, over time, the muscles around the heart become atrophied, resulting in enlarged ventricles. Once atrophy sets in, because the heart muscle only has a finite length to which it can be stretched, it can no longer stretch, then it begins to pump ineffectively and the ineffectiveness of the heart muscle reflects in what is referred to as cardiomyopathy with secondary congestive heart failure. At that point, the heart is unable to push the blood away from the ventricles (heart chambers) and the blood/water backs up into the lungs and accumulates as fluid, and then shortness of breath develops. If not treated quickly it can result in what is referred to as pulmonary edema (acute congestive heart failure), and the result of which, when it is not treated quickly and acutely, is immediate death. In the less dramatic way, the enlarged heart sets in and the person suffering from it begins to develop lassitude, inability to walk down the block without stopping several times, inability to sleep at night on one pillow and constant coughing at night. That condition is referred to as nocturnal coughing. All these are signs that the heart is failing. If the person gets to a physician quickly, the condition can be discovered and treatment can be started with appropriate medication to prevent the aforementioned acute condition from occurring.

Another organ that suffers immensely from the effect of hypertension is the kidney. Hypertension damages the kidney, resulting in kidney failure. The way that happens is that the pressure rises within the vessels that run through the substance of the kidneys. All the different tissues of the kidney need blood vessels of different sizes to carry blood and oxygen to them. As the pressure rises within the kidneys, there are structures within the kidneys referred to as glomeruli (the filtering system of the kidneys) and the glomeruli need to be fed blood and oxygen. As the blood pressure rises, these very delicate blood vessels begin to rupture. They are rupturing without the individual realizing that that is occurring. After a while, these vessels rupture and die out and the tissues that they are responsible to bring blood and oxygen to will no longer be there and, because, these areas of the kidneys die. Eventually, the person loses so many glomeruli that the kidneys cannot function properly (renal insufficiency). Once the glomeruli die, the kidneys can fail suddenly. Once the kidneys fail, waste materials accumulate within the body, resulting in swelling of the legs with smelly breath and salty skin, and a condition referred to as chronic renal failure with uremia develops. At that point either peritoneal dialysis or hemodialysis on a chronic basis must be used to clean the blood free of toxic materials to maintain life. If a man is fortunate enough that he can get a kidney transplant, and the transplant succeeds then he can go back to normal kidney function and a normal life. Therefore, high blood pressure that goes untreated can damage the kidney to the point of kidney failure. Typically, the kidneys fail slowly, losing function in a gradual way.

Another organ that is very sensitive to the effects of hypertension is the eye. When the blood pressure rises in the body, the pressure also rises within the vessels in the eyes. The vessels inside the eyes are quite fragile and because they can be damaged easily. The damage that occurs in the vessels inside the eyes cause different degree of leakage to occur inside the eyes. If left untreated, blindness is usually the result. Hypertension is also associated with an increased incidence of glaucoma, a common disease in men and in particular in men of color.

The brain is another organ that suffers the effects of hypertension. Hypertension causes different degrees of damage in the brain. Over time, the effects of elevated pressure cause plaques to develop within small vessels and large vessels of the brain. The damages that occur within the small vessels result in multiple small vessel infarctions. That condition inevitably leads to the condition referred to as multi-infarct syndrome. Multi-infarct syndrome is the most common cause of senility in men in the world (organic brain syndrome). This condition affects hundreds of millions of men in the world over (maybe more than one billion men). This is so common because several hundred millions men suffer from hypertension in the world; most of them are either going untreated or being improperly treated. In the United States there are roughly 65 million individuals who suffer with hypertension, and of that number only about 40 percent seek medical attention, but sadly only about 20 percent get their blood pressure controlled to about 140/90, and 140/90 is not good blood pressure control.

The incidence of hypertension is quite high among men of color. Black men and women of color in general are more prone to the development of early senility due to untreated hypertension or poorly treated hypertension. Elevated blood pressure can cause three different types of major strokes to occur (cerebrovascular accident). The first type of stroke is called ischemic stroke; the second type of stroke is hemorrhagic stroke; and the third type of stroke is embolic stroke. Ischemic stroke occurs because of chronic narrowing of the affected vessel with plaques and/or the rupture of plaques within the affected vessels, resulting in bleeding, with clot formation acutely closing off the vessel, cutting off blood flow, resulting in a stroke. Elevated blood pressure causes hemorrhagic stroke to occur due to chronic damage that takes place affecting the vessels, resulting in acute rupture of those vessels, causing hemorrhage to occur inside the brain. Hypertension-associated embolic stroke can occur because of hypertensive heart disease with enlargement of the heart. This can cause atrial fibrillation to develop, and if the atrial fibrillation remains untreated with anticoagulants such as Heparin or Coumadin to prevent clot formation, then the clot might become dislodged from the atrium to the brain, causing an embolic stroke. Frequently hypertension is intertwined with obesity, diabetes mellitus, and elevated lipids in men. These conditions interplay in a significant percentage of men. Sixty two percent of black American men are obese. Sixty-nine per cent white men are obese. Sixty-five per cent of Hispanic men are obese.

Seventy-three per cent Mexican American men are obese. Thirty-four per cent Asian men are obese and sixty-one per cent American Indians/Alaska Natives are obese.

The over all incidence of elevated cholesterol in men in the USA is fifty per cent.

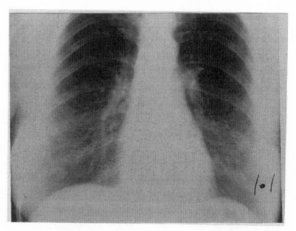

Figure 1.1—Male chest x-ray, normal

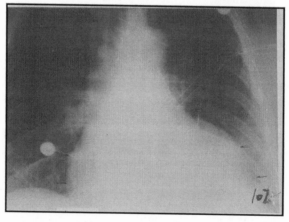

Figure 1.2—An abnormal chest x-ray in a female patient with hypertensive cardiovascular disease, showing heart failure because of chronic hypertension with secondary coronary artery disease, leading to an enlarged heart and heart failure, with arrow showing enlarged border of the right heart and arrows showing enlarged border of the left heart with pleural effusion (fluid in lower left lung).

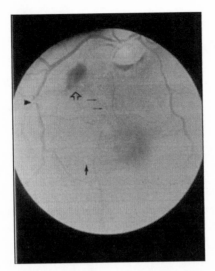

Figure 1.3—*Showing different degrees of abnormalities in the eye of a hypertensive patient (hypertensive retinopathy). Small arrow showing silver wiring; big arrow showing hard yellow exudates; open arrowhead showing hemorrhage; arrowhead showing A-V nicking.*

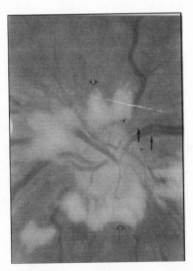

Figure 1.4—*Showing different types of abnormalities in the eye of a hypertensive patient (hypertensive retinopathy). Small arrows showing early papilledema, one big arrow pointing to engorgement of (larger vessel). The other big arrow pointing to arterial attenuation (smaller vessel): open arrowheads showing cotton wool exudates.*

TREATMENT OF HYPERTENSION IN MEN

IF THE BLOOD pressure in a man is 138/88, he is overweight, and he has a family history of hypertension (that is, either his mother or his father has hypertension), then the approach to that upper normal limit of blood pressure is to repeat the blood pressure during an office visit in about one month.

If in the second visit, the blood pressure is again 138/88, and then the treatment is a 2-4 grams sodium, 90 grams protein, 160 grams carbohydrate, 31 grams fat diet per day along with exercise to try to lose the weight and thereby prevent the blood pressure from creeping up even higher.

The usual daily American diet contains an average of 7 grams of sodium. The diet of black American men, Hispanic men and Asian men is likely to contain on the average 10 grams of sodium. That is so because in the case of the black men, they eat a lot of the so-called soul food and other types of salt-rich foods. The salt adds taste to these foods. The same is true for Hispanic men. As for Asian men, they use a lot of soy sauce as part of a cultural habit. White males eat a lot of salt because they consume a lot of fast foods, and these typically are rich in salt and if one is accustomed to eating food that is salty, no matter what type of food one eats one tends to add more salt to it in order to satisfy one's taste for salt. They are many black men, Hispanic men, Mexican American men, Asian Men, American Indian Men/Alaska Native men and poor white men who live under substandard economic conditions exposing them to economic conditions that cause them to eat manyfast foods; because that is the type of foods, they can afford to buy. Fast foods, in general, are of poorer quality. To enhance taste, a lot of fat and salt are added. Therefore, fast foods end up containing much more salt than would normally be the case. The poorer the men the more likely they are to eat a diet of poorer quality. Since the diet is of poor quality, a lot of spices and salt are added in order to enhance the taste and make the foods more palatable. These foods are bad for the human body in particular when eaten on a regular basis. So, when the statement is made that the poorer the individuals, the poorer the quality of foods they eat, that is a statement of fact, because the foods that are of higher quality cost much more money and poor folks are not able to afford them. They can only eat what they can afford to buy. They have many other bills that they have to pay, and many of them have children they have to support, etc., etc.

In the US, the richest country on the planet, about 38 million individuals live on the brink of hunger every day. Even before Hurricane Katrina, 14 millions children were going to bed at night hungry and state in the US with the most people going hungry is Texas according to recent reports.

Worldwide, 800 million people suffer from hunger. Every day 25,000 people die of hunger in the world. A total of 9 million people die yearly because of hunger in the world. Therefore, when people are poor, they eat what ever they can find to stay alive.

The DASH Diet (Dietary Approaches to Stop Hypertension) recommends eating nuts, legumes, seeds, fruits and vegetables four to five times, along with low fat dairy intake. The result shows lowering of both systolic and diastolic blood pressures (Source: *Internal Medicine News*, June 1, 2003). Therefore, adherence to a good diet is very important as both prevention and management of hypertension.

Treatment of high blood pressure should be started early. Once the blood pressure reaches 140/90 in a salt-sensitive man, treatment with medication ought to be started, particularly if the man is obese. The best and most effective medication for hypertension is a water pill (diuretic). It does not matter what the racial make-up of that man is, so long as his kidneys are functioning. Water pills work to control high blood pressure by preventing salt from being reabsorbed by the kidneys back into the blood stream, taking water with it, which results in raising the blood pressure. Some of the common diuretics that are available in the United States are Hydrochlorothiazide, Dyazide, Moduretic, Lozol, Maxzide, Lasix, Bumex, etc. All these medications are effective in removing salt and water from the body. The cost of Hydrochlorothiazide at 25 mg per day is low (30 generic tablets cost $10.00). However, if one were to buy a more expensive medication, the blood pressure would be treated much less effectively (using it as mono-therapy meaning by itself) and yet the man would spend four times more money for that medication. (A good example is Procardia XL 30 mg, which costs $41.00 taken one tablet per day). Another example is Zestril 10 mg (30 tablets cost $33.29), and yet because it is an angiotensin-1-converting enzyme (ACE) inhibitor (meaning that it needs the presence of an elevated level of renin to be effective in bringing down the blood pressure), it does not work at all in people with low renin to treat hypertension. Zestril and other ACE inhibitors such as Capoten, Vasotec, etc. are great medications to treat hypertension when used in some white males who have high renin and in people who are both diabetic and hypertensive to treat micro-albuminemia. These medications are also extremely effective in the treatment of congestive heart failure and certain cardiac arrhythmias.

The mechanism of hypertension in men who have high renin is different from that in men who have low renin. The most effective medications for the treatment of hypertension in men, must contain a thiazide diuretic without regard to race, so long that the men have normally functioning kidneys.

There is a new renin inhibitor approved by the FDA recently to treat hypertension.

The name is Aliskiren (Tekturna) it blocks renin directly to decrease blood pressure.

Water pills work to control high blood pressure by preventing salt from being reabsorbed by the kidneys back into the blood stream, thereby taking water with it, resulting in a decrease in the blood pressure. Here are some of the common diuretics that are available in the Unites States for treatment of hypertension:

1. Hydrochlorothiazide
2. Dyazide
3. Moduretic
4. Lozol
5. Maxzide
6. Lasix
7. Bumex
8. Microzide, etc.

Lasix and Bumex, however, are loop diuretics and they are not really very appropriate for treatment of hypertension, as explained next. All these medications are effective in removing salt and water from the body. There is a substance made by the human kidney called renin. renin, once made by the kidneys, enters into a biochemical reaction leading ultimately to another substance called aldosterone, which causes salt retention leading to water retention, which in turn causes expansion of water within the intravascular compartment, leading to elevation of blood pressure. That system is called the renin angiotensin-aldosterone system. However, black men, Hispanic men, Asian men and some white men have low renin in their blood as a genetic fact. So prescribing medications that work to attack the renin angiotensin system to decrease blood pressure in these men is not very effective. Furthermore, these medications have many side effects and are very expensive. Examples of these medications are beta-blockers, such as Inderal, Lopressor, Tenormin, Toprol XL Coreg, to name a few, and ACE inhibitors such as Capoten, Zestril, Prinivil, Accupril, etc. Beta-blockers are excellent medications for treating angina, migraine headaches, cardiac arrhythmias, congestive heart failure, etc., in people of all ethnic make-ups and work very well in these circumstances. However, they do not work in men who have low renin to decrease blood pressure and should not be prescribed for that purpose in these men. In fact, according to the ASCORT study, beta-blockers do not work to decrease blood pressure in men of any racial background. Therefore should not be used in the routine treatment of hypertension. Some

ACE inhibitors work only slightly to lower blood pressure in men who are salt-sensitive and have low renin, and therefore ought not to be used to treat high blood pressure in these men. However all angiotensin II receptor antagonists (ARBS) work to decrease blood pressure by blocking the renin angiotensin-aldosterone system in all men no matter their ethnic make up. The only situation in which a beta-blocker might have some effect in a salt-sensitive person in controlling hypertension is if the person is under stress and is secreting a lot of adrenalin—the beta-blocker might transiently shut off the sympathetic system in that setting to decrease the blood pressure. However, when a salt-sensitive low-renin-secreting person's kidneys fail and the person develops chronic renal failure, the renin level goes up, and then a beta-blocker becomes a necessity in the treatment of hypertension because the renin level is always elevated in chronic renal failure.

Another situation, in which the beta-blocker might work to decrease blood pressure, even though the man may be classified as salt-sensitive with low renin, is in renovascular hypertension. When plaque or fibrous substances within the vessels obstruct the circulation of the kidneys, then the renin level at that point is elevated. In that circumstance, beta-blockers would work via the renin angiotensin-aldosterone system and the beta-receptors within the kidneys to decrease the blood pressure.

As has been just stated, ACE inhibitors are very good medications in the treatment of the blood pressure in non-salt-sensitive Caucasian males and in the treatment of cardiomyopathy with associated congestive heart failure in all individuals regardless of their ethnic background.

ACE inhibitors can be used with caution in men with chronic renal failure to treat high blood pressure, because in that setting, the renin level is high. The reason for the caution is because ACE inhibitors can cause an increase in the BUN serum potassium, and the elevated serum potassium is a major problem unless the patient is on chronic dialysis, in which case the potassium can be removed during dialysis.

As just mentioned, the second most common form of hypertension in men is renovascular hypertension, which represents about 2%. of the total hypertension population in the US. The cause of Reno vascular hypertension is a blockage or stenosis in an artery carrying blood to the kidney as an individual ages, plaques develop within the blood vessels carrying blood to the kidney. The result is elevation of renin, causing a state of elevated renin level in the blood and secondary elevation in blood pressure. In renovascular hypertension, frequently a sound referred to as a bruit can be heard over the flanks of the patient's abdomen using the stethoscope. However, in a certain percentage of patients with Reno vascular hypertension, a bruit is not heard. In this situation, either the so-called Capoten test or renal angiography has to be done to determine whether renovascular obstruction exists or not.

The most commonly prescribed Angiotensin-Receptor Blockers (ARBS) are:
Cozaar
Diovan
Aceon etc;

The ARBS work to decrease blood pressure by blocking the entire renin-angiotensin pathway and in so doing decrease the production of aldosterone and prevents salt retention.

Medications such as Procardia, Adalat, Verapamil, Cardizem, Norvasc, etc., are called calcium channel blockers. They work to decrease blood pressure by relaxing the smooth muscles inside blood vessels. They are expensive, but they are excellent medications to treat hypertension even in men, when used in combination with water pills. They ought not to be used as monotherapy to treat hypertension in anyone with the slightest trace of African blood running through their veins, or anyone with low-renin-type hypertension, which means several billion people the world over. Alpha-blockers such as Hytrin or Cardura are also good medications and can be used along with water pills to treat hypertension in men. Clonidine in either pill or patch form is a very good medication to use along with water pills to treat hypertension in men. Aldomet and Hydralazine also are very effective medications when used with water pills in men to treat hypertension. Many other medications can be used in combination with water pills to treat hypertensive men. Whenever the kidney senses that, the blood pressure is dropping regardless of the reason why the blood pressure is being brought down it is the kidney's job to hold onto salt in the body to maintain the blood pressure for the safety of the body. This is a physiological phenomenon that occurs in all human beings but this is more so in salt-sensitive individuals such as men of color and Asian men. Men of color and Asian men have low-renin-type hypertension, also referred to as high-volume hypertension, and always be conscious of the amount of salt in their foods. Wherever salt goes, water always goes with it and this is a physiological fact. If an individual is both hypertensive and diabetic, then it is appropriate to prescribe an ACE inhibitor for that person along with any other combination of antihypertensive medications, to a condition called microalbuminuria. (Microalbumin can cause damage to kidney tubules, which can, in turn, lead to kidney failure.) Care must be taken to first document the presence of microalbumin in the urine of hypertensive/diabetic men before prescribing an

ACE inhibitor for his because 75% of diabetics do not have microalbuminuria. Oftentimes, the opponents of the water pill put forth the argument that water pills cause potassium loss in the urine, thereby decreasing the serum potassium level, which can be dangerous. The truth is that a middle-aged or younger adult eats roughly 80 mg of potassium in his or his diet by eating fruits, drinking juice, etc., and that is clearly enough for these individuals to remain in potassium balance. Further, medications such as Moduretic, Dyazide, Maxzide, etc., contain triamterene, which prevents potassium loss in the urine. Still further, potassium chloride can be prescribed by mouth along with the water pills, if on testing the blood, the potassium is found to be low. It is the standard practice to prescribe potassium supplement for any elderly patient on water pills, to prevent low serum potassium. Elderly men frequently eat a diet that contains less than 80 mg of potassium per day. In addition, elderly men have a higher propensity of losing potassium in their urine when taking water pills. For these, and all the other aforementioned reasons, when an elderly person is on water pills and particularly if that elderly person is on Digitalis, close attention must be paid to the serum potassium, and potassium replacement ought to be provided to prevent potassium loss, which by itself can cause severe cardiac dysrhythmias. The argument that water pills causes blood sugar to rise is in fact a false argument, because replacing potassium restores insulin receptor sensitivity, which then keeps the blood sugar at a normal level. The benefit of having well-controlled blood pressure far outweighs the questionable slight increase in cholesterol that might be seen in some rare instances in individuals taking water pills. All that needs to be done is to advise the individual to stay on a low-fat diet and monitor the serum cholesterol as often as possible. The incidence of high blood pressure is on the decrease in white males but is on the increase in men of color and is continuing to increase steadily in that group of men.

The new concept that must be understood and kept in mind in the treatment of hypertension is that all human beings are salt sensitive and therefore be treated with a salt removing diuretic as part of the medications used to effectively treat hypertension. Source: JAMA Volume 289, No 19 May, 21, 2003. The JNC-7 report.

There is a rare tumor of the adrenal gland called pheochromocytoma that secretes substances called catecholamines that cause a characteristic elevation in blood pressure. Because 95% of the time when a person has high blood pressure, it is due to the so-called essential hypertension, it is more cost effective to do a few simple tests following a complete physical examination and start treatment for the blood pressure. It is inappropriate to do extensive and expensive tests before trying treatment with antihypertensive medications in a man with hypertension. The basic tests that are necessary in the initial evaluation of a hypertensive man include:

1. Complete blood count
2. Blood chemistries, such as blood sugar, blood urea nitrogen, serum electrolytes, serum creatinine, lipid profiles such as cholesterol, triglycerides, high-density lipoprotein, low-density lipoprotein
3. Urinalysis
4. EKG
5. Chest x-ray

The tests for pheochromocytoma are expensive and very tedious to do. It requires serum catecholamines; 24 hours urine catecholamines and a specific diet must be adhered to for several days before these tests can be done. It is simpler to do an abdominal CT scan to evaluate the adrenal glands looking for abnormality, rather than doing these very extensive blood tests looking for pheochromocytoma, which is quite rare. Most of the time, people with pheochromocytoma have sustained elevated blood pressure rather than the blood pressure that goes up and down as is being taught in medical schools and residency training.

To determine the extent of damage that the hypertensive state has done to the different end organs of hypertensive men, a series of basic tests ought to be done. The end organs are:

1. The brain,
2. The heart,
3. The eyes,
4. The kidney.

These basic tests are not only reasonably inexpensive but they are clinical rationales for doing them. The CBC is able to tell whether a person is anemic or not, and in renal failure associated with long-time hypertension, the red blood cell count is low because the kidneys are damaged and are not able to make erythropoietin. Erythropoietin is a hormone made by the kidneys to stimulate the production of red cells by the bone marrow, which is the organ within which red blood cells are made in an adult. The urinalysis is abnormal in kidney disease associated with hypertension. When high blood pressure damages the kidneys, the urine specific gravity is low. The urine is likely to have protein in it and the urine sediment when examined with the microscope is likely to have substances called casts, indicating intrinsic kidney damage. In the blood chemistry tests, the BUN, the creatinine, the serum potassium and the bicarbonate may all be abnormal in high blood pressure-associated kidney disease. If the blood sugar is elevated, that means the patient, in addition to having hypertension, may also have diabetes mellitus. The serum lipids such as cholesterol, triglycerides, LDL, are elevated and if the person is hypertensive, the blood sugar is elevated, and the man happens to be obese, that is very important; that is called syndrome X or metabolic hypertension. This a very serious condition during which there is an interplay between obesity, hypertension, hyperlipidemia and diabetes in the same individual. That is a very deadly combination that needs to be handled extremely expertly and carefully. The chest x-ray is important to determine whether the heart is enlarged or not, or whether the lungs have fluid in them, a condition known as congestive heart failure. If the heart is enlarged, it gives the physician a very good idea as to how long the person has been hypertensive. The electrocardiogram (EKG) is very important, in that it allows the physician to have an idea as to the different types of damage that the high blood pressure may have caused to the heart muscle over a long period.

These basic tests having been done, then the physician has sufficient information at hand to organize a sensible, rational, safe and cost-effective treatment plan for the hypertensive patient. Examining the eyes using the ophthalmoscope allows the physician to see the fundi of hypertensive men, which shows small blood vessels in the eyes, and if found to be damaged, reveals that these men have been hypertensive for a long time and most probably without effective treatment.

For men to keep their blood pressure normal, in addition to appropriate medications such as diuretics, they must eat a diet that is low in salt, fat, and carbohydrates and high in fiber, protein, vitamins, iron and minerals. They also must control their weights and they must exercise regularly.

Men must endeavor to exercise regularly, stop smoking, and abstain from abusing alcohol, if they are to decrease their incidence of high blood pressure. These measures can lead to decreasing some of the adverse consequences of high blood pressure such as stroke, heart attack, and kidney failure. All these factors contribute to the black man's decreased median survival of 68.7 years as compared to the white man's median survival of 75 years. There is a need for a change of lifestyle of men to help decrease the incidence of hypertension. That change in lifestyle is not always realistic because of the poor economic circumstances of black men, Hispanic men, Native American men and poor white men. The stress brought on by a multitude of problems associated with poverty plays a major role in the elevation of blood pressure in poor men and if it is not diminished, it makes it that much more difficult for these men to control the elevation of their blood pressure. Poverty imposes a great deal of stress upon poor men and the stress contributes to the elevation of blood pressure. Hypertension is one of the leading cause of morbidity and mortality in men, but education and an understanding of this most serious disease can delay its onset by many years and can decrease its incidence in men. Hypertension is the same disease in all men without regard to race or creed. All men who suffer from essential hypertension are salt sensitive to one degree or an other and, must be given a thiazide diuretic as their main medication for hypertension. Doing otherwise guarantees the development of major difficulty in controlling their blood pressure. Treating these men's blood pressure with a proper regimen goes a long way in decreasing their death rates by preventing the multitude of hypertension-associated complications. Treating black men, Asian men and men of color in general who are likely to be salt sensitive and have low renin with the proper second anti-hypertensive or when necessary a third anti-hypertensive medication such as Calcium channel blocker or Angiotensin-II Converting Enzyme Antagonist is curtail, if one expects to properly control the blood pressure in these individuals. It is time that the medical community stops fostering the covert false notion of **racialism** in treatment of hypertension. Hypertension is colorblind. It knows no skin color or racial differences, and affects every one in the same adverse way. Hypertension is an easily treatable disease if the right medication or medications are provided for the right men under the right clinical circumstances. The result would be that this most easily treatable disease would be treated much more effectively, thereby preventing its devastation of men.

CHAPTER 2

STROKE IN MEN

ONE OF THE LEADING DISEASES that kills men is stroke. In the year 2002, there were a total of 5,400,000 people with stroke in the US and 2,400.000 of them were men. More than 730,000 individuals suffer a stroke every year in the US, 500,000 of these strokes are first strokes and 200,000 are recurrent strokes. 88 percent of these strokes are ischemic, 9 percent are intracerebral hemorrhage and 3 percent are sub-arachnoid hemorrhage.

In 2002, 327,000 men had stroke in the US. During that same period of time, 277,000 white males had stroke or 2.3%, 50,000 black males had stroke or 4.0%, 2.6% Mexican American males had stroke, 2.4% Hispanic or Latino males had stroke, 2.4% Asian males had stroke and 4.6% American Indians/ Alaska Natives had stroke.

In the U.S., every 44 seconds someone suffers a stroke and every 3.3 minutes someone dies of a stroke. In 2002, 162,672 individuals died of stroke. 1 of every 15 individuals who died in the U.S. in 2002 died of Stroke. In the year 2002, 52,959 white males died of stroke and 7,828 black males died of stroke. Stroke is the third leading cause of deaths in the U.S. after heart disease and cancer.

Every year 275,000 people die of strokes in the U.S. About 7.6% of the individuals who suffer ischemic strokes and 37.5% of those who suffer a hemorrhagic stroke die within 30 days. There are 4,600,000 survivors of strokes in the U.S. and 2,300,000 of them are men.

The 2002 overall death rates for stroke were 56.2. The death rates for white males in 2002 were 54.2, 81.7 for black males. The 1999 rates of death from stroke for Hispanics were 40.0, 52.4 for Asians/Pacific Islanders and 39.7 for American

Indians/Alaska Natives. Source: Heart Disease and Stroke Statistics Update American Heart Association, 2005. Both the incidences of stroke and the death from stroke are significantly higher for black men as compared to white men.

Black men/men of color have higher prevalence of small vessel strokes (19% black men vs. 6% white men), intracranial senses (19% black men or men of color vs. 6% whites), and lacuna strokes (10% black men or men of color vs. 2.7% whites) ("Heart and Stroke Statistical Update," American Heart Association, 2002).

The prevalence of hypertension in black men or men of color is 68% vs. 30% in white men. About 49% of black men or men of color in the U.S., as compared to 19% of white men, have two or more risk factors for strokes, such as cigarette smoking, hypertension, diabetes, obesity and coronary artery disease.

The most common risks for stroke are
1. Hypertension
2. Diabetes mellitus
3. Obesity
4. Arteriosclerosis
5. Hyperlipidemia (high cholesterol)
6. Tobacco smoking
7. Atrial fibrillation
8. Primary polycythemia
9. Secondary polycythemia
10. Essential thrombocythemia
11. Sickle cell anemia
12. Hypercoagulable state
13. Thrombophilia
14. The Obstructive sleep Apnea Syndrome
15. Serum B12 deficiency
16. Serum Folic acid deficiency
17. Elevated Homocysteine level
18. Decreased protein C level
19. Decreased protein S level
20. Decreased anti thrombin III level
21. Taking birth control pills
22. Taking any estrogenic hormone
23. Elevated Lipo-protein-a level
24. Elevated anti-phospholipin antibody

25. Elevated circulating lupus anticoagulant
26. Hematocrit level 40% or greater in patients with chronic renal failure can cause stroke to occur
27. Hematocrit level greater than 34% in patients with sickle cell anemia can cause stroke to occur
28. Hyperviscosity state in patients with multiple myeloma can cause stroke to occur
29. Nephrotic syndrome
30. AIDS
31. Factor V Leiden mutation
32. Prothrombin G20210A mutation
33. Migraine with aura

The total yearly health cost of stroke in the US is 56.8 billion dollars.

What is a stroke?

A stroke is when an obstruction of blood flow occurs within the blood vessel, preventing blood flow to an area of the brain. Consequently, that area of the brain becomes damaged. That damage, results in what is called a stroke. Another terminology frequently used to describe a stroke is cerebrovascular accident.

That obstruction of blood flow can be caused by either plaques within a vessel or by clot from the heart brought through the vessel by the bloodstream to the brain. Another type of stroke is when a vessel inside the brain ruptures and leaks blood inside the brain. The rupture of a vessel in the brain is either due to a vessel filled with Atherosclerotic plaques or the elevation of blood pressure within the vessel, which causes the membrane of that vessel to rupture, and leaks blood into the brain, leading to a stroke. That type of stroke is called a hemorrhagic stroke. Brain aneurysms, which are a meshwork of vessel malformations due to genetic defects, can rupture and leak blood into the brain when the blood pressure is too high. Aneurysms of the brain can rupture, causing a hemorrhagic stroke within the brain, whether the blood pressure of the individual is elevated or not. Another frequent cause of bleeding into the brain is hemangiomas, or arteriovenous malformations. These are a group of small arteries and veins in a mesh, which form an abnormal network of vessels, which can bleed easily in the brain, leading to hemorrhagic stroke. There is a form of stroke called a transient ischemic attack (TIA). In TIA, there is a transient occlusion of a small vessel by a clot or a clump of platelets, which are trapped within the vessel, preventing free flow of the blood to pass to deliver oxygen to that part of the brain. That temporary lack of oxygen to the brain causes a clinical condition, which can temporarily lead to loss of consciousness, seizures, weakness, lassitude, and a feeling of being sick, which sometimes can last for several hours or several days. Frequently these men have what is called pre-syncope or a full-blown syncopal episode because of the TIA. That condition occurs usually in the setting of what is referred to as multi-infarct syndrome, which is the result of many years of either poorly treated or untreated hypertension. In multi-infarct syndrome, different parts of the brain deep within it are affected with that condition. For men ages 65–69, the prevalence of TIA is 2.7% and for men ages 75–79 the prevalence of TIA is 3.6%

The most common types of stroke or cerebrovascular accident include are:
1. Atherosclerotic or ischemic stroke—88% of all strokes.
2. Lacunae stroke.
3. Embolic stroke, which represents 24% of all strokes.
4. Hemorrhagic stroke represents—10% of all strokes.
5. Ruptured aneurysms.
6. Bleeding arteriovenous malformations.
7. Transient ischemic attacks.
8. Subarachnoid hemorrhage—3% of all strokes.
9. Occlusion of carotid arteries by plaque, causing stroke to occur because of lack of blood flow to the brain.

In men, atherosclerotic-type strokes and hypertension-associated strokes are the two most common types seen. Stroke is one of the leading diseases that cause the death of men and more men die of stroke than women. The combination of salt sensitivity, salt retention and water retention and the elevated high blood pressure that results from it, is partly responsible for such a high incidence of strokes in salt sensitive/low-renin men such as black men, Hispanic men, Asian men, Native American men and many white men.

Atherosclerotic disease of the brain occurs in a very large percentage of men. The reasons for that high percentage of brain atherosclerotic disease in men comprise of:
1. Hypertension
2. Obesity
3. Diabetes mellitus
4. Hyperlipidemia/high cholesterol
5. Tobacco smoking
6. Alcohol abuse
7. The different stresses associated with life including discrimination of different types, poor economic conditions, poverty, lack of education, poor health, etc., and all the other bad things that some men have

to cope with, which include poor diet rich in fats, salt and carbohydrates; all these bad things contribute to the development of strokes.

Even men who are rich and have all the best of everything, face the same fate if they don't take good care of themselves as far as the development of stroke is concerned. Obesity, diabetes mellitus, hypertension, stress and domestic turmoil also can affect men of good financial means, good education and good professions.

The human brain is in total control of all activities associated with being a human being. The ability of the brain to control what humans do differentiates the human animal from all other animals.

The following outlines in part some of the things that the human brain is in control of:

1. The ability to think
2. The ability to gather information and process such information logically and rationally to formulate judgments rightly or wrongly.
3. The ability to breathe
4. The ability to see
5. The ability to hear
6. The ability to smell
7. The ability to feel
8. The ability to taste
9. The heartbeat and other crucial functions of the heart
10. Lung functions
11. Hunger
12. Lack of desire for foods
13. Thirst
14. Lack of desire to drink
15. Sleep
16. Insomnia
17. Happiness
18. Unhappiness
19. Moods
20. Good moods
21. Bad moods
22. Elation
23. Motivation
24. Lack of motivation
25. Hardworking habits
26. Laziness

27. Neatness
28. Sloppiness
29. Anger
30. Aggressive behavior
31. Antisocial behavior
32. Pleasant and friendly behavior
33. Lying as a habitual behavior
34. Honesty
35. Dishonesty
36. Criminal behavior and other antisocial behaviors
37. Sexual orientations/preferences
38. Sexual desires
39. Erectile function
40. Ejaculatory functions and sexual satisfactions
41. Bowel functions
42. Urinary functions
43. Chewing
44. Swallowing
45. Sneezing
46. Coughing
47. Yawning
48. Lying down
49. Sitting
50. Bending
51. Standing
52. Walking
53. Running
54. All other motor body functions
55. Writing
56. Reading
57. Speaking
58. In short the brain is in control of all bodily functions

Different parts of the human brain are in control of these different functions, so when the brain is damaged by a stroke, accidents of one type or another, by infections or other abnormalities that interfere with its normal functions, one or several of these vital functions become impaired in one way or another.

Hypertension causes strokes through three basic mechanisms: 1) Increased blood pressure in the vessels within the brain causes the inside part of these vessels to become damaged, and over time, the damaged areas of these vessels trap platelets and other material as they pass through with the blood. A nidus of these different materials develops within these vessels and the result is plaque formation. The formation of plaques within these vessels leads to narrowing of these vessels, impeding blood flow. Superimposed on the plaque frequently is a clot which can acutely close off a vessel, resulting in a cerebrovascular accident stroke. A plaque within a vessel can cause a stroke through different mechanisms:

(a) The plaque can cause the vessel to become narrowed impeding blood flow and oxygen delivery to a particular part of the brain. (b) The plaque that seats inside that vessel can break off, causing either an embolus or a clot to start forming, resulting in a stroke as has just been outlined. 2. Another mechanism through which hypertension causes stroke is acute intracerebral bleeding secondary to very elevated blood pressure causing rupture of a blood vessel, resulting in bleeding within the brain. Bleeding inside the brain can result in coma because of edema (swelling) within the brain, and if the coma lasts too long, then the result can be death of the affected man. 3. Another type of stroke syndrome that occurs in men who have been hypertensive for a long time, and in particular if the blood pressure has not been treated or not treated properly as aforementioned, is multiple small vessel infarctions of the brain.

The following are radiological examples of strokes.

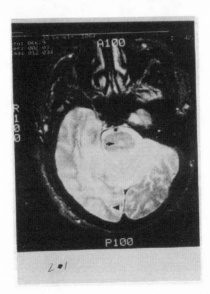

Figure 2.1—MRI of the brain in the patient with hypertension: small infarct in the pond (arrow) and right occipital white matter (arrowhead).

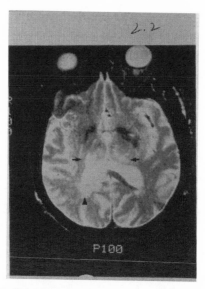

Figure 2.2—MRI of the brain in patient with hypertension: infarction of thalamus (arrows) and right parietal white matter (arrowhead).

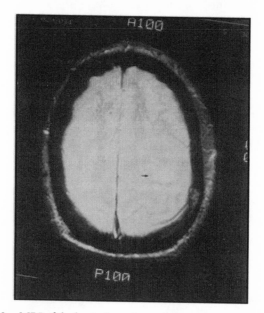

Figure 2.3—MRI of the brain in patient with hypertension: left parietal small infarction (arrow).

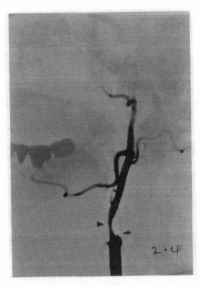

Figure 2.4—Atherosclerotic disease of carotid arteries in patients with hypertension causing transient ischemic attacks (pre-stroke syndrome). Carotid angiogram: occlusion of internal carotid artery at its origin (arrow); narrowing of proximal internal carotid artery (arrowhead).

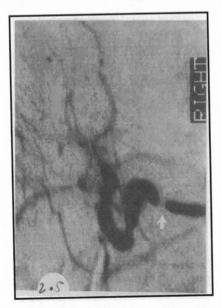

Figure 2.5—Cerebral angiogram 95% occlusion of internal carotid artery in a patient with hypertension (arrow).

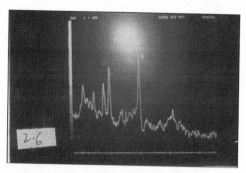

Figure 2.6—SPECT MRI of the brain of a man with Alzheimer's disease showing hypoperfusion of the frontal lobe of the brain.

These small vessels are located deep inside the brain and supply blood to very vital structures within the brain. That condition is associated with early memory loss resulting in organic brain syndrome. Multiple small vessel infarctions are second only to Alzheimer's disease as a cause of senility. In fact, it is probably more common than Alzheimer's in terms of causing senility because there are so many more hypertensive patients than people who have Alzheimer disease. It is not uncommon to see 40-year-old men who have been hypertensive since their 30s or 20s who are having difficulty remembering very simple things because of multiple small vessel infarctions of the brain, as seen on brain MRI (magnetic resonance imaging). (CT of the brain does not show that syndrome very well.)

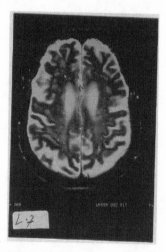

Figure 2.7—MRI of the brain of a man with Alzheimer's disease and longstanding hypertension showing multiple small vessel infarctions of the brain.

In evaluating poor memory loss in 40-to 60-year-old hypertensive men, the following needs to be done:

1. A complete history and physical examination by a competent internist or primary care physician or neurologist
2. CBC with differential
3. Blood chemistry
4. Urinalysis
5. Thyroid tests such as T4, TSH, and T3
6. B12 level
7. Complete lipid profile
8. VDRL
9. HIV test
10. Chest x-ray
11. EKG
12. Brain CAT scan and if normal, an MRI of the brain
13. A thorough neurological examination by, as already stated, a neurologist or an internist or family practitioner
14. If the aforementioned tests are normal and the neurological examination is normal, then a SPECT scan of the brain must be done to look for hypo perfusion in the frontal lobe of the brain. (Hypoperfusion in the frontal lobe of the brain is seen in Alzheimer's disease on SPECT MRI of the brain.)
15. Ultrasound of the carotid arteries (these arteries are located on the left and the right side of the neck and carry blood to the brain)

Each one of these tests is done for a particular reason.

The history gives the physician a profile as to what sorts of things or conditions the patient may have been exposed to. The physical examination allows the physician the opportunity to find abnormalities that may shed light on the poor memory. The complete blood count tells the physician if the white blood cell count is either too low or too high. Both too low and too high white blood cell counts may be associated with conditions that might explain the memory loss. It is important to realize that there is a difference in the level of white blood cell counts in Caucasians as compared to black men and other men of color. The normal white blood cell count in white men is 4,500 to 10,000. In black men, the normal white blood cell count is from 3,500 to 10,000. In black Caribbean men and Ashkenazi Jewish men the normal WBC may be as low as 2.500. If the WBC is found to be 3,500 or even lower in a man of immediate African ancestry and the differential count is normal then there may not be a need to do anything further. The red blood cell count tells the physician whether the poor memory is due low red cell count (anemia) or too high red blood cell count (polycythemia). When the red blood cell count is too low, oxygen cannot be delivered easily to the body's vital organs including the brain. Poor oxygen delivery to the brain is one of the causes of poor memory (organic brain syndrome). When the red blood cell count is too high, such as in polycythemia, high viscosity of the blood results in stasis within the vessels, making it difficult for oxygen to get to the brain for proper functioning. The thicker the blood, the more difficult it is for oxygen to get to the memory center in the brain for good memory to occur. The platelet count, which is part of the CBC, is also very important. If the platelets drop to less than 20,000 (normal platelet count is 130,000 to 400,000), spontaneous bleeding can occur anywhere in the body, including the brain. Bleeding in the brain can result in serious brain malfunction including poor memory. If the platelet count is too high, 750,000 to 1,000,000 or greater, both stroke and bleeding can occur within the brain, resulting in poor brain functioning including poor memory. (this occurs only if the high platelet count is associated with a myeloproliferative disorder, such as Polycythemia Vera, Essential polycythemia, or Chronic Myelogenous leukemia). Abnormalities in the differential blood count may indicate many different abnormalities, including leukemia or lymphoma, both of which frequently affect the brain, resulting in poor brain functioning. The blood chemistry and its component parts are very important in determining whether a person's poor memory is due to abnormality or abnormalities of the body's chemistry. Abnormalities in the electrolytes can cause poor brain function. The electrolytes are sodium, potassium, chloride and bicarbonate. Severe acidosis (too low bicarbonate) or severe alkalosis (too high bicarbonate) can lead to abnormalities that can cause brain abnormalities and brain malfunction. Too high blood sodium (a condition called hypernatremia), the normal sodium being 135 to 140, can cause brain malfunction, including confusion, to occur. Too low blood sodium, 110–120, can cause confusion, poor memory, and, at times, seizures to occur. One of the frequent abnormalities in the blood chemistries that can cause brain malfunction is too low blood sugar, known as hypoglycemia. The normal blood sugar is between 60 and 112. When the blood sugar falls to less than 60 or lower, that situation can lead to confusion, poor memory or seizure. Starvation is a common cause of low blood sugar. Medications such as blood sugar-lowering pills and insulin are the most common medications that frequently cause too low blood sugar to occur. When the blood sugar is too high, 400 or greater, it can lead to a condition called diabetic ketoacidosis, which can cause severe brain malfunction and, if not treated quickly and properly, can cause the person to go into coma and die. What happens in diabetic ketoacidosis is that the person is unable to use sugar as fuel, due to lack of insulin; therefore, fat is being used as fuel, resulting in breakdown products of fat, which are ketone bodies. These ketone bodies are toxic to the body, leading to severe brain malfunctioning, including confusion and sometimes seizures. There is another condition involving high blood sugar called non-ketotic hyperglycemia, which frequently can lead to coma if left untreated for very long. In that condition, there is no high level of ketones, but the blood sugar rises very high, and sometimes greater than 2,000, and frequently in men who never before had trouble with elevated blood sugar.

High blood sugar acts as a diuretic. The affected man passes a large quantity of urine daily and experiences extreme thirst. After a while, the volume of urine that he passes is far in excess of the fluid he takes in, resulting in severe dehydration, including dehydration of the brain, causing coma to develop, and death if left untreated.

When the kidneys are malfunctioning, many abnormalities can be detected in the blood and in the urine, but some of the earliest and most important abnormalities that can be seen when the kidneys start to fail are:

1. High BUN
2. High creatinine
3. High potassium
4. High phosphate
5. Low bicarbonate
6. Anemia
7. Too much protein in the urine
8. Low 24-hour urine creatinine clearance

When the kidney fail, waste products, which are very toxic, cannot be removed from the blood, resulting in malfunctioning of the brain including confusion and seizures.

Another important series of blood chemistry tests that are used by physicians to detect diseases in the human body are the liver function tests. In particular, liver function tests such as serum calcium, serum phosphate, serum LDH, serum SGOT, serum SGPT, GGTP, serum uric acid, serum bilirubin, and alkaline phosphatase and prothrombin time. Abnormalities seen in these different tests may indicate association with different diseases such as hepatitis, cancer involving the liver, etc. Complete liver failure causes mental confusion and, at times, seizures. If the urinalysis is abnormal, it may indicate infection in the bladder or kidneys. If sugar is found in the urine, it may indicate diabetes mellitus. If a acetone is found in the urine, that may indicate dehydration or the presence in the body of the condition called diabetic ketoacidosis as afore-mentioned, seen in people who are diabetic, when the diabetes is out of control. If protein is found in the urine, it may indicate different degrees of kidney failure. When sediment of the urine is examined under the microscope, different crystals may be seen in association with kidney stones. Materials called casts of different types may be seen in these sediments representing association with different diseases of the kidneys. Prominent among these diseases include urinary tract infection, kidney stone, sickle cell disease, cancer of the bladder, cancer of the kidney. In the males, these same diseases may be present if blood is seen in the urine, that is, if he is not menstruating.

When the kidneys fail, urine output ceases and different degrees of mental confusion can be seen and if dialysis is not carried out to cleanse the blood of toxic substances, coma may ensue, which may result in death. Blood tests to evaluate the functions of the thyroid glands are very important. Both hypothyroidism (low function of the thyroid gland) and hyperthyroidism (high function of the thyroid gland) can cause mental aberration, resulting at times, in memory loss, confusion and many times, coma.

Low Vitamin B12 can cause a multitude of problems, such as numbness, pain and needle symptoms over the legs and the fingers. Memory loss and neurological damage can occur because of low B12. If the B12 level remains low for five years or more, permanent brain and neurological damage are certain to occur. Many conditions that can cause low Vitamin 12. Among them are:

1. Pernicious anemia
2. Infestation with fish tapeworm
3. Malabsorption of B12
4. Atrophic gastritis
5. Blind loop syndrome
6. Vegetarian diet resulting in low B12 and a stroke.
7. Chronic inhalation of Nitrous oxide

and more recently, a condition has been discovered—the low B12 syndrome as it occurs in the elderly population. It is, therefore, very important to do a B12 level when evaluating a person for memory loss. It is also important if one has evidence physically that a person is suffering from B12 deficiency and the B12 level comes back normal, to do a urine or blood test for methylmalonic acid. It is a very sensitive test because if someone has B12 deficiency the methylmalonic acid will be elevated. Folic Acid deficiency can also cause stroke to occur because, low folic acid cause elevated homocysteine level which can cause clotting to develop any where in the body including the brain resulting in a stroke. Any men taking hormonal treatment, such as Lupron to treat prostate cancer, can develop deep vein thrombophlebitis, pulmonary embolism and stroke because, estrogenic hormone can cause anti-Thrombin III level to go down resulting creating a state of hypercoagulability in the blood causing clotting to develop any where in the body including the brain. Low folic acid level in the blood causes a rise in the level of homocysteine which in creates a state of hypercoagulability which can cause stroke to occur. Low protein S and protein C also causes a state of hypercoagulability and the potential for clotting in the human body to occur including in the brain-causing stroke. Elevated levels of circulating Lupus anticoagulant and anti-phospholipin antibody in the body also create a state of hypercoagulability with the potential for causing clotting anywhere in the body including the brain. Elevated Lipoprotein—a can cause stroke to occur, because the Lipoprotein can competitely displaced plasminogen, resulting in the clotting of fibrin. It can also displace heparin creating a hypercoagulable state which can cause clotting to occur anywhere in the body including the brain.

Nephrotic syndrome can cause stroke, because in nephrotic syndrome both protein C and protein S are lost in large quantity in the urine and end result is hypercoagulability of the blood which can cause clotting to occur in the and anywhere else in the body. AIDS in its advanced stage can cause a series of neurological problems and among these problems is stroke because AIDS frequently causes a protein losing nephropathy to develop, resulting in the lost of protein S in the urine. When that happens, clotting can occur anywhere in the body, including the brain.

Hyper viscosity can occur in multiple myeloma and the viscosity of the blood is so very high that it cannot pass through the blood vessels easily to deliver oxygen to the brain which, in turn can cause stroke to occur. In polycythemia Vera the thickness of the blood With hematocrit of 60% or greater, the circulation of blood through the brain is impeded prevent free movement of oxygen within the brain thereby creating a situation for stroke to occur. In polycythemia Vera as well as in essential thrombocythemia, the elevated platelet can lead platelet aggregation causing stroke. In sickle cell anemia, stroke occurs quite frequently because the malformed shape of the red blood cells as well as the stickiness of these cells along with the cells to blood vessels damage that the sickling syndrome causes etc, creates the formula for the easy development of stroke in people who are afflicted with sickle disease. Hyperlipidemia/hycholesterol cause can cause stroke to occur, because the deposition of cholesterol inside blood vessels leads to atherosclerotic plaque formation, resulting in narrowing of blood vessels inside the brain impeding free movement of blood and oxygen causing stroke.

The Obstructive Sleep Apnea Syndrome is established as disease entity when an apnea-hypopnea index of 5 or higher events occur in 1 hour. When that happens, it is reported that that is associated with stroke and deaths of many of the affected individuals. The possible reasons reported to account the high incidence of stroke and death from that syndrome is

1. Acute hemodynamic changes during episodes of apnea
2. Decreased cerebral blood flow
3. Paradoxical embolization
4. Hypercoagulability of the blood
5. Hypoxia-related cerebral ischemia
6. Atherosclerosis (source New England Journal of Medicine VOL. 353 NO 19 November 10th, 2005)

Obesity with a BMI greater than 30 is highly associated with the development of stroke. Diabetes mellitus is a high risk for stroke because, the elevated blood sugar damages blood vessels in the brain resulting, in narrowing of vessels and causing local inflammation within vessels resulting in atherosclerotic plaque formation which predisposes to the development of stroke.

Atrial Fibrillation can cause stroke because, when the atrium is fibrillating, the blood inside it remains stagnant and the stagnant blood can form clots. When the atrium begins to contract again, it can send a piece of the clot through the stream to brain causing a stroke. That is why people with atrial fibrillation are treated with blood thinner such as Coumadin, Heparin or Aspirin in some cases.

Tobacco smoking can cause stroke because the nicotine and other materials that damage blood vessels. Once the blood vessels are damaged, atherosclerotic plaques develop causing narrowing of blood vessels impeding blood flow to brain causing stroke.

A test for syphilis, using the RPR or VDRL, is very important because syphilis, when involving the brain, can cause severe brain damage resulting in memory loss, etc. The VDRL test is used to detect syphilis in the human body, if it is positive, it is very important to do the confirmatory blood test, FTA-ABS (Fluorescent Treponema Antibody-Absorption Test). In true syphilitic infection, that test stays positive for life. When neurosyphilis is suspected, then CT scan ought to be done, and if the CT scan appears normal, then a lumbar puncture ought to be done to examine the cerebrospinal fluid for the presence of syphilis.

In the evaluation of poor memory (organic brain syndrome) the HIV Type I or Type II test is very important and ought to be done. Frequently, in AIDS, loss of memory is a presenting symptom. That is due either to HIV infection of the brain tissue itself or infections of the brain such as toxoplasmosis, cryptococcus of the brain or herpes infection of the brain, etc.

In evaluating poor memory or organic brain syndrome, the chest x-ray is very important because the chest x-ray may show evidence of cancer in the lungs, which if allowed to spread to the brain, can result in memory loss, confusion and, at times, coma. There are many infectious processes that can be seen in the lungs on chest x-rays which may affect the function of the brain, resulting in poor memory, confusion and sometimes coma.

Doing an electrocardiogram in evaluating a patient with poor brain function is important because the EKG may show evidence of recent myocardial infarction during which the patient may have become hypotensive and that situation may have affected brain function transiently. The EKG may show cardiac arrhythmias or other rhythm abnormalities that may interfere with proper pumping of the heart, preventing adequate oxygen delivery to the brain, causing transient ischemic attack and its associated brain malfunctions.

When a man presents either to the emergency room or to the doctor's office with symptoms of brain malfunction manifesting as acute confusion or acute memory loss that could at times be due to a syncopal episode. Syncopal episode can be brought on by a number of different things, among them malfunctioning of the heart, which can oftentimes be seen on an EKG or 24-hour Holter monitor.

When a man presents with symptoms that are consistent with stroke, several things need to be done. A thorough history ought to be taken from the patient if he is able to speak, and if he cannot speak, the history should be taken from a family member. The next thing to do is to carry out a complete physical examination. It is crucial that the patient's airway is quickly evaluated to be certain he is breathing properly and that he has control over his saliva to prevent aspiration.

It is also crucial that all precautions are taken to watch out for seizures that can occur because of the damage to the brain. Oxygen ought to be administered, IV access ought to be established, and a Foley catheter ought to be inserted. Blood must be drawn for blood tests such as CBC, SMA20, PT, PTT, ANA, ESR, B12, serum folic acid, lipid profile, serum Lipoprotein—a level, serum homocysteine level, serum immunoglobulin levels and serum protein electrophoresis.

Other tests that need to be done are chest x-ray, EKG, and urinalysis and a brain CT.

In acute stroke, the CT scan of the brain is used right away to see whether there is blood within the substance of the brain or whether the brain is swollen or whether the ventricles of the brain are pushed to one side or another, or whether there is a brain tumor. Any one of these findings can cause symptoms consistent with a stroke. Sometimes evidence of old strokes can be seen on the same brain CT scan. When contrast material is injected into the patient's blood stream, through an arm vein, more can be seen within the brain, such as metastatic brain tumor or fungal infection such as toxoplasmosis, as seen in patients with AIDS. Frequently, nothing is seen on a non-contrast brain CT in someone who has an acute stroke. That is not to say that the person does not have a stroke. It simply means it takes one to two weeks to see evidence of a non-bleeding stroke on a brain CT, but doing it eliminates the presence of both acute bleeding and brain tumor. Elimination of these findings in the brain when someone presents with an acute stroke is not only important in diagnosing the cause of the acute stroke, but it also allows the treating physician the possibility to proceed with such a thing as a lumbar puncture to rule out subacute bleeding. It also allows the treating physician to use medications such as tPA (tissue plasminogen activator), heparin and aspirin, if he or he thinks that that in an evolving stroke. Heparin or tPA can help to prevent an acute stroke in that setting. The CAT scan of the brain does all these things, in addition to being a diagnostic instrument. MRI of the brain can be used to evaluate the brain immediately after a stroke and it will show the acute stroke or whatever else may be causing the patient's neurological symptoms.

Once the initial evaluations of the patient are completed, blood must be drawn for CBC, PT, PTT SMA20 (blood chemistry profile), lipid profile and urinalysis.

Depending on the severity of the stroke, a Foley catheter may be inserted into the bladder to insure that the patient can pass his urine and to monitor his urine output.

If the blood pressure is very high, heparin ought not to be used to avoid bleeding into the brain.

In that case, the blood pressure must be brought down very carefully to avoid worsening the stroke or to prevent the precipitation of a new stroke by dropping the blood pressure too fast.

If bleeding in the brain has been ruled out, then the patient ought to be given 325 mg of aspirin to chew and swallow. If he is not able to do these things, he then can be given the aspirin in suppository form rectally.

The decision that must be made is whether he should be given heparin intravenously or whether he should be given tPA IV in an attempt to dissolve the clot that is causing the stroke.

These are very difficult decisions and can only be made by the treating physicians who are at the bedside.

Then one might ask why not does an MRI right way on everybody who has a stroke, bypassing the need for a brain CT? For one thing, the brain MRI is very expensive; it costs about $1,500 with contrast and $950.00 without contrast.

Brain CT with no contrast costs about $520. Another reason is that not every community hospital has MRI available and not everybody is suitable for an MRI study. Some people are claustrophobic, they just do not want to go into the MRI machine and some people are too obese to fit into an MRI machine. The maximum weight that can fit in the MRI machine is about 300 lbs. Sometime in the future they might be able to make a machine that can fit these individuals. Further, open MRI is now available which may be easier for individuals who are claustrophobic to be able to undergo the MRI test. In addition, there are certain individuals who have metals implanted in them due to a previous accident or other surgical procedure, making them unsuitable for the MRI machine.

The list of metals found in the body that can prevent an MRI from being done is quite long, but the most important ones include:

1. Aneurysm and hemostatic clips
2. Biopsy needles
3. Carotid artery vascular clamps
4. Halo vests
5. Heart valve prosthesis
6. Intravascular coils, filters and stents
7. Ocular implants
8. Orthopedic implants, materials and devices
9. Otologic implants
10. Pellets and bullets
11. Penile implants
12. Vascular access ports, etc., as published in the literature

Some of these devices may be dislodged by the magnetic field of the MRI machine, with possible disastrous consequences.

All of the above tests and procedures may be necessary, at any one time, in any patient who presents with a stroke. Men of color are at higher risk of having strokes as compared to other men because of their higher incidence of hypertension, obesity, and diabetes mellitus. Black men are five times more likely to have a stroke and dying from that stroke, as compared to white men. Some of the predisposing factors of developing a stroke in men:

1. Men of color are many times more likely to be hypertensive than do white men and hypertensive men of color are less likely to seek medical care for their hypertension. When treatment is given, it is less likely to be appropriate and, therefore, less effective. Some of these men often time do not follow medical advice properly and eat a diet too rich in salt, all of which contribute to a worst out come.

2. The incidence of obesity is quite high among men. Approximately 27.6% of men (or 27,480.000) in the United States are obese and obesity plays a major role in the elevation of blood pressure. 28.2% White males is obese, 27.9% Black males is obese, 27.3% Mexican is obese, 25.4% Latinos is obese, 7% Asians is obese and 31.3% American Indians/Alaska Natives are obese. Over all, there are 63.120.000 obese adults in the US and there are 134,750,000 obese/overweight adults in the U.S. 5.290.000 of that number are adolescents. There are 3.890.000 obese children in the U.S.

3. The high salt content of the diet that men like to eat plays a major role in the elevation of the blood pressure and its devastating propensity in causing stroke.

4. Another factor that plays a role in an increased incidence of stroke in men is stress. Many minority men are under stress because of their poorer educational status, their poorer economic status, their poorer social status and their overall poorer living conditions, which cause a constant state of stress, resulting in elevation of hormones, such as epinephrine and norepinephrine. These can cause a rise of blood pressure with subsequent development of stroke.

Until the aforementioned conditions are improved, the incidence of stroke in men the world over can be expected to continue unabated. Men can decrease their incidence of dying from stroke by decreasing the amount of salt, fat, and carbohydrates in their foods and by exercising.

Stress is something over which men may or may not have control. Men have more control over the foods that they eat and the quantity of food they eat. It is a known fact that the poorer the individual, the less likely it is that he or she is able to afford the proper nutritional types of foods that are necessary to maintain good health. Sometimes it is not so much the quantity or quality of the food itself, but a combination of poor quality, high quantity and poor preparation. The way one prepares one's food goes a long way in keeping one healthy. Although a person may not be able to afford good quality foods, there are many simple things that can be done to prepare the foods in a healthier way. One should be careful to avoid some of the negative consequences of eating foods that are too salty, greasy, or too studded with carbohydrates. Stroke is a leading cause of long-term disability in the US. Among individuals who had ischemic stroke who were 65 years or older, 6 months after the stroke:

50%   had some hemiparesis.

30%   were unable to walk without some assistance.

26%   were dependent in activities of daily living.

19%   had aphasia (cannot speak).

35%   had depressive symptoms.

26%   were institutionalized in nursing home.

(Source: J stroke Cerebrovascular Dis 2003; 12:119–26)

Stroke is a very financially costly disease. In 2005, it is estimated that 56.8 billion dollars will be spent on the treatments of stroke in the US.

Treatments of strokes include aspirin, Aggrenox, heparin, tPA, control of hypertension and physical therapy with rehabilitation therapy. These are used in different stages of the stroke syndrome. Treatments for TIA, include Aspirin 81 mg per and Aggrenox 1 tablet twice per day.

One of the important things to do for the stroke patient is to provide his with prophylactic anticoagulant treatment with either Coumadin or heparin to prevent DVT (deep vein thrombophlebitis). Stroke causes the patient in many instances to be come immobilized which, in turn can cause the patient's blood to become stagnant resulting in DVT.

Patients who suffer hemorrhagic strokes ought not to be given anticoagulation to prevent DVT or pulmonary embolism because that type of treatment would cause more bleeding into the brain.

In these cases, a sequential compression device ought to be used in their legs to prevent DVT and a inferior vena cava filter ought to be placed in their inferior vena cava to prevent the migration of clot into the lung, which can cause pulmonary embolism.

Every year in the US, 2.5 million people have DVT (clot in the leg) and 600,000 people develop pulmonary embolism (Source: *Internal Medicine World Report*, Vol. 18 No. 6, and June 2003). Every year, 200.000 individuals die of pulmonary embolism in the US. 60,000 people die each year with the diagnosis of pulmonary embolism discovered only at autopsy. 10 per cent of deaths that occur in the hospital occur because of pulmonary embolism in the US 3% of DVT occurs on the outpatient. 20% of individuals who develop DVT had been hospitalized the previous 90 days.

In summary, it is clear that diet, weight management, proper controls of blood pressure, blood lipid, blood sugar and screening for thrombophilias and providing appropriate preventive treatments when indicated are all important factors in the prevention of stroke and in the prolongation of the lives of men.

CHAPTER 3

HIGH CHOLESTEROL IN MEN

IN 2002, 927,448 INDIVIDUALS DIED of cardiovascular disease in the United States making CVD the number one cause of death in the US. 433,825 of these individuals who died were men. Worldwide 17 million people die of CVD every year.. Coronary artery disease (plaques inside the vessels around the heart) has many risk factors including:

1. Hypertension
2. Hyperlipidemia
3. High triglycerides in the blood
4. Elevated low-density lipoprotein in the blood (LDL)
5. Low high-density cholesterol in the blood (HDL)
6. High cholesterol in the blood
7. Family history of early heart attack, especially where a parent died of heart attack in his or her early 40s to mid-50s
8. Cigarette smoking
9. Diabetes mellitus
10. Elevated lipoprotein A
11. Elevated homocysteine level
12. Elevated hs-CRP (C reactive proteins)
13. Obesity
14. Type A personality

15. Stress associated with work, bigotry, racism, illiteracy, poverty and poor economic status
16. Alcoholism

There are 50,400,000 (50.4%) men with high cholesterol in the U.S. and high cholesterol is one of the leading risk factors for coronary artery heart disease.

51.0% White males have high cholesterol.

37.3% Black males have high cholesterol.

54.3% Mexican-American males have high cholesterol.

25.6% Total Hispanics have high cholesterol.

26% American Indians/Alaska Natives have high cholesterol.

27.3% Asians/Pacific Islanders have high cholesterol.

The different types of abnormal lipids that can be found in the blood of men are:

1. Hyperlipidemia
2. High cholesterol
3. High triglycerides/high cholesterol
4. High low-density cholesterol (LDL)
5. Low high-density cholesterol (HDL)
6. High cholesterol/LDL ratio
7. High VLDL cholesterol

All these abnormal lipids are transmitted genetically from parents to their children to one degree or another.

According to a recent report that appeared in the *New England Journal of Medicine*, Vol. 342 No. 12 (March 23, 2000), four new markers of inflammation were found to be predictors of future development of coronary heart disease. These are hs-CRP, serum amyloid A., interleukin-6, and sICAM-1. According to the authors, the hs-CRP was the most sensitive predictor when found to be elevated.

Hyperlipidemia (too much fat in the blood) is, generally speaking, a genetically transmitted disease. If a person's mother or father has too much fat in his or her blood, this trait is likely to be transmitted to his or her children, resulting in hyperlipidemia, which can lead to the development of coronary heart disease resulting in heart attack and possible early death. Hyperlipidemia is categorized as.

1. High blood cholesterol
2. High blood triglycerides
3. High low-density lipoprotein
4. Low high-density lipoprotein
5. Cholesterol/HDL ratio which is LDL/HDL greater than 7.13.

In a man, if the LDL/HDL ratio is greater than 5.57, that is a high risk..

Each one of these different components of hyperlipidemia represents an independent risk factor when abnormal, resulting in coronary heart disease.

Normal blood cholesterol is from 130 to 200 mg/dl. Normal blood triglycerides are 60–150 mg/dl. Normal HDL is 35–80 mg/dl. Normal LDL is less than 130 mg/dl. Normal cholesterol/HDL less than 3.4. Normal LDL/HDL is less than 2.8—these ratios are for men. In men, cholesterol/HDL ratio is less than 3.27 and the LDL/HDL less than 2.34.

Most members of the public believe that blood cholesterol level is the only thing that matters when dealing with abnormal fat levels in the blood. This is wrong, because a person may have perfectly normal total blood cholesterol and yet have significant hyperlipidemia, predisposing that person to coronary artery disease. Be aware that the quick cholesterol test may be misleading if normal. Normal blood cholesterol by itself is not enough to tell if a person has abnormal genetically transmitted lipid. There are five basic cholesterols in the blood:

1. Total cholesterol
2. High-density lipoprotein (HDL)
3. LDL cholesterol
4. Triglycerides
5. VLDL (Very low-density lipoprotein)

HDL is the cholesterol that takes the regular cholesterol from the blood, carries it into the bowel and the colon, mixing it with stool, and carries it out of the body. If the HDL is low, less than 45 mg/dl, then there is not enough of it in the blood to complex with bad cholesterol to remove it from the body. This is a genetic abnormality transmitted from parents to children. More appropriately, these lipid abnormalities are called hyperlipoproteinemias. When both the fasting total cholesterol and the LDL are elevated, that is type 2a hypercholesterolemia.

When the fasting total cholesterol, the LDL cholesterol, and the triglycerides are elevated, that is type 2b hypercholesterolemia. When the total cholesterol is high and if the triglycerides are very high, that is type 3 hyperlipidemia. When the triglycerides are very high and the VLDL is high, that is type 4 hyperlipidemia. High chylomicrons, high VLDL, high triglycerides and cholesterol manifest type 5 hyperlipidemia.

Type 1 hyperlipoproteinenemia is manifested by high chylomicrons.

Secondary hyperlipoproteinemia is seen in association with several medical conditions, such as diabetes mellitus, hypothyroidism, uremia, and nephrotic syndrome, alcoholism with acute or chronic pancreatitis, ingestion of oral contraceptive, etc.

First, high triglycerides and VLDL may be evident on the skin and under the eyes as deposits (xantomas). Second, VLDL, triglycerides, and high cholesterol may be high in diabetic men who develop ketoacidosis. Third, high triglycerides, high cholesterol, diabetes mellitus, and hypertension may be present persistently in obese men (Syndrome X).

The use of birth control pills or ingestion of any estrogen-containing pills can raise the level of VLDL and triglycerides. One of the dangers of taking estrogen-containing pills is the possibility of high level of lipids. It is important to know the lipid level in a person before he or he starts taking estrogen pills. If a man has an elevated lipid level, estrogen-containing medication may be harmful to his health by increasing the blood lipid further, predisposing that individual to heart attack, stroke, phlebitis, pulmonary embolism, etc.

Alcohol abuse is also associated with elevated lipids in the blood, such as triglycerides and in particular high very-low-density lipoprotein and chylomicrons. Type 5 hyperlipidemia and sometimes Type 4 hyperlipidemia may be associated with increased alcohol abuse. Type 5 hyperlipidemia may cause acute pancreatitis, which is a serious medical condition and if left untreated can be fatal.

Hyperlipidemia causes coronary artery disease because in a high lipid state, lipid is deposited within the lumen of coronary arteries, causing gradual narrowing of these vessels and resulting in coronary occlusive heart disease. When the vessels around the heart are narrowed, the condition called angina pectoris frequently develops. Angina pectoris is manifested by chest pain, because of lack of oxygen delivery to the heart muscle. As just stated, the pain occurs when tissue is deprived of oxygen, causing a series of substances, called kinins, to be secreted in and around that tissue, which causes the burning pain to occur. A good example of what kinins are is what one develops in a blister in one's finger or toe. If one bursts the blister right away, the liquid that forms within it causes a burning sensation to occur in the finger or toe because that liquid contains kinins.

High lipoprotein—a is also associated with coronary heart disease. A high level of homocysteine level is also associated with coronary heart disease. Both conditions are genetically transmitted and can cause thrombosis to occur anywhere in the body.

When one is having a heart attack, what happens frequently is that the clot forms acutely. The plaque within the vessels cracks and bleeds or a fissure develops within the vessel resulting in clot formation. The clot closes the vessel, acutely cutting off blood flow to the part of the heart muscle for which that vessel is responsible for delivering oxygen, and the result is an acute heart attack. The muscle which is damaged may die acutely due to lack of flow of blood to it. Cardiac dysrhythmias can develop, resulting in all sorts of rhythm disturbances such as atrial arrhythmias, ventricular tachycardia and ventricular fibrillation, etc., which can lead to the death of the individual who just had the heart attack. If a person presents to the emergency room with acute chest pain and a physician administers tPA acutely to dissolve the clot based on the symptoms and the EKG findings, the death of the involved muscle can be prevented. This can frequently result in the survival of the patient by preventing the heart attack from occurring. It is safe to say that from the time that the patient presents with the symptoms up to several hours later, in certain circumstances, the tPA can still be of value if administered.

In 2002, 7,100,000 men had coronary heart disease in the US. During that same time period, 252,760 men died of CHD. There is a high rate of cardiovascular-associated deaths in men due to the following factors:

1. High blood pressure
2. Obesity
3. High lipids in the blood
4. Smoking
5. Diabetes mellitus
6. Poor diet with too much fat, carbohydrates and salt. Thirty four percent of men are obese in the United States and obesity is a major risk factor for coronary artery disease.
7. Stress associated with racial discrimination, gender discrimination, poverty, poor education, poor economic status, marital problems, raising children and caring for a family, etc.

All these factors together play a major role in the causation of an increased rate of coronary artery disease in men.

The following is a list of the things that an individual can do to decrease the incidence of coronary occlusive disease secondary to high lipids:

1. Maintain an ideal weight.
2. Exercise regularly.
3. Do not abuse alcohol.
4. Eat plenty of fruits and vegetables.
5. Prepare the foods only with vegetable oils.
6. Avoid butter, if possible.
7. Use skim milk.
8. Remove the skin from the chicken to remove as much fat as possible.

9. Use margarine that is low in fat.
10. Avoid red meat as much as possible.
11. Decrease ingestion of pork, bacon, sausages, egg yolks—all these foods are too rich in fat.
12. Avoid too much simple carbohydrate-containing food because carbohydrates are converted into fat in the liver, which ultimately results in fat deposition in the tissues, resulting in obesity.
13. Cut down on foods such as cakes because they have too much sugar in them.
14. Avoid fast foods as much as possible because they contain too much fat, carbohydrates, etc.
15. If you know that you have high cholesterol, then you should minimize your ingestion of lobster, crabs, shrimps, and oysters because they contain high cholesterol.
16. Also, avoid foods, such as coconuts and avocado that have too much cholesterol.
17. Eat foods with high fiber, such as collard greens when prepared without ham, hocks, hock tails and bacon. Avoid putting these things in the collard greens. Vegetable oil, a little bit of hot sauce, and a little bit of wine make the greens taste just as good.
18. Eat foods with complex carbohydrates, such as yams, plantain, sweet potato, and green bananas. These foods are very high in cellulose, which results in fiber. They have good vitamins in them and satisfy hunger and yet they will not make you gain weight, because the human body is not capable of breaking down complex carbohydrates. People in the Third World eat these types of food and they largely do not suffer from the same degree of obesity as men in the United States. The incidence of high lipids is quite low in the Third World because a lot of vegetables and greens are eaten, not having the same access to fast foods. All fat-containing foods that are eaten in the United States and other developed countries predispose their inhabitants to all sorts of diseases such as cancer, coronary artery disease, and diabetes.
19. Use vegetable oils that contain polyunsaturated fat to cook your foods.

The diet of men in the United States is too rich in fat, salt and carbohydrates. Poor men do not have time to exercise because of their substandard economic situation, which is not their fault but that of the social and economic situations that they find themselves. I Treatments of hyperlipidemia:

Some of the most important parts of the treatment of high cholesterol, high triglycerides and hyperlipidemia in general are diet, exercise and weight loss. However, once the cholesterol reaches a level at which the diet is not sufficient, then the clinical thing to do is to provide the patient with medication. There is a series of medications around referred to as Statins or HMG-CoA reductase inhibitors, and they are

Zocor
Lipitor
Mevacor
Pravachol
Lescol XL
Crestor
Vytorin

The Statins wok to lower cholesterol by blocking Hydroxymethylglutaryl-coemzyme A reductase (HMG-CoA reductase) which is the rate-limiting enzyme for the production of cholesterol in the liver. In doing so, the statins reduce liver cells content of cholesterol and stimulate the receptors for low-density lipoprotein cholesterol (LDL-C) which makes it easier to remove LDL-C from the blood.

Bile acid-binding resins such as Cholestyramine and Colestipol prevent bile acids from entering into the circulation of the liver and are diverted into the lower gastrointestinal tract to be removed with the stools out of the body. That process allows for the lowering of LDL cholesterol and increase HDL. The usual dose of Cholestyramine is 8–12 grams two or three times per day by mouth. The usual dose of Colestipol is 10–15 grams 2 or 3 times per day by mouth.

Lopid (gemfibrozil) decreases triglycerides and VLDL (very low-density lipoprotein) and increases HDL. The usual dose of Lopid is 600 mg by mouth 2 times per day. Tricor (fenofibrate) is also used to treat patients with high triglycerides. It lowers triglycerides and VLDL and increases HDL. The usual dose of Tricor is 145 mg or 48 mg daily by mouth. It is important that these fat-lowering medications and in particular the Statin be taken ½ hour after dinner every night and the reason is that fat is circadian, which means there is more fat in the blood at night. The more fat there is in the blood at the time the Statin is being taken, the better the chances of removing the fat from the bloodstream or the better the chances of blocking the liver's ability from producing more cholesterol. Zetia works to lower cholesterol from the blood by preventing the absorption of cholesterol by the small intestine.

It is important to realize that these medications work best when given in the evening because cholesterol works via the circadian system. That is to say, the cholesterol level is highest in the evening. The usual daily doses of these medications are 10–20 mg, or 20mg-40mg a half hour after dinner nightly for
Lipitor 10–40 mg
Mevacor 20–40 mg
Zocor 20–80 mg
Pravachol 40mg
Vytorin 10/10 mg, 10/20 mg, 10/40 mg, 10/80 mg (a combination of Zetia and Zocor)
Lescol XL is 80mg
Crestor 5–10mg
Zetia works to lower cholesterol by preventing its absorption from the small intestine.
The usual dose of Zetia is 10 mg per day.
Tricor works to decrease triglycerides by blocking its absorption into the blood stream.
The usual dose of Tricor is 48 mg, 54 mg, 145 mg and 160 mg per day.
All anti lipid medications work best when taken ½ hour after dinner. This so because fat is circadian, meaning the highest level of lipid in the human blood stream is at night, in particular ½ hour after dinner. The best time to take anti lipid medications is when there is more fat to block from absorption into the blood stream. Taking anti lipid medications in the morning does not work.
These medications are quite expensive, but they are very effective in bringing down the cholesterol, LDL, and triglycerides and raising the HDL, thereby decreasing incidence of coronary disease. All these medications, and in particular the HMG CoA reductase inhibitors, can cause mild liver function test abnormality and for that reason it is important to monitor the liver function tests every six weeks to every two months in men who are taking these medications. It is very important to emphasize that these medications must be used in conjunction with a low-fat, low-carbohydrate diet along with a good exercise program.

Another known side effect of these medications is muscle and joint pain. In some cases, the muscle breakdown can lead to rhabdomyolysis, which, if not recognized quickly and treated, can lead to kidney failure.

Niacin is also a very good medication to treat high cholesterol.

The usual starting dose is 500 mg at bedtime.

The maximum dose of Niacin is 2000 mg at bedtime. Niacin has many side effects and prominent among them are flushing and diarrhea, etc.

Along the same line, it has been shown that drinking one or two glasses of wine at night, either red or white, with dinner, increases the level of the HDL (the good cholesterol). It is not advisable that men drink or abuse alcohol, but these studies clearly show that moderate ingestion of alcohol, in particular red wine, seems to have a significant advantage in increasing the level of the HDL cholesterol.

Diet plays a major role in the prevention of obesity and the prevention and control of hypertension. Diet also plays a major role in both preventing and controlling the levels of cholesterol and triglycerides in the blood. The so-called soul food that black men and other men of color like to eat so much is a legacy of slavery some 500 hundred years ago. However, soul foods have too much fat, carbohydrates, and salt, and are too spicy. These foods taste good, but they are unhealthy. Therefore, it is fine to eat them every now and then; but when a man eats them on a daily basis, it increases his chances of becoming obese and raising his blood pressure and his cholesterol. A combination of obesity, high blood pressure and high level of fat in the blood is responsible in part for the high incidence of coronary artery disease, stroke and deaths of men in the United States. To prevent these things from happening, the diet men eat clearly must be modified. Diet is very ethnic in its origin. People of different ethnic backgrounds have different tastes for different foods, and that is fine, except that one has to understand that everything has to be done in moderation. If a man eats fat and salt-laden foods too often, that man is likely to pay the consequences with an increased incidence of coronary artery disease, hypertension and stroke. Poor men in large measure suffer from these conditions because of poor living conditions, poor diet and overall poor economic conditions. An understanding of these issues and doing the things that are necessary either to modify or change them, will go a long way to prevent or decease the high incidence of hyperlipedimia/high cholesterol and coronary heart disease seen in men in the US.

CHAPTER 4

OBESITY IN MEN IN THE UNITED STATES

OBESITY IS A SERIOUS MEDICAL PROBLEM. Morbid obesity is a frequent cause of disability in men.

There are 68,590,000 or 68.8% overweight/obese men in the US.

There are 134,750,000 overweight/obese individuals in the US.

Obesity is associated with about 440,000 deaths annually in the US.

Over weight is defined as a BMI of 25.0 or higher. Obesity is defined as a BMI of 30. or greater. BMI (body mass index) = weight in kilograms divided by height in meters squared (kg/m²)

Table I—Ideal Weights Table

MEN HEIGHT FEET	INCHES	SMALL FRAME	MEDIUM FRAME	LARGE FRAME
4	10	102–111	109–121	118–131
4	11	103–113	111–123	120–134
5	0	104–115	113–126	122–137
5	1	106–118	115–129	125–140
5	2	108–121	118–132	128–143
5	3	111–124	121–135	131–147

5	4	114–121	124–138	134–151
5	5	117–130	127–141	137–155
5	6	120–133	130–144	140–159
5	7	123–136	133–147	143–163
5	8	126–139	136–150	146–167
5	9	129–142	139–153	149–170
5	10	132–146	142–156	152–173
5	11	135–148	148–159	155–176
6	0	138–151	148–162	158–179

Taken from "The Third World Tropical Diet Health Maintenance and Medical Management Program," 1992 By Valiere Alcena, MD, FACP

Table II—Modified classification of overweightness on obesity by BMI

	Obesity Class	BMI kg/m2
Underweight		<18.5
Normal		18.5–24.9
Overweight		25.0–29.9
Obese	I	30.0–34.9
	II	35.0–39.9
Extremely Obese	III	>40

BMI = body mass index (Source: Obese. Res. 1998; 6:515–2095.)
Another method of measuring obesity is calculating body mass index (BMI: weight/height^2, kg/m^2).

69.4% white males are overweight/obese.
62.9%black males are overweight/obese.
73.1% Mexican American males are overweight/obese.
65.2% Hispanic males are overweight/obese.
34.5% Asian males are overweight/obese.
61.7% American Indians/Alaska Natives are overweight/obese.

The overall cost of health problems associated with obesity in the U.S. is 100 billion dollars per year.

Obesity, when it is not associated with malfunction of the endocrine system, is always the result of eating too much of the wrong foods. The foods are foods that are too rich in fats, salt, and simple carbohydrates and too low in protein.

The most effective diet is a diet that is low in simple carbohydrates, fats and high in protein. Source:

THE THIRD WORLD TROPICAL DIET HEALTH MAITENANCE AND MEDICAL MAGEMENT PROGRAM WRITTEN BY VALIERE ALCENA M.D. F.A.C.P PUBLISHED BY ALCENA MEDICAL COMMUNICATION INC, Copyright© 1992, ISBN 0–9633365–0-9

A diet low in fat high in protein and low in simple carbohydrates is good diet that can lower weight, blood sugar and cholesterol. The question is, can this diet help men to maintain the weight they have lost long term.

When a man eats foods that have too much fats and carbohydrates, when the body is unable to break them all down, the rest of them are stored in the liver where they are distributed to different tissues of the abdomen, the hips, the thighs and other parts of the body. The fats and carbohydrates that are broken down are used as fuel to provide needed energy for proper functions of the body.

In order for this process to work properly, one needs a well-functioning basal metabolism. The basal metabolism is a process through which the body burns calories that are ingested in the body. If the basal metabolism is high, one burns calories too fast and stays thin. If the basal metabolism is too low, one burns calories too slow and stays fat. Slow basal metabolism, when not associated with medical problems such as hypothyroidism, is always the result of a genetically transmitted abnormality, which is passed on from parents to offspring.

There are several medical conditions that are associated with obesity, among them are:

1. Hypothyroidism
2. Syndrome X
3. Metabolic Syndrome
4. Primary Cushing's Syndrome (when the adrenal gland secretes too much hormone)
5. Secondary Cushing's disease (associated with long term steroid treatment)
6. Gigantism is a condition causes a person to become overgrown, due to over active pituitary gland.

If a man is obese, and is not suffering from an endocrine condition and is not taking steroids or estrogen replacement medication, then the man is obese because of a combination of low basal metabolism in association with ingestion of too much of the wrong foods. Foods that contain too much simple carbohydrates when eaten in excess can lead to obesity. According to the recent literature, the human gut contains about 100 trillions bacteria and some species of these bacteria have the ability to transform certain food materials into fat to be stored for future use and through this mechanism obesity can develop.

Time will tell if this hypothesis is true or not.

In the United States of America, many factors interplay in causing this high degree of obesity. For instance, the diet industry spends somewhere from 40 to 50 billion dollars a year selling the different products and types of dietary programs that these industries are involved in. The medical profession devotes very little time and resources in the prevention and treatment of obesity. The food industry spends somewhere around 36 billion dollars a year advertising the different food products and agricultural materials they produce and encouraging people to eat more. The main reason why the medical profession in the United States spends very little time in the prevention and management of obesity is that insurance companies could not care less about obesity and will not pay physicians to provide medical care for obese patients. The federal and state governments are not doing very much either, because those two governments spend only somewhere around 50 thousand dollars a year on nutritional and other educational programs addressing obesity, which is a pitiful gesture. In the U.S., 100 billion dollars are spent to treat obesity and its different complications. The different medical complications associated with obesity include:

1. Breast cancer
2. Colon cancer
3. Prostate cancer
4. Pancreatic cancer
5. Heart disease
6. Adult-onset diabetes
7. Gall Stones
8. Cholecystitis
9. Pancreatitis secondary to Gall Stones
10. Hypertension
11. Stroke
12. High cholesterol

13. Deep Vein Thrombophlebitis

14. Pulmonary embolism secondary to deep vein thrombophlebitis etc.

Many factors interplay in the excessive degree of obesity seen in men. The main factor is low basal metabolism. Low basal metabolism is inherited from parents to offspring. Genetic traits are adaptable, penetrating and "transmittable." Obese men the world over inherited the obesity gene, from their ancestry. That gene is disseminated among these men and their children. The human race and all is its original DNA genetic traits began in Africa around 60,000 years ago. Source: *The* Journey *of Man, A Genetic Odyssey, Princeton University Press, 2002.*

Another factor that plays a significant role in the development of obesity in men is the food they eat. Men who live in the third world who, by necessity, are forced to eat a meager diet are less obese than men who live in the developed countries, such as the United States. In the third world, men eat plenty of fresh fruits, green vegetables, grains, yams, plantains, bananas and less red meat, and plenty of fish. These men exercise more because they often have to walk long distances to the farm or the marketplace and they walk to the river to fetch water, etc. Some of them spend long hours working under the hot sun in the farms and some work long hours in sweatshops. Still others work at home doing all sorts of chores around their houses. All these activities cause them to lose calories, which is quite important in maintaining their weights. A combination of these factors leads to less obesity in these men who live in the third world. Nevertheless, they still carry the gene and are able to pass it on even though they themselves manage to work off the extra fat that was to be deposited into their tissues as predetermined by their hereditary trait. In addition, it must be understood that if a man is fat, he is likely to give birth to a fat baby, even though the baby may not be fat at birth. Because of the low basal metabolism gene, the baby will grow to become a fat adolescent and a fat adult. The foods that men in the third world eat are high in protein, low in fat, high in vitamins and fibers and low in carbohydrates. That combination of foods contains high complex carbohydrates. Examples of high complex carbohydrates foods include

1. rice
2. bagels
3. pretzels
4. pasta
5. yams
6. sweet
7. plantains

8. potatoes
9. dumpling
10. corn
11. cereals
12. breads
13. whole grains
14. tortillas
15. waffle
16. grits
17. millet
18. oats
19. wheat germs
20. granola
21. cornmeal
22. shredded wheat
23. flour etc.

High complex carbohydrates when eaten, is broken down very slowly in the body and provides a lower but longer level of energy. That is what makes them ideal food products, in that a person can eat high complex carbohydrates to satisfy hunger and provide vitamins and fiber for regular gastrointestinal functioning, particularly for proper bowel movements. Therefore, they cannot lead to an increased level of calories, which can cause a person to become obese. On the other hand, simple carbohydrates, such as sugar-containing foods, when eaten can be broken down in the liver and some of them distributed into the tissues and muscles, resulting in obesity in individuals who consume them in large quantities.

The aforeoutlined foods, when prepared in vegetable oil, either boiled or broiled and not fried, satisfy hunger, provide needed vitamins such as Vitamin A, Vitamin K, the B Vitamins, including B6, B12, etc. All of them are important nutrients for the body.

As just mentioned above, adult-onset diabetes mellitus is closely associated with obesity. What is the relationship between the onset diabetes mellitus and obesity? When a man is obese, his fat cells are resistant to the effect of insulin, creating an insulin-resistant state in his body. In this setting, the insulin cannot penetrate these fat cells to bring about the metabolism of sugar. Consequently, blood sugar rises. The rising blood sugar creates all sorts of symptoms, which are very disturbing to the affected man. Since the insulin has difficulty entering into the fat cells, it remains elevated in his bloodstream. The high insulin level, in turn, forces the obese man to crave for sweets-containing foods to satisfy his craving for sweet, resulting in a vicious cycle. The more obese a man is, the higher the level of insulin in his bloodstream. The higher the level of insulin in his bloodstream, the more he craves sweets-containing foods, which are high in simple carbohydrates and rich in calories. The more he eats the calorie-rich foods, the fatter he becomes, raising his blood sugar even higher.

Obesity is associated with Atherosclerotic heart disease, in that the persistent high level of insulin that is present in the bloodstream of the obese man causes plaques to develop within vessels throughout his body, including the coronary arteries around the heart. When these arteries are occluded, blood flow is impeded, preventing proper oxygen delivery to the muscles of the heart, causing pain in the chest to occur. Because there are plaques in the coronary arteries, sudden closure of one or several of these coronary arteries can result in a heart attack and, frequently, death of that man can occur.

Obesity as just outlined is quite common in men. Obesity is very highly associated with hypertension, which is also quite common in men. When a man is obese, the obesity is frequently associated with diabetes mellitus, hyperlipidemia, and hypertension. That combination of diseases is frequently referred to as syndrome X, or more recently renamed as metabolic hypertension. (Syndrome W is used as well to refer to that condition.) Men of color retain more salt in their bodies than do other men and, because, these men retain more fluid, and the fluid retention causes elevation in their blood pressures. When an obese man loses weight, frequently his blood pressure decreases and the need for medication decreases proportionately.

Obesity is commonly associated with stroke. Many of the conditions that are frequently seen in men who are obese, such as diabetes mellitus, hypertension and hyperlipidemia, are also seen in men who suffer from stroke, and frequently the underlying reason for the stroke seen in these men is the obesity. The reason why obesity, diabetes, hyperlipidemia and hypertension are associated with stroke is that all these conditions can cause atherosclerosis to occur. Once vessels in the brain develop plaques, these vessels become narrowed, thereby preventing the proper flow of blood and oxygen to the brain tissues. When one of these vessels becomes acutely closed, a stroke is usually the result.

Obesity is frequently associated with breast cancer in men. The type of breast cancer seen in that group of men is extremely aggressive and very resistant to treatments, resulting in a high percentage of deaths.

Osteoarthritis of the lower back, knees, and ankles is frequently seen in obese men. The obesity causes a great deal of mechanical stress on these areas of the body, resulting in wear and tear, causing severe pain, and suffering in these obese men.

Men who are obese feel the pressure of society, which seems to favor thinner men. That negative attitude causes these men to become depressed a great deal of the time. Depression is more common in obese men than in thin men. Obese men have difficulty in finding girlfriends, they have difficulties in finding jobs, and they face discriminations of all sorts, in a society obsessed with thinness and beauty and handsomeness. Obesity is a serious medical problem with significant impact on the overall health of men who are afflicted with it.

The result of obesity, these men suffer from psychosocial deprivation, economic deprivation and the interplay of these problems results in unnecessary early death from heart disease, cancer, hypertension, diabetes mellitus, and stroke and kidney failure.

To avoid these problems, these men must fight against obesity by eating a diet low in fat, low in salt, low in carbohydrates and high in protein, in green vegetables, in fruits, in non-shellfish, in chickens, veal, and low in red meats, in sausages, in bacon, in pork, ham, in egg yolks and low in breads, and cakes. In general, fast foods are not healthy because they contain too much fat, salt and carbohydrates, all of which can contribute to obesity when eaten in excess.

It is important for men to exercise at least three times per week. It is not necessary to spend money going to different exercise centers to exercise. These centers charge plenty of money and poor men cannot afford to pay to go to these exercise centers. For those who can afford to go, it is OK, and they are likely to benefit. Walking one hour daily helps to burn off significant calories. Aerobic exercise, push-ups, bicycling, gardening, walking the dog, and other forms of exercise can all contribute to decrease a man's weight.

The drain on the pocketbooks of these men because of the so-called diet programs is enormous. These programs are expensive and, according to the U.S. Government, have questionable motives in saying that they are trying to help these men to lose weight. In summary, these programs may be medically dangerous if entered into without proper medical supervision.

Every year 100 billion dollars are spent in the US to treat obesity and its multitude of associated medical problems. (Source MMWR, Vol. No, 36, Sept. 13, 2002DC/NCHS). Every year about 400.000 adults in the US die because of obesity and its associated medical problems.

Learning a new way to prepare foods and a change in the eating habits of men from the so-called soul food and fast foods will go a long way in helping obese men to lose weight without participating in expensive and potentially dangerous diet gimmicks that are designed to make money for the people who are pushing these programs. Men ought to pay attention to basics and adhere closely to a healthy lifestyle of exercise, good diet, low alcohol consumption and frequent visits to the physician's office for proper health screening. Understanding these facts and taking the necessary precautions are the best ways to go about solving the problems associated with obesity and its devastating consequences on men.

CHAPTER 5

DIABETES MELLITUS IN MEN IN THE USA

Five percent of the world population of 6,553,332,067 or 32,766,670 has diabetes mellitus type II according to the CDC.

In Europe, 8% of the adult population is diabetic, and 60,000,000 of the adults are prediabetic according to the International Diabetes Federation.

There are 304,000,000 people in the USA and there are 21,000,000 people in the U.S. with diabetes mellitus. 7% of the US population has diabetes and 54,000,000 individuals are prediabetics and most of them don't know they have it according to the CDC. Every year 1 million individuals develop type 2 diabetes in the US.

Diabetes mellitus can be prevented according to the DREAM study (Diabetes REduction Assessment with ramipril and resiglitazone Medication) published in Lancet if individuals at high risk for diabetes are treated with Rosiglitazone (Avandia).

Avandia works by making fat cells more sensitive to insulin thereby preventing the blood sugar from being elevated in the blood stream and decreasing the level of insulin in the blood.

About 1.7 million individuals in the US have type 1diabetes. 11.6% Blacks men in the U.S. have diabetes mellitus. 9. 2% white males have diabetes mellitus. 13.9% Mexican American men have diabetes. 9.4% Hispanics men have diabetes. 6.3% Asian males have diabetes mellitus. 16% American Indians/Alaska Natives men have diabetes mellitus. 15% American Indians/Alaska Natives getting medical care from the Indian Health Services have diabetes.

Diabetes mellitus has increased 600% in the United States since 1958 and it is estimated that the incidence of diabetes mellitus will rise by 35% in the next ten years. The worldwide incidence of diabetes mellitus was 171 million in the year 2000 and it is estimated that in the year 2030, the worldwide incidence of diabetes mellitus will be 366 millions.

The genetics of diabetes mellitus Type II works out that way. Roughly, one-half of the first-degree relatives of diabetics are said—according to recent reports—to have or will develop abnormal glucose tolerance, and about one-fourth will become diabetic. Another way of stating the genetics is that about 4/10 of siblings of diabetics and 1/3 of the offspring of diabetics have the propensity to become diabetic.

Type I diabetes is a different disease altogether from Type II diabetes and it is said to be caused by either an autoimmune phenomenon, autoimmune disease or some sort of a viral disease, but no one is quite sure. Type I diabetes usually starts in childhood.

The number of annual deaths due to diabetes in the year 2002 was 73.249.

In the year 2002, 28.110 white males died of diabetes mellitus and 5.207 black males died of diabetes mellitus.

The risk of death is roughly two times higher more in diabetic men than in non-diabetic men. The incidence of death from diabetes mellitus is 27% higher in black males as compared with white males. Diabetes mellitus was the sixth leading cause of deaths in the U.S. in 1999.

What is diabetes mellitus?

Diabetes mellitus is a condition in which the body is incapable of using sugar as a fuel due to lack of insulin. Three basic abnormalities cause diabetes to develop:

1. Lack of insulin secretion from the pancreas
2. Abnormal insulin secretion from the pancreas, and
3. Insulin resistance.

In the first instance, the beta cells of the Islets of Langerhans of the pancreas have been destroyed either by an autoimmune process or by viral organism resulting in a total lack of insulin in the body, sometimes since early infancy or childhood, resulting in juvenile diabetes. In the second, the pancreas still has the ability to produce insulin, but needs to be forced to secrete it. In the third instance, the pancreas simply cannot make any more insulin, period. That is Type II diabetes. In the third instance, insulin has to be given either subcutaneously or intravenously. That is called insulin-requiring diabetes mellitus type II.

The normal blood glucose is from 65 to about 116 mg/dL. Diabetes mellitus is a condition in which the blood glucose is higher than normal, when the blood glucose is drawn following a period of fasting for about 8 to 12 hours. As just mentioned, the normal blood glucose is between 65 to 116 mg/dL. If the fasting blood sugar remains abnormally high (126 or more) on more than three occasions, an individual can be said to have glucose intolerance and most probably is suffering from diabetes in its earliest form.

Another way to test the blood of an individual to see if he or he is diabetic is for the physician to order what is called a two-hour post-prandial glucose test. (Post-prandial means after eating.) Two hours after eating a meal containing sugar, a tube of blood is drawn from the individual and if the blood glucose is elevated, between 140 mg/dL and 190 milligrams per deciliter or (mg/dl), then that individual is said to have glucose intolerance or early diabetes mellitus. The genetic locus for insulin-dependent diabetes mellitus is on chromosome 6. The genetic locus for non-insulin dependent diabetes mellitus is unknown. Usually insulin-dependent diabetes (juvenile diabetes) or type I diabetes, occurs before age 40. On the other hand, non-insulin-dependent diabetes (Type II diabetes) occurs after 40, although there are exceptions. Most of the time however, insulin-dependent diabetes mellitus appears before age 20, but it can occur later in life. Non-insulin-dependent can also occur in late teens and early adulthood. It can happen both ways, but ages 35 to 40 are usually the cut-off point for someone to present with Type I diabetes mellitus. If a man is age 35 or over, the diagnosis is most likely going to be adult-onset diabetes, or Type II diabetes. If a man is below age 35 or for that matter below age 20, the diagnosis is most likely going to be insulin-dependent diabetes or type I. Again, there are crossovers and there are exceptions. Recently, a group of obese adolescents ages 10–19 has been reported to have Type II diabetes mellitus.

There are different types of Type II diabetes mellitus. The most common type is due to the inability of the pancreas to secrete insulin. Other types are due to insulin resistance because of obesity. Often, in people who have chronic pancreatitis, the pancreas may ultimately fail, resulting in Type II diabetes mellitus. Cushing's disease can cause chemically induced secondary diabetes, although it can be transient.

Endocrine pancreatic failure occurs in obese men resulting in type II diabetes. That happens because the pancreas over secretes insulin because of insulin resistance, which the obese state causes. In obesity, the insulin is not able to penetrate the fat cells; the result is that the pancreas keeps secreting insulin as though there is a need for it, and after an extended period, it uses up its store of insulin.

Steroids can cause blood sugar to rise in men who have occult or pre-diabetes. Alcoholics who suffer from chronic pancreatitis can also develop diabetes mellitus as result of pan-pancreatic failure.

Men who have occult diabetes mellitus or pre-diabetes can develop overt diabetes with markedly elevated blood sugars when under stress or when these men become infected.

Stress causes an excess secretion of adrenalin, which works counter to the effect of insulin, allowing a rise in blood sugar.(adrenalin is an anti-insulin hormone). Men who are known diabetics, when under stress, experience a rise in their blood sugars, necessitating an increase in the doses of their insulin.

What is happening in the body of a man that causes his to become diabetic?

The pancreas is an organ that is located on the left side of the abdomen. The pancreas has several functions to perform within the body for proper health. Among these functions is the secretion of insulin.

What is insulin?

Insulin is a hormone that is produced by the pancreas. The beta cells of the pancreas produce insulin.

How is the pancreas able to produce insulin?

The pancreas is able to produce insulin by means of a group of cells located within the area of the pancreas referred to as the Islands of Langerhans. These cells have the ability to produce the hormone called insulin. Once produced, the insulin is secreted into the bloodstream.

What is the role of the insulin in the body?

The job of the insulin is to metabolize (breakdown) sugars and other carbohydrates, so that the body can use them. The insulin actually forces the glucose into cells where it is used for the multitude of functions that are necessary for the body to function properly.

Sugar plays two functions in the human body under the influence of insulin.

1. Sugar is used as a fuel for the body to function properly. The human body gets the bulk of its energy from the breakdown of sugar under the influence of insulin.

2. Sugar is needed in order for the blood to carry oxygen to the different tissues and organs of the human body, and most importantly the brain. Without sugar, human beings cannot carry the appropriate amount of oxygen to the brain, which is needed to remain alert. Insulin is needed to push the sugar into these tissues and organs for proper body functions.

When the body is not able to use sugar because of lack of insulin, it is forced to use fat for fuel. Fat is a very bad fuel to be used for energy because it is not effective. When one uses fat it produces breakdown products called ketones, bodies that are very toxic when dumped into the bloodstream. The accumulation of these ketone bodies in the body because of the inability to use sugar is a condition known as ketoacidosis, which can be life-threatening if it goes unrecognized and untreated.

There exists another common type of diabetes mellitus Type II that is due to hemochromatosis. Hemochromatosis is a condition described in the chapter on anemia in that book. Hemolytic anemias cause iron overload and secondary hemochromatosis. The gene for primary hemochromatosis is located on the long arm of chromosome 6 on the HLA locus. More recently, a genetic test has been developed that identifies the gene called C282Y. That gene is known to cause hemochromatosis. Many individuals who have Type II diabetes believe that they inherited the diabetic gene that was passed on to them by their parents, when in fact; it is the hemochromatosis gene that was passed on to them, which results in their iron overload. The excess iron accumulates in the pancreas, damaging the area where the beta cells are produced and preventing it from being able to make enough insulin, resulting in hyperglycemia and a form of Type II diabetes.

The percentage of men who have hemochromatosis is not well known. However, it used to be thought that primary hemochromatosis was a disease seen mainly in European Caucasians and Scandinavians, which turned out not to be altogether the case. There are black men, Hispanic men and Asian men who have genetically transmitted primary hemochromatosis, although many of these men are negative for the C282Y gene. Yet many more genes that cause primary hemochromatosis are yet to be discovered. The C282Y gene that causes hemochromatosis has been identified in a black woman by the author (Valiere Alcena, MD, FACP, et al, "Prevalence of Iron Overload in African-Americans: A Primary Care Experience; A Clinical Observation," *Prestige Medical News, Feb, 7th, 2003*.

More genetic research needs to be done to try to determine the locations of the gene that causes hemochromatosis in non-Caucasian men. The serum ferritin test, which when high may mean that a man has hemochromatosis, costs about $60 and is routinely available.

Clinically, hemochromatosis is manifested the same way in non-Caucasian men as it is in Caucasian men, although the severity is more intense in Caucasian men, as evidenced by the fact that the number of homozygous patients seen in clinical practice is greater in the Caucasian population. What used to be called African Iron Overload Syndrome is in fact really primary hemochromatosis with the same clinical manifestations as seen in white males.

How does the iron cause destruction of the pancreas that results in the development of diabetes mellitus?

Iron is a very toxic material, which when broken down releases free radicals in the body, resulting in severe tissue damage. It is the free radicals that are released from iron when broken down that cause the damage to tissues in the body. In the case of the pancreas, these free radicals damage the pancreas because the iron is located within the pancreas. The breakdown of iron causes the release of these free radicals, which gradually destroy the beta cells that are responsible for the production of insulin. Once the pancreas is damaged by the breakdown of iron, elevated blood sugar begins to develop and the result is a form of Type II diabetes mellitus as previously mentioned.

Other early signs of diabetes mellitus in men may include recurrent fungal toenails infection, fingernail infection, recurrent paronychia (infection in the bed of the nails), recurrent groin fungal infection, blurry vision, thirstiness, infertility, lack of libido, numbness in toes and fingers. All of these may also be due to occult or overt diabetes, etc.

Some of the overt signs of diabetes in addition to the above listed ones are urinary frequency, excessive consumption of fluid, dryness of the mouth, weight loss and frequent urinary tract infection.

Diabetes is a very complicated and complex disease that affects all organs in the human body one way or another. However, the organs that suffer most from the devastation of diabetes are the so-called end organs. These end organs consist of:

1. The eyes
2. The heart
3. The kidneys
4. The brain
5. The peripheral vascular system
6. The peripheral nervous system

Other organ systems that are frequently affected by diabetes mellitus, causing severe pain and suffering, are the nervous system, causing peripheral neuropathy with pain, numbness, and coldness in the toes, feet and fingers. If severe enough, diabetic neuropathy can cause the affected man to be unable to walk. The skin is one of the most frequently affected organs in patients with diabetes. Diabetes affects the colon by causing constipation. Diabetes affects the stomach by causing gastroparesis with frequent indigestion, bloating, and burning in the stomach. Diabetes affects the urinary system by causing urinary retention.

The eyes are affected by diabetes because of the series of damages that the elevated blood sugar causes to take place inside the eyes.

These damages result in bleeding within the eyes, a condition called diabetic retinopathy (see figures 1 and 2).

Diabetic retinopathy is a condition that if left untreated can lead to blindness. The treatment for diabetic retinopathy is laser surgery.

The heart is affected by diabetes by causing hardening of the arteries, known as atherosclerosis. Atherosclerosis causes narrowing of the coronary arteries, resulting in ischemic heart disease, which causes angina pectoris and frequently results in myocardial infarction (heart attack).

The kidneys are affected by diabetes through damage to the kidney tubules and glomeruli, resulting in diabetic nephropathy of different degrees. Diabetic nephropathy can cause protein loss, microalbuminuria and, ultimately, nephrotic syndrome. The result of that constellation of abnormalities is elevated serum BUN, creatinine, potassium and renal insufficiency, which usually results in end-stage renal failure. End-stage renal failure is treated with dialysis.

The brain is affected by diabetes by way of atherosclerosis of the arteries inside the brain, causing narrowing of these vessels and preventing easy flow of blood and oxygen, which can result in strokes.

These are some of the acute symptoms that may signify that a person is diabetic:

1. Weight loss
2. Thirstiness
3. Blurred vision
4. Urinary frequency
5. Frequent tiredness and a feeling of unwell ness, which, if very non-specific, may be due to diabetes mellitus.

If these symptoms are not recognized, and the diagnosis is established and treatment is begun, then the patient may go on to develop diabetic ketoacidosis, which can lead to a comatose state and, ultimately, death.

There is a subgroup of diabetes called hyperosmolar nonketotic diabetes mellitus. It is a condition in which the individual loses so much water that the blood sugar can exceed 1,000 and sometimes 1,500 to 2,000. nanogram/dL Because the person has lost so much water that the brain becomes dehydrated, the patient can go into a coma without having diabetic ketoacidosis. That is a very serious condition and if it is not recognized right away and treatment given with appropriate and careful fluid replacement and insulin, then the person may develop acute kidney failure because of marked dehydration, and death can result.

Some of the late signs and symptoms of diabetes are.

1. Blindness
2. Chronic kidney failure
3. Coronary artery disease
4. Recurrent leg and feet ulcers with frequent loss of lower limbs 5. Peripheral neuropathy
6. Sexual impotence
7. Loss of libido
8. Gastroparesis.
9. Infertility
10. Constipation
11. Recurrent fungal infections of the skin, sinuses, etc.

Another frequent problem that develops is urinary tract infection because diabetes damages the smooth muscle and nerves within the bladder, causing poor contraction of the bladder, preventing complete excretion of urine. The residual urine that stays in the bladder serves as a culture medium allowing for bacterial growth, and the result is recurrent urinary tract infection and all its many potential complications.

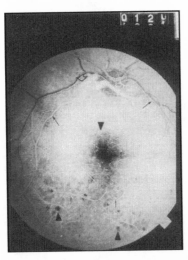

Figure 5.1—Showing different degrees of abnormalities in the eye of a patient with diabetes mellitus (diabetic retinopathy); Fluorescein angiogram shortly after injection of dye in patient's eye. Dye in arteries (white) and just starting to enter veins (large arrow). White area off NH is neovascular tuff (open arrow). White spots are hemorrhages (arrow heads). Tiny white dots are microaneurysms (small arrow).

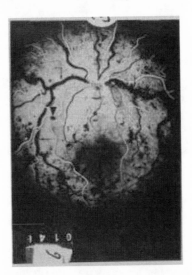

Figure 5.2—Showing different degrees of abnormalities in the eye of a patient with diabetes mellitus (diabetic retinopathy). Large arrows showing dilated veins. Arrowheads showing hemorrhages inside the eye.

Why is the incidence of diabetes mellitus so high among men?

The answer lies partly in the fact that 68% of adult males are obese/overweight in the US and obesity/overweightness has a high association with diabetes mellitus.

Both obesity and certain forms of adult-onset diabetes mellitus are genetically transmitted diseases and it is therefore not surprising that these two diseases are so closely linked and so highly prevalent in men. Obesity causes a state of insulin resistance to exist, meaning that in the natural situation the insulin that the obese person's pancreas secretes has a great deal of difficulty penetrating the fat cells to carry out proper metabolism (breaking down) of sugar. When that happens, the blood sugar stays above normal in the blood, causing a state of glucose intolerance, which is the earliest form of diabetes mellitus.

Another possible explanation for that high incidence of diabetes mellitus in men is stress. When added to the underlying obesity, stress associated with racial discrimination and its multitude of related problems, as well as the problems associated with daily living in the United States, makes it clear why minority men's and other poor men's blood sugars are so much higher and so much more difficult to bring under control as compared to the blood sugars of well to do white males. When an individual is under stress, that person secretes adrenalin in excess, and adrenalin is an anti-insulin hormone. Another way of saying it, is that adrenalin prevents the insulin from doing its work, which is to break down sugar. The result is that the sugar level rises. Any other type of stressful situation, such as an acute heart attack, an acute infection such as urinary tract infection, pneumonia, or any accident can cause the level of adrenalin to go up, resulting in an elevation of blood sugar.

The dietary habits of some men play a major role in their being overweight and play a major role in their being insulin-resistant. These men eat a diet that is rich in fat and simple sugars. In poor men, poverty plays a major role in their inability to afford better foods. Therefore, they eat the foods they can afford. The types of foods that they can afford are frequently of poor quality. Even when the food is of very good quality, the way in which it is prepared makes it too rich in fat and carbohydrates.

Food tends to be very ethnic in character. The foods that men of color like to eat—so called soul food—has its origin in Africa and the legacy of slavery. During slavery, slaves were not able to eat higher-quality foods. Therefore, they compensated by preparing the foods in a way to make it more palatable by curing it with a fruit called "sour." that fruit is very juicy and is a bitter orange.

When plenty of salt, hot pepper and other spices are added, the food is more palatable and its taste improves but not necessarily in quality. That is the legacy of the so-called soul food, which is frequently eaten by some men, but is detrimental to their health. White men and Asian men eat these foods less frequently, and when they do, they eat them as delicacies.

Fast foods like hamburgers, cheeseburgers, hot dogs, fried chicken, spareribs, pizza, etc., have proliferated in U.S. society and are easy to purchase. Young men of all ethnic backgrounds eat these foods very often, they are getting fat, and many of them are developing type II diabetes. Those foods, although popular, are definitely not very nutritious and certainly not particularly healthy. It is perfectly fine to eat fast foods if done infrequently, but if one makes it a habit to feast on these foods on a regular basis, then the health consequences can be dire indeed.

Obesity and diabetes are intertwined, and as just outlined, they are both genetically transmitted diseases and interact together. When they interact together in the same man, it makes it much more difficult to provide medical care for such a man who is both obese and diabetic.

Insulin is a hormone that the body needs in order to break down sugar, to provide energy, and to carry oxygen to the brain and tissues in the body. Stress causes a person to secrete a series of other hormones called counterregulatory hormones, which includes adrenalin and nor-adrenalin. When secreted in large amounts as described above, adrenalin and nor-adrenaline can negate the effect of insulin, making it much more difficult to lower a person's blood sugar. Most of these counterregulatory hormones, including Cortisol, have effects that would counter the insulin's ability to do its work properly in the body.

An obese man has a good deal of difficulty using insulin because the obesity state renders his insulin-resistant. Men who are obese and diabetic and living under stressful conditions have a constant interplay of over secretion of adrenalin as well as an inability for insulin to penetrate the fat cells in order to lower their blood sugars. All these factors make the management of their diabetes extremely difficult.

What can men do to decrease their incidence of diabetes and what can those men who are genetically predetermined to develop diabetes do to delay the onset of that disease?

The first thing for men to do is to learn about their family health history. They should ask questions about their parents and their grandparents who might have been diabetic. They should also find out if their siblings are diabetic. If the mother or the father died at an early age, they ought to inquire from their aunts and uncles whether diabetes existed in the immediate family. If they have access to the treating physician who cared for their parents, they ought to inquire as to the health records of their parents to ascertain whether the physician treated their parents for diabetes. Knowing the family history may in many instances save lives. If either parent has diabetes, or more so, if both parents are diabetic, then these men must be ever so careful and must see their physicians for frequent evaluation of their blood sugars. Having that knowledge can go a long way in helping these men take the necessary precautions to delay the onset of diabetes and its devastating complications.

Some of the precautions that men need to take to decrease their chances of becoming diabetic and, if already diabetic, to better control their blood sugars include:

1. Eat a diet rich in fruits, vegetables, protein, high in complex carbohydrates, and low in fat, simple sugar and salt.
2. Exercise regularly to burn calories, thereby decreasing weight and increasing insulin-sensitivity, which in turn decreases blood sugar.

The increase in insulin sensitivity decreases the level of insulin in the blood, which in turn decreases the obese man's appetite and decreases the craving for carbohydrate-containing foods. High insulin levels in the blood of obese men are part of the reason why these men have such a craving for carbohydrates, resulting in a vicious cycle. The more obese a man is, the more insulin-resistant he becomes, and the more insulin-resistant he is, the more he feels a need to eat carbohydrate-containing foods. Insulin is an anabolic hormone, meaning that the more insulin is injected exogenously into the obese diabetic, the more the obese diabetic man eats and the more obese he becomes. The only way to break that vicious cycle is to treat the obese diabetic with a strict dietary program that can decrease the weight and thereby increases the insulin sensitivity. If possible, the best way to treat the obese diabetic man is with oral hypoglycemic agents and diet. Use insulin to treat the obese diabetic man only when it is necessary.

There is a long list of oral hypoglycemic agents available on the market to treat men with type II diabetes.

The following is a partial list of these medications.

1. DiaBeta
2. Glucotrol
3. Glucotrol XL
4. Amaryl
5. Actos
6. Glucophag
7. Glucophage XR
8. Glucovance
9. Diabinese,
10. Januvia

Type I diabetes is treated only with insulin; because the pancreas of men with type I diabetes is not able to secrete any insulin at all.

The following oral hypoglycemic agents, Glucophage, Glucophage XR, and Actos, work to lower blood sugar by increasing insulin sensitivity and uptake from the blood to cells and tissues. Glucovance, which is a combination of Glucophage and Glyburide, on the other hand, works by both stimulating the pancreas to secrete insulin while facilitating insulin uptake in the blood to cells and tissues to lower the blood sugar. Because of that, these oral hypoglycemic agents can be used in conjunction with insulin, as well as with other oral agents to control blood sugar.

DiaBeta, Glucotrol, Glucotrol XL, Amaryl and Diabinese work to lower blood sugar by stimulating the pancreas to secrete insulin into the blood-stream to control blood sugar. In addition to controlling blood sugars, all these agents work to allow the body to properly use sugar as fuel for normal body functions.

There are some Type II diabetics who are insulin-requiring, meaning that they need insulin in order to survive, because the pancreas is no longer able to produce insulin in any amount. On the other hand, there is another group of diabetics who are non-insulin-requiring, meaning that they still have enough beta cells left in their pancreas that can be stimulated by oral agents to secrete insulin into the bloodstream to break down the sugar as just described. The way one finds out which group of diabetics is insulin-requiring and which group is not, is by trial and error.

The different doses of oral hypoglycemic agents used to treat diabetics are as follows:

The usual starting dose of DiaBeta (glyburide) is 2.5 mg-5 mg each morning with breakfast; a maximum dose of 20 mg per day divided into 10 mg twice per day can be used.

The usual dose of Glucotrol (glipizide) is 5 mg each morning with breakfast, but a maximum dose of 40 mg can be given per day in divided doses. The usual dose of Glucotrol is 5 mg with breakfast each morning, but a maximum dose of 20 mg per day can be given in divided doses to control the blood sugar. The usual starting dose of Amaryl is 1–2 mg per day with breakfast. A maximum dose of 8 mg per day may be used in divided doses to control the blood sugar. The usual dose of Actos is 15–30 mg per day. A maximum dose of 45 mg can be used to control the blood sugar. The usual dose of Glucophage (metformin) is 500 mg three times per day, but a maximum dose of 2550 mg per day can be used to control the blood sugar. The usual dose of Glucophage XR (metformin) is 500 mg with supper, but up to 2000 mg with supper may be used to control the blood sugar. The usual starting dose of Glucovance is 1.25 mg DiaBeta with 250 mg of Glucophage (1.25/250 mg), but 5/500 mg twice per day of Glucovance may be used to control the blood sugar. The usual dose of Diabinese is 250 mg per day, but up to 500 mg per day can be used to control the blood sugar.

The dose of these hypoglycemic agents must be decreased significantly in elderly men to prevent hypoglycemia; because the elderly man is more likely to have fewer fats on his body and is also less likely to eat a good diet. These two factors, along with the long-acting effects of the agents, can cause severe and prolonged hypoglycemia in elderly men if the doses of these medications are not well monitored.

Januvia works by inhibiting the dipeptidyl peptidase-4 (DPP-4) for 24 hour after ingestion. The usual dose Januvia is 100 mg per day by mouth.

Another important factor to consider when treating elderly men or men of any age with type II diabetes with oral hypoglycemic agents is the status of their kidney functions. The state of renal insufficiency, which is very likely the older a man becomes, dictates that less insulin is needed to maintain the normoglycemic state. That is so because 15% of the body's sugar is metabolized (made in the kidneys), and as the kidneys become sick and insufficient, the less able they are to produce that amount of sugar, making the need for insulin less, therefore the need for oral hypoglycemic agents or exogenous insulin is much less.

There are many different insulin preparations available to treat diabetes mellitus, some of them, such as Humulin N or NPH, are long-acting, and some of them, such as Humulin R regular insulin, are short-acting. Some insulin preparations are intermediate-acting. There is also a mixture of regular insulin with long-acting insulin called Novolin 70/30, Humalog Mix 75/25, Humalog and more recently Levemir FlexPen with a 24 hour ½ life. The patient's physician and the patient determine the types of insulin that are appropriate for his.

The following is a list of some of the insulin preparations.
1. Humulin N
2. Lantus
3. Humulin R
4. NovoLog
5. Novolin 70/30
6. Humalog
7. Levemir FlexPen

In the acute setting, in a man who presents with elevated blood sugar, dehydration, thirst and other associated acute symptoms of diabetes, he must be treated inside a hospital with fluid replacement, electrolyte replacement, and either IV regular insulin drip or subcutaneous insulin to bring the blood sugar down and correct the dehydration and the electrolyte abnormalities. If he presents in diabetic ketoacidosis, he must be treated with IV fluid, and regular insulin either intravenously or subcutaneously. If he is in shock, and cannot perfuse his skin well, the regular insulin must be given intravenously to assure its entry into the bloodstream to bring down the blood sugar and correct the ketoacidosis.

The management of diabetes mellitus and its associated problems is very complex and it takes an experienced physician to properly treat them. A diet poor in simple sugar, carbohydrates, in association with exercise and weight management are crucial and necessary parts in the treatment of diabetes mellitus.

Type I diabetes mellitus (juvenile diabetes) is treated with insulin, diet, exercise and weight management. Oral agents that work to control the blood sugar by stimulating the pancreas are not appropriate in the treatment of juvenile diabetes because there is no insulin in the pancreas for these oral agents to secrete in the bloodstream.

In the hospital setting, blood sugar is tested several times per day and insulin dosages are adjusted according to the level of sugar in the blood.

At home, there are different types of blood sugar meters available commercially for patients who are diabetic to test their blood sugar, which allow them to adjust their insulin dosages or the dosages of their oral hypoglycemic agents on instructions from their physicians.

Men who are diabetic ought to have their eyes examined to be certain that they do not have diabetic retinopathy. They also ought to see the podiatrist in order to have proper foot care and avoid cuts in their toes that can lead to diabetic ulcers with the potential for the loss of a limb.

The reason why diabetic men do not heal very easily is due in part to poor circulation, which is secondary to the damage that diabetes causes to veins, arteries and smaller vessels in their feet, which results in poor blood and oxygen delivery to tissues in their extremities.

Another reason why diabetic men don't heal easily is that when a cut occurs, the polynuclear white blood cells of the diabetic man don't migrate well towards the site of the cut. The result is the development of infection.

It is a good idea also for the diabetic man to get in contact with the American Diabetic Association to become familiar with all the different programs that are available to them. In addition wearing a bracelet on their arms identifying themselves as diabetics is a very good idea so that they can be easily identified as diabetics in the event that they become ill in the street or on the job, either because of hypoglycemia (low blood sugar) or hyperglycemia (high blood sugar).

In such a case, the bracelet will show that the wearer is diabetic. He can be quickly given a piece of candy, a glass of orange juice or soda while waiting for medical help to arrive in the event of a hypoglycemic reaction. It is also a good idea for diabetic men to always carry in their pocketbooks a candy bar so that in the event that they feel dizzy and weak or feel like they are going to develop a hypoglycemic episode which consists primarily of dizziness, sweatiness, or a feeling of impending doom, they can prevent the hypoglycemic episode by eating the candy bar.

Hypoglycemia (low blood sugar) that occurs on a repeated basis is very dangerous because sugar is needed to carry oxygen into the brain. When the patient is having repeated episodes of hypoglycemia, the brain is being deprived of oxygen. In other words, when the diabetic person feels sick, it is best for his to ingest sugar because it is easy to bring the blood sugar down. On the other hand, it is much more difficult to treat the condition of low blood sugar or hypoglycemia. In particular, hypoglycemia associated with oral agents that the man might be taking must be treated in a hospital setting because it could take days to raise the level of the blood sugar that is because the half-life of some of these hypoglycemic agents can be quite long.

Diabetes mellitus, while not a curable disease, is definitely a treatable disease. There are plans underway for pancreatic transplants and if these become successful, then the disease can, at that point, be considered curable. Insulin pumps are also already in use. These pumps add a great deal to the treatments of diabetic men requiring insulin.

There is research underway to try to determine the cause of Type I diabetes and the hope is that someday, the answer to these problems will be found. Meanwhile, it is important for diabetic men to learn as much about diabetes mellitus as they can, and in the case of diabetic men who are obese, it is important that every effort is made to get the excess weight under control to help better control their diabetes.

In the year 2002, the over all death rate from diabetes mellitus in the US was 25.4 %

The death rate for white males was 28.6% while the death rate for black males was 49.4%

Deaths from heart disease in individuals with diabetes mellitus are about 4 times higher than the death rates from individuals without diabetes.

The cost for the over all treatments of diabetes was $132 billion in 2002. (Source the Burden of Chronic Diseases and Their Risk Factors, CDC/NCHS, Feb, 2004)

CHAPTER 6

HEART DISEASE IN MEN

HEART DISEASE IS THE LEADING cause of death among men of all ethnic groups in the U S. There are a total of 70, 100,000 individuals who have cardiovascular heart disease (CVD) in the U.S. There are 32.500.000 males with cardiovascular disease in the US, representing 34.4% of all men. 34.3% white males have cardiovascular disease. 41.1% black males have cardiovascular disease. 29.2% Mexican American males have cardiovascular disease. There are 27,000,000. individuals with cardiovascular disease who are 65 years old or older in the US. There are more 16,000,000 people in the US with coronary heart disease. 7,100,000 of them have had heart attacks. There are 6,400, 000. individuals who suffer from angina pectoris (chest pain). In the year 2002, there were 543,00 men who presented to hospital in the US with Acute Coronary Syndrome (unstable angina).

Every year 452,000 people die of ASHD in the US.

There are 4,900,000 individuals who have congestive heart failure in the US, and there are 500,000, new cases of congestive heart failure every year. (Source National Health and Nutrition Examination Survey NHANES1999–2002) 2,400,000 men suffer from congestive heart failure in the US. Every year, there are 1.1 million heart attacks in the U.S. and 450,000 of them are recurrent heart attacks (Source: *Morbidity and Mortality: 2002 Chart Book on Cardiovascular, Lung and Blood Diseases*. Bethesda, Maryland National Heart, Lung and Blood Institute, May 2002). Every day 2,600 people die of cardiovascular disease in the U.S.; that represents on an average one death every 33 seconds. In the year 2000, there were 2,400,000 deaths in the U.S. from different causes and 1,415,000 of these deaths were due to cardiovascular disease of different types. Each year over 500,000 people die of coronary heart disease in the U.S. Cardiovascular heart disease is the number one killer in the U.S. The total number of deaths due to cardiovascular disease in the year 2002 was 927,448. 375,392 white males died of cardiovascular disease in 2002. 48,993 black males died of cardiovascular disease in 2002.(source CDC/NCHS;2002) It is estimated that there were 7,100,000 males with coronary heart disease in the U.S. in the year 200, and during that same period of time, 4,100,00 of these men have had myocardial infarctions. 252,760 of these men died of coronary heart disease in 2002. Of the men who died of coronary heart disease, 223,262 were white males and 24,322 were black males. 25% of men die within a year after suffering a heart attack. Half of men under age 65 who have had a heart attack die within 8 years after suffering the first heart attack from coronary heart disease. 50% of men who died suddenly due coronary heart disease had no previous symptoms of coronary heart disease. (Source: Heart Disease and Stroke Statistics 2005 Update American Heart Association.)

The prevalence of coronary heart disease in men in the U.S. is 8.4% in white males, 7.4% in black males, 5.6% in Mexican-American males, 4.8% in Latino males, 5% in Asian males and 3.6% in American Indians/Alaska Natives. In the year 2002, of all deaths from coronary heart disease 51.1% were of men.

The estimated direct and indirect total cost of cardiovascular heart disease in the year 2005 in the U.S. is 393.5 billion dollars. (Direct costs include hospital, nursing home, physicians/other professionals, drugs/other, medical durables, home health care. Indirect costs include lost productivity/morbidity, lost productivity/mortality.) (Source: *Heart Disease and Stroke Statistics*: 2005 Update, American Heart Association.) In the year 2002 433,825 men died of CVD in the US. Of that number, there were 375,393 white males and 48,993 black men. 49.4% of deaths from coronary heart disease occurred in men and during that same period of time 53.5 % of deaths from cardiovascular disease occurred in men. Cardiovascular disease is the number one killer of men in the U.S. Every year more than half a million men die from cardiovascular disease, one death per minute. The cost of direct and indirect cost of coronary heart disease is projected to be 151.6 billion dollars in 2007.

Why is there such a high incidence of coronary artery heart disease and death from CAD in men in the USA?

The reasons are:

1. Sixty eight percent of men (68.590.000) is obese/overweight in the USA.

2. In the USA, 31.5% of men or 29, 400,000 million suffer from hypertension.

3. Black men and men of color in general are less likely to receive early treatments for hypertension than white men, making the total number of problems associated with CAD in black men and men of color in general more numerous and more advanced at presentation.

4. The diet that men of color eat contains more fat than the diet that white men eat.

5. Men of color are more likely to ignore their symptoms of shortness of breath, chest pain and other cardiac symptoms, such as palpitations.

6. Black men and other men of color are less likely to get proper medical attentions when they show to the emergency room seeking medical help. Some of the health care professionals giving care in the emergency rooms lack the necessary cultural sensitivity to provide the medical care that black men and other men of color need to treat they many serious presenting medical problems. Often these medical conditions are already in advance stages and in desperate need of the most competent care.

7. Black men and other men of color are less likely to be offered cardiac catheterization to evaluate them for the likelihood of coronary artery disease. When these men are found to have coronary occlusive disease, they are less likely to be offered coronary bypass to treat their coronary artery disease. Men of color live under conditions that oftentimes are more stressful than do white men, such as supporting and raising a family on meager income and working two jobs to try to pay bills. While poor white men face some of these same economic problems, they do not have to deal with constant indignities of daily racial discrimination and harassment of different types. These multitudes of responsibilities and the psycho-socio-economic problems create an unhealthy situation, which predisposes the black men, and other me of color to a constant stressful way of being that creates a perfect formula for the development of coronary heart disease and heart attacks and sudden death.

8. The combination of obesity, hypertension, diabetes mellitus, hyperlipidemia and insulin resistance, referred to as syndrome X or metabolic syndrome plays a major role in the causation of coronary artery disease in men.

The diet of most men of color is less healthier than that of white men, because in part the economic situation of that subgroup of men is poorer; creating a lifestyle that predisposes them to poorer cardiac health. The diet that this subgroup of men eats frequently is too rich in fats, carbohydrates and salt and too poor in protein and fibers. Such a diet is guaranteed to create the development of many serious medical problems including heart disease. The cholesterol level of men of color is higher than that of white men. Obesity is more prevalent in men of color than in white men. The incidence of hypertension is higher in men of color than in white men. Stress as a psychological state is more prevalent in men of color than in white men. The incidence of cigarette smoking is higher in men of color than in white men, percentage-wise. The incidence of alcohol abuse, percentage-wise, is higher in men of color than in white men. The percentage of IV drug abuse is higher in men of color than in white men. All these factors contribute in one form or another to make the overall cardiac health of these men bad. The result is that the overall rate of heart disease morbidity/mortality is higher in men of color. When men of color of present to emergency rooms as previously mentioned with symptoms of heart disease, they are less likely to get proper medical care as compared to white male patients. Their pain is usually attributed to other factors. They are less likely to be assigned to a coronary care unit and they are less likely to be offered cardiac catheterization, angioplasty or coronary bypass. The individuals who receive the quickest attention and receive highest priority in the health care system in the USA are the white males. That is so in part because, more often than not, the physicians making the rulings as to who gets what type care are white male doctors in training (interns, residents and fellows). These young physicians work at the front line in the emergency rooms and inside the hospitals.

In community hospitals where there are no training programs, the attending physicians see their own patients and control the quality of the care given.

The availability of health insurance plays a major role in the type of care that is offered to some men when they present seeking health care. For instance, according to recent report, 45.8 million individuals do not have health insurance in the US and many of them are poor people. White males have better access to health care than black males. White males live longer than black males and men of color in general. The median survival for white males is 75.1 years and the median survival of black American males is 68.6 years, a difference of 6.5 years in favor of white American males.

The bottom line is that taken together, white American males live 6.5 years longer than black American males and this is not due to genetic inheritance but rather this due to a multitude of economic, educational, professional, racial and psychosocial advantages that the white males enjoy over the black males in the US.

Risk factors for coronary heart disease in men include:
1. Hypertension
2. Obesity
3. Diabetes mellitus
4. Poor dietary habits
5. Hyperlipidemia (high cholesterol, high triglycerides, high LDL, low HDL, high cholesterol/HDL ratio)
6. High lipoprotein A in the blood
7. High lipoprotein A in conjunction with high LDL in the blood
8. High homocysteine level in the blood
9. Alcohol abuse
10. Stress
11. Type A personality
12. Tobacco smoking
13. Hereditary predisposition
14. Poverty etc.

How does hypertension cause cardiovascular heart disease?

Hypertension takes various routes in causing heart disease. First, the fact of having a high pressure within vessels while the blood passes through those vessels causes the lumen of the vessels to be damaged. The areas of the blood vessels' lumen that get damaged trap debris as the blood passes through them and platelets and lipid particles settle onto the damaged areas inside the vessels, resulting in the formation of a nidus. Once a nidus is formed, then more of such materials are deposited on these areas, resulting in formation of plaques. The plaques grow larger and larger, causing narrowing of the vessels, particularly in the coronary arteries. The narrowed coronary arteries prevent blood and oxygen delivery to heart muscle, causing symptoms of coronary heart disease.

Another mechanism through which hypertension causes cardiovascular heart disease is when the blood pressure remains so high for a long time, and remains untreated for a long time, that the heart muscle becomes hypertrophied (enlarged). The enlarged heart in time becomes unable to pump blood properly and fails, resulting in congestive heart failure. The reason why the enlarged heart fails is because muscle fibers have a finite stretch ability, and once the muscle fibers of the heart are stretched to the maximum, then the heart becomes like a big floppy bag with very poor function, resulting in the development of many serious and disabling symptoms of cardiovascular disease, including cardiac rhythm abnormalities.

Diabetes mellitus has a high association with coronary artery heart disease.

How does diabetes mellitus cause cardiovascular disease?

The high level of blood sugar in the circulating blood damages blood vessels, including the vessel around the heart, namely the coronary arteries. Once the effects of diabetes damage the lumen of the coronary arteries, then plaques easily form, resulting in coronary disease and the symptoms of coronary heart disease. Sorbitol is a sugar whose level becomes quite elevated in uncontrolled diabetes and Sorbitol has a very toxic effect on different vessels in the body as well as different peripheral nerves in the body, causing a multitude of vascular and nerve damage.

Obesity has a high association with the development of coronary artery heart disease.

How does obesity cause cardiovascular heart disease?

Obesity is associated with coronary heart disease by being associated with diabetes mellitus, hyperlipidemia and hypertension. Some prefer to call that metabolic syndrome, metabolic hypertension, syndrome W or syndrome X. A sedentary life style is highly associated with obesity, increasing the evidence of coronary heart disease. In addition, obesity is associated with coronary heart disease because obesity creates a state of insulin resistance in the human body. The insulin resistance results in an elevated level of insulin in the circulation of the human body. That excess insulin works in a negative way to cause more plaques to develop in arterial vessels of these obese patients. In other words too much insulin in the circulation is arthrogenic. The higher the level of circulating insulin, the higher the likelihood that affected men might develop coronary occlusive disease. The more obese a man is, the more insulin-resistant he is likely to be, and the more insulin-resistant he is, the higher the level of circulating insulin is in his blood.

Once plaques form in these arteries, the vessels' narrowing process begins, leading to all the possible problems associated with that process.

How does eating a poor diet contribute to a high incidence of Atherosclerotic heart disease in men?

The fat-rich diet leads to higher lipid levels and its propensity to causing coronary artery heart disease. The higher carbohydrate-containing diet results in obesity, and its propensity to the development of heart disease. The high salt in the diet that men eat contributes to the development of hypertension and all of its effects in the causation of high blood pressure in men. The high carbohydrates content in the diet of men is also associated with both the development and poor control of diabetes mellitus, which ultimately contributes to the development of coronary artery heart disease. Having high cholesterol and high triglycerides (hyperlipidemia) is a genetically transmitted condition from parent or parents to their children. However, diet plays a major role in how high the level of cholesterol, triglycerides and low-density lipoprotein goes. The high-density lipoprotein (HDL) goes up with exercise and moderate intake of wine, 2–3 glasses of red or white wine or 1–2 drinks of hard liquor per day. It is said that it is not the alcohol in the wine that causes the increase in HDL; rather, it is the substances found in the skin of the grapes that are used to make wine. These substances are also found in olives and green peas. Apparently, these substances play some role in vasodilatation of vessels, which is an important factor in reducing the formation of coronary occlusive disease. The French, however, show that the effect of alcohol on decreasing the stickiness of the platelets is important in preventing clot formation. It is not altogether clear whether white wine has a similar effect.

There are five parts to the clinically lipid profile:
1. Cholesterol
2. Triglycerides
3. High-density lipoprotein
4. Low-density lipoprotein
5. HDL/cholesterol ratio

Each one of these five parts of the lipid profile, when abnormal, is a risk factor for the development of coronary heart disease. The cholesterol is abnormal when it is too high, greater than 200 (there are certain situations in clinical medicine when too low cholesterol is also abnormal, in particular in malabsorption. The triglycerides are abnormal when the level is too high. The HDL is abnormal when it is too low. The low-density (LDL) is abnormal when it is too high. The ratio of HDL to cholesterol is abnormal when it is too high

Poor and lower-middle-class men in the U.S. have limited income, so their food-buying power is also limited to buying foods that are poor in quality. Consequently, the health benefit of these foods is limited. These foods satisfy hunger, but have very little nutritional values. Foods such as bologna, bacon, sausages, pig feet, cow feet, cheeseburgers, pizza, Tacos, hamburgers, chitterlings, and collard greens cooked with ham hogs are greasy and too rich in fats and salt to have any substantial nutritional value. As just stated, these foods do satisfy hunger and that is a positive thing, but in the end they can cause high cholesterol, they can contribute to obesity, they can contribute to high blood pressure, all of which can lead to the development of coronary artery disease and all its bad consequences.

Foods such as pork, beef, eggs, ham, lobster, shrimp, crabs, oysters, cheeses, avocado, coconut, etc., are rich in cholesterol and when eaten in large quantity and too frequently can cause elevation in blood cholesterol.

How does the high fat level in the foods that some men like to eat cause them to have a high incidence of coronary artery disease?

Once the lipid level is high in the blood, regardless of how it gets there, it causes plaque to form. Once plaque is formed, coronaries become narrowed, resulting in coronary artery heart disease, all its associated symptoms, and other consequences. Fifty thousands four hundred (50,400,000) American men have high cholesterol.

The breakdown of these different men racially who have high cholesterol is 51% white men, 37.3% of black men, and 54.3% of Mexican-American men, total Hispanic men 25.6%, total Asian/Pacific Islanders 27.3% total American Indians/Alaska Natives 26.% (Source: National Health and Nutrition Examination (NHANES) 1999 to 2000. Circulation, 2003; 107: 2185–2189. Low-fat diet and exercise decrease the bad cholesterol level and increase the level of the good cholesterol.

How can high level of lipoprotein—A in the blood causes a heart attack to occur?

Lipoprotein—A is a large lipoprotein, which is made by the liver and secreted into the blood. When the level of lipoprotein—a is elevated in the blood, if the LDL cholesterol is also elevated, the two work synergistically to bring about the development of plaques within the coronary arteries around the heart, resulting in coronary artery heart disease on the one hand. On the other hand, when the lipoprotein—a level in the blood is elevated, and yet the LDL level is normal, the elevated lipoprotein—a by itself can cause a clot to develop in the coronary arteries without the formation of plaques, resulting in an acute myocardial infarction. This reaction occurs because lipoprotein—A competes with plasminogen displaces it, overwhelming it and rendering it helpless in preventing clots from forming. (The main role of plasminogen is to prevent fibrin/clot from forming.) In addition, lipoprotein—a attaches itself to heparin, cells and tissues creating a state of hypercoagulable state making clot formation to occur spontaneously, which can cause death to occur.

About 20% of the U.S. population have elevated lipoprotein—A.

High homocysteine level in the blood is toxic to blood vessels and can cause both plaques to form inside vessels in the body. High homocysteine level in the blood can also cause a clot to form anywhere in the body spontaneously.

Alcohol abuse can cause coronary artery occlusive disease to develop, because when alcoholics are drunk, they frequently become agitated. The agitated state creates a hyperdynamic situation, resulting in rapid heart rate and elevation of blood pressure. This transient but frequent high blood pressure causes two things to happen: 1. The high blood pressure damages the inside of coronary arteries, resulting in plaque formation and eventual narrowing of these vessels; 2. The frequent elevation of blood pressure causes enlargement of the heart, resulting in hypertensive heart disease, which in time causes congestive heart failure. Another form of heart disease that frequently develops in alcoholics is alcoholic cardiomyopathy.(enlargement of the muscles and the different chambers of the heart). The toxic effect of alcohol itself causes that damage to muscles of the heart to develop. The result of the alcohol-associated heart disease is congestive heart failure and cardiac arrhythmias of different types and severities.

Stress can cause heart disease to develop via several mechanisms:
1. Stress causes the level of adrenalin in the blood to rise.
2. The rise in the level of adrenalin causes the blood pressure to rise.

3. The rise in adrenalin can also cause both acute heart attack as well as cardiac arrhythmias to develop, with lethal consequences, at times.

Type A personality (an aggressive and restless person who is always on the go) is associated with the development of coronary heart disease via some of the mechanisms just outlined.

Tobacco smoking can cause coronary occlusive disease because of the effects of nicotine on the coronary vessels, resulting in the development of plaques inside these vessels.

Heredity is associated to a very high degree with coronary heart disease. If a man's mother or father had coronary heart disease or died of a heart attack, chances are he also is at high risk of encountering the same fate, if appropriate medical care is not sought by his to forestall the likelihood of his developing CAD.

Poverty is associated with an increased incidence of coronary artery heart disease because all the factors just outlined are seen in greater number in poor men than in men who have good financial means.

Many of the 45.8 million or so people in the USA who have no health insurance are men. Many of these men are employed, and yet they have no health insurance because they simply do not have enough money to pay for it. According to a recent report, there are 19 million children in this country who are poor and live below the poverty level and most of those children are children of color. Roughly, 14 million children in the USA go to bed hungry every night. Many of these children are young boys who have no health insurance and because, their overall health status is poor. When people are poor, they are concerned about being able to find the bare necessities of daily living, such as where to find foods to eat. Finding healthy food to eat does not enter into the equation of their lives. They are concerned about being able to afford the light bill, to keep the place lit. They are concerned about being able to pay for the crude oil or gas bill, making sure that the home will be kept warm in the winter so that they do not freeze to death. These are important and essential factors in the overall health status of men. Worldwide, twenty-five thousands people die of hunger every day and six millions people die of hunger every year. Hunger causes malnutrition and causes anemia due to lack of protein to make red blood cells, which, in turn can lead to high cardiac out put congestive heart failure etc.

When men are poor, however, the state of their poverty is associated with a greater number of poor health habits, all of which can lead to the development of major medical problems such as hypertension, high cholesterol, obesity, diabetes mellitus, cancer, Atherosclerotic heart disease, cardiovascular heart disease, heart attack, congestive heart failure, stroke, osteoarthritis, etc. Men who are not poor and consequently don't live in poverty do suffer from these medical problems as well, but, because they are more likely to have health insurance, and can see a physician with ease, these problems are dealt with quicker and more efficiently.

Poor men and most men of color tend to go to physicians with diseases of all sorts when these diseases are already in their advanced stages. They frequently ignore their symptoms and go to physicians when the medical problems are frequently more challenging to deal with.

Symptoms of coronary artery disease and heart attacks in men are.

1. Chest pain is often the most common symptom of atherosclerotic heart disease
2. Shortness of breath
3. Pain in the left shoulder radiating down the left arm, associated with numbness and shortness of breath.
4. A combination of the aforementioned three symptoms
5. Worsening of these symptoms on exertion
6. That complex of symptoms is often referred to as angina pectoris
7. Irregularity, rapid heartbeats and too slow heartbeats is referred to as bradycardia/tachycardia
8. When the chest pain is associated with dizziness, sweating and shortness of breath, it can often mean not just angina but often that the patient is in the process of having an acute heart attack
9. Shortness of breath along with accumulation of fluid in the lungs and ankles can be a result of cardiovascular disease and a particular condition known as congestive heart failure

How to diagnose cardiovascular heart disease

To arrive at a diagnosis of cardiovascular heart disease in a person, the physician must:

1. Take a good history.
2. Carry out a good physical examination.
3. Do an electrocardiogram (EKG).
4. Follow up with a chest x-ray.

Based on these tests, the physician may institute a treatment protocol involving beta-blocker, nitroglycerin and aspirin, if there is no contraindication to aspirin. Then arrangements can be made for the man to undergo a stress test, provided, he is not having active chest pain. If the cardiac stress test, along with an echocardiogram, suggests the possibility of a coronary occlusive disease, i.e., atherosclerotic heart disease, then he can be referred to a cardiologist for a cardiac catheterization. In the acute setting, when the patient presents to an emergency room, all of those just mentioned, namely the history, the physical exam, the EKG, the chest x-ray can be done in an emergency room setting to begin the process of evaluating the patient's symptoms for an acute cardiac event. In evaluating the patient with chest pain in the ER, a new blood test (troponin-1) can be done. Troponin-1 is a substance that is secreted by heart muscle that has just become damaged. That test becomes elevated within six hours of an acute myocardial infarction, and remains elevated for about two weeks. The troponin-1 is therefore quite sensitive to help the physician to pick up an acute myocardial infarction. The normal troponin-1 is 0–0.4NG/ml.

The other blood tests that are available to assist the physician to ascertain whether the patient has had a myocardial infarction or is having a myocardial infarction, are the creatinine phosphokinases referred to as CPK. The total normal CPK is usually from 30 to 174 U/L i.e., (unit per ml). There are three different types of CPK that are measured in clinical practice

1.   MM CPK, which comes from skeletal muscle
2.   BB that comes from the brain mostly
3.   MB CPK, which comes from heart muscle mostly

Few other conditions can cause the MB fraction of the CPK to go up, such as Duchene's muscular dystrophy

Dermatomyositis

Myoglobinuria

Polymyositis

Rhabdomyolysis

Reye's syndrome

Rocky Mountain spotted fever—these can cause slight elevation in the MB fraction of the CPK

In acute heart attack where there is heart muscle damage, the MB CPK is elevated. In most laboratories, the normal MB is as high as 4–5%. Most hospital laboratories are set up to do electrophoresis on the CPK MB fraction. The CPK MB electrophoresis is read as either positive or negative. If it is positive for MB, then you get the total MB level to follow. The first cardiac enzyme to rise when an acute heart attack has occurred is the troponin-1; it rises 1–6 hours after heart muscle damage. Ordinarily the CPK is tested three times during an acute hospitalization for an acute heart attack. Usually the total and MB CPK go up between 12 and 24 hours and start coming back down in 24–48 hours.

There are two other enzymes in the blood whose levels go up after a heart attack and there are lactic dehydrogenase (LDH) and the (SGOT) Serum Glutamic Pyruvic Transaminase. Of these three blood enzymes, the first to go up following a heart attack is the CPK, then the SGOT and then the LDH. The first to go down after a heart attack again is the CPK, followed by the SGOT, followed by the LDH. It usually takes the troponin-1 about two weeks to go down to normal.

There are classic abnormalities that are seen on the EKG tracing when an acute myocardial infarction is about to occur, or has just occurred, hours before the person presents either to the emergency room or to the doctor's office. What is often seen is what is referred to as coronary insufficiency. The EKG might show what is called inversion of the T-wave on different parts of the EKG along with ST depression. A classic example is called ST elevation, an elevation of the ST segment of the EKG from the base line. Physicians are able to map out the circulation of the heart, as it relates to coronary artery, based on the 12-lead EKG. For instance, in a myocardial infarction occurring in the inferior wall of the heart, one expects to see abnormalities in leads 2, 3 and AVF. If it is happening in the lateral wall, then one sees abnormalities in leads 1, AVL and maybe V1, V2. If it is taking place in the anterior wall of the heart, then one can see findings in lead leads V1-V6. The right coronary artery supplies blood and oxygen to the inferior wall of the heart and the left anterior descending coronary artery supplies blood and oxygen to the left part of the heart, so on and so forth.

It is very important for a physician to know how to read an EKG properly in order to know if a person is just about to have a heart attack or just had it hours before. That is very important because by infusing tPA (tissue plasminogen activator) in an individual's blood, the clot that is occluding the involved coronary artery causing the myocardial infarction can be dissolved, thereby preventing the heart attack from taking place. Up to six hours after a heart attack has occurred, if the patient presents to the emergency room tPA can still dissolve the clot that has caused the heart attack thereby opening up the vessel and preventing further muscle damage, limiting the severity of the heart attack, which can sometimes help to save the life of the patient. Oftentimes, the history as to when the patient started to experience chest pain, shortness of breath, sweating or just severe pressure in the chest, along with the EKG finding, is all that is needed to indicate that heart attack is occurring.

If the EKG findings and the history are not consistent with a myocardial infarction, then the man may be having an angina, unstable angina, or pre-infarction angina (Acute coronary Syndrome). How a physician is able to determine if a man has had or is having a myocardial infarction, angina, unstable angina, or pre-infarction angina (Acute coronary Syndrome) is based on the experience and clinical judgment of the physician, along with the findings on the EKG and the cardiac enzyme blood tests.

Every year, a significant percentage of men get admitted to intensive coronary care units complaining of chest pain, which in fact, were not having cardiac-related chest pain or myocardial infarctions. On other hand, many men get sent home because the physicians, either in the emergency rooms or in their offices, saw these men or did not think they had heart-related chest pain, resulting in these men having heart attacks at home and sometimes dying because.

The literature is full of articles indicating the fact that men, and in particular men of color, receive less attention when they present to an emergency room with chest pain as compared to their male counterparts. As stated above, black men and other men of color also are referred less often for invasive cardiac tests, such as cardiac catheterization, to determine whether they have coronary occlusive disease to explain their complaints of chest pain.

To underline that issue even more strongly, the recent literature shows that the lifetime risk of heart attacks at age 40 is 1 in 3 for men. Even as late as age 70, the incidence of coronary artery disease and heart attack is 1 in 4 for men. It is also important to realize that cardiovascular disease is the number one cause of death in men, and the number one cause of death in the U.S.

Several possible scenarios exist when a man presents to the emergency room with chest pain:

1. A man is seen for the complaint of chest pain, evaluated and sent home and instructed to see his physician for follow-up or is referred to a medical clinic for follow up.

2. A man is seen for complaint of chest pain evaluated and admitted for further evaluation and observation on a telemetry unit.

3. A man is seen for chest pain, evaluated and the physician feels that the man has pre-infarction or unstable angina (Acute coronary Syndrome) and is admitted for treatment in the coronary care unit. In that case, he will be treated with heparin, aspirin, nitroglycerin, a beta-blocker and oxygen.

4. In addition, three sets of cardiac enzymes and troponin-1 tests are ordered. An EKG is taken also for three days to be sure that a myo-

cardial infarction has not occurred. In the setting of number 1 and 2 above, an echocardiogram may be done to rule out acute myocardial infarction or other causes of chest pain such as mitral valve prolapsed, myocarditis, pericarditis, etc.

5. A man who presents with chest pain and other symptoms of a heart attack and is found to be having a heart attack by EKG findings and sometimes by the first elevated CPK value or the troponin-1 value is admitted to the coronary care unit and given coronary care unit care for an acute myocardial infarction. That particular man who is found to be having a heart attack is a candidate to receive tPA if there is no contraindication. As mentioned above, in that particular setting, the tPA can be lifesaving in that it can dissolve the clot that is causing the heart attack to occur, thereby allowing blood flow and oxygen to go to the affected muscles of the heart, limiting the amount of damage that is being done to the heart muscles.

If a myocardial infarction is ruled out, after three sets of enzymes and an EKG that is unremarkable, then further decision has to be made as to how to proceed in evaluating that person. One common approach is to do a nuclear Adenosine or MIBI stress test, Persantine MIBI test or a stress echocardiogram. If any one of these tests is negative, then the assumption is that the patient does not have severe coronary occlusive disease. That patient is frequently sent home and taken off acute myocardial-type medications such as beta-blockers and nitrates. These tests, though they are excellent, are not 100% foolproof. There have been situations when a nuclear imaging test of the heart was normal, and yet the patient went on in a matter of days or weeks to have a heart attack. What can be said is that if the nuclear stress test or the stress echocardiogram is negative, the patient probably does not have major occlusive coronary heart disease. These stress tests can miss a 30–40% occlusion of a coronary artery. For several reasons a fissure or crack can occur in a 30–40% plaque inside a coronary artery, causing bleeding and clot formation resulting in closure of that vessel and an acute heart attack. Human beings carry in their mouths anaerobic bacteria that produce enzymes that can cause that fissure or crack to occur in a coronary. It is said that certain species of mycoplasma bacteria can contribute to the development of coronary artery disease. It may be wise to test the blood for the presence of the antibody to mycoplasma. And if the antibody test is positive, then erythromycin can be used to treat these people. When a man has only a 30–40% occlusion of a coronary vessel, that vessel has not had sufficient time to develop collateral vessels, so when that suffers an occlusive incident, there are no collateral vessels in the immediate vicinity to protect the affected myocardium and keep it alive. So in that setting a 30–40% coronary occlusive disease is worse than an 80% occlusion in that the 80% occlusion has had plenty of time to develop collateral vessels, which can protect the heart muscle in the event of a heart attack to keep the heart muscle alive.

The other scenario is that if the patient continues to have chest pain and yet there is no clear evidence of acute myocardial infarction, then that patient is a candidate to be taken immediately to cardiac catheterization in order to visualize the vessels around the heart, to see if indeed the patient has major coronary occlusive disease. It is not safe to do a stress test on someone who is having active chest pain.

Doing the regular treadmill stress test in evaluating someone for coronary insufficiency has some value, but because it has such a high incidence of false positivity and also such a high incidence of false negativity, it has become less and less appropriate in the setting of acute evaluation of chest pain. Especially in men, there is a very high incidence of false negative treadmill stress test. For that reason, nuclear cardiac imaging has replaced the treadmill stress test. The regular treadmill stress test is appropriate for a younger individual in the 35-to-40-year-old bracket who is being evaluated to fly planes, or race a car, starting a jogging program or something of that sort.

As just mentioned there are several sensitive stress tests available to evaluate the heart:

1. The MIBI Myoview stress test.
2. IV Persantine or IV Adenosine.
3. IV Dobutamine
4. Resting Thallium distribution stress test.
5. Stress echocardiogram

Any one of these tests can be used to evaluate the heart. In certain circumstances, a gated blood pool, known also as MUGA, is done in evaluating the heart.

The Persantine MIBI stress test and Adenosine stress test are suitable for individuals who are able to exercise. Roughly two days prior to having these stress tests, certain medications and certain beverages have to be stopped. Among them are beta-blocker medications—to name a few, Tenormin, Atenolol, Metoprolol, Propanolol; Coreg, etc. Some calcium channel blockers need to be stopped, as well, such as Cardizem, Nifedipine, and Verapamil, etc. Certain medications such as Aminophylline and Theophylline must be stopped. Beverages such as coffee, tea, and any caffeine or decaffeinated beverages ought to be stopped prior to having these tests done. The cardiac nuclear department has a long list of things that men cannot do that they give out prior to having these tests done, so men know precisely what not to do. This is done because it is important that the heart is able to pump forcefully without interference. The higher the heart rate during exercise, the more stress there is on the heart, and the more stress there is on the heart the better the evaluation of the heart. Anything that suppresses the contractile effort of the heart has a negative impact on the evaluation of the result of the stress test. People who are going to have the Persantine stress test also ought to take certain precautions as mentioned above. If the patient is taking Dipyridamole, which is still being used in certain settings, that medication must be stopped before undergoing a Persantine stress test.

The MIBI nuclear stress test or the Adenosine stress test is done in such a way as to be able to tell both angina and/or previous myocardial muscle damage. The Sestamibi test or the thallium test has the same clinical properties as potassium. This being the case, potassium will only be picked up by live heart muscle as a physiological fact. Taking advantage of that known fact, the physician injects the MIBI substance into the blood of the man being tested, and after it mixes with his own blood, that minute nuclear material functions as a tracer in his blood to allow for the stress test to be carried out. The entire process is computerized, allowing color pictures of the heart to be taken along with many other important values such as the ejection fraction of the heart.

These nuclear cardiac stress tests enable cardiologists to differentiate between normal heart muscles, scarred heart muscles and heart muscles that are not receiving sufficient blood and oxygen. During the exercise, the area of the heart that is supplied by the plaque-containing coronary artery does not receive sufficient blood and oxygen, resulting in an area of emptiness or lightness as compared to the rest of the pictured heart muscles. Because at rest the oxygen demand is less, that same area when pictured again normalizes; then that is an area of poor blood flow made worse by the stress of the work imposed on the heart by the stress, simulating the natural phenomenon referred to as angina or coronary insufficiency. Physicians can in fact tell exactly which coronary artery or arteries are diseased with plaques based on the result of the MIBI stress test.

On the other hand, if the abnormal area remains unchanged, both at rest and during exercise when pictured, it means that that person has had a previous myocardial infarction, either known or unknown. The reason why the area remains unchanged, showing an area of defect, is because the muscle that is showing as a defect is scarred and is dead muscle. Dead tissue cannot pick up potassium, and Sestamibi and thallium have some of the same chemical properties as potassium, as previously mentioned.

Another nuclear stress test that is frequently employed to diagnose occlusive coronary artery disease is the Persantine MIBI stress test. That test is suitable for individuals with infirmities that prevent them from being able to exercise on a treadmill. Some of these are men who suffer from arthritis of the lumbar spine or arthritis of the knees, they are markedly obese, or they have had a stroke or they are somewhat more advanced in age and they are not able to exercise. The difference between the regular MIBI stress test and the Persantine MIBI stress test is that Persantine is given to the person undergoing the test to dilate the coronary arteries acutely. The acute dilatation causes the heart to beat very fast, resulting in a stressful situation for the heart. The result is the same as exercising on the treadmill to raise the heart rate. Another advantage of the Persantine stress test is that beta-blockers and calcium channel blocker medications can be continued while the patient is having the test. The findings discussed under the heading MIBI stress test are the same as the Persantine stress test and has the same meaning. If the stress MIBI is negative, that is evidence that the man who was tested probably does not have significant occlusive coronary artery disease. That is, however, not always the case; though these stress tests are very sensitive tests, every now and then there can be a false negative test.

If the person continues to have chest pain, then the right thing to do is first to do an abdominal ultrasound to evaluate the gall bladder, because gall bladder disease, such as gallstones, can cause chest pain that is similar to chest pain seen in coronary heart disease. Interestingly, medications such as nitroglycerin, which relieves angina chest pain, can also relieve gall bladder disease pain, confusing the whole situation. Gall bladder disease due to gallstones is quite common among men, in particular men who are 30–40 years old, obese and fertile. Men of color are more likely to develop obesity and therefore more prone to develop gallstones. Also, men of color are more likely to be carrying abnormal hemoglobins, which predispose them to a higher propensity to the formation of gallbladder disease. They are more likely to form bilirubin stones. Sickle cell hemoglobin, hemoglobin C, beta thalassemia, alpha thalassemia, and different combinations of these abnormal hemoglobins cause hemolysis, resulting in the formation of bilirubin gallstones. It is the dumping of bilirubin in the bloodstream that ultimately leads to bilirubin gallstones causing gall bladder disease to be so frequently seen in that subgroup of men who suffer from hemolytic anemia of different types.

If the abdominal sonogram is negative, ruling out gallstones, then an upper G.I. series must be done to look for diseases such as hiatal hernia with or without reflux esophagitis or ulcers of different types and degrees in the stomach. Any one of these can cause chest pain similar to the chest pain caused by coronary artery heart disease. Hiatal hernia with reflux is frequently seen as a cause of severe chest pain. That particular condition is called GERD (gastroesophageal reflux disease). Frequently, the physician does not have the luxury of waiting to do an evaluation of the gallbladder or the stomach in a man who is having pain in the chest with negative stress test. In that case, he must go directly for a coronary angiogram to be certain that coronary artery disease is not the cause of the pain. It would be rather dangerous to wait to do a prolonged G.I. work-up while the patient is having pain that could be risking the possibility of a heart attack while the patient is waiting for these tests to be done. As just stated, before undertaking that invasive procedure, however, the physician must be sure that all other possible causes of chest pain have been ruled out, including mitral valve prolapsed, which can be seen on echocardiogram, and costochondritis, which can be detected on physical examination. Pulmonary embolism must also be ruled out by doing ultrasound of the extremities, with d-Dimer blood test or by doing a lung scan. Other tests to do are ESR and ANA to rule out inflammatory processes such as myocarditis, pericarditis and pleuritis. Chest x-ray ought to be done to rule out pneumonia, which can also cause chest pain. If he has fever, then a series of viral blood tests ought to be done to rule viral disease as a cause of the fever and chest pain.

Costochondritis is a condition that causes pain in the ribs and upper chest wall, and when the physician touches these areas with the examining finger, they are tender. Conditions such as arthritis or bursitis of the left or right shoulder with radiating pain down the arm must also be considered.

Chest pain can also be due to cancer of the lung, and therefore a chest x-ray must be done to rule out that possibility.

There are many conditions that cause chest pain, but the point is that the physician must keep an open mind and properly evaluate for these possibilities before proceeding to more invasive tests to explain the chest pain. It is neither too expensive nor too time consuming to do these things. As just stated, before offering a man cardiac catheterization, a thorough medical evaluation must first be completed, unless he continues to have chest pain and the clinical impression is that he faces an impending myocardial infarction; naturally the physician ought to proceed immediately to do a cardiac catheterization..

Ordinarily, cardiac catheterization for the possibility of coronary occlusive disease is undertaken when a man has a positive stress test and he has failed medical management and also the patient is of an age where cardiac catheterization will not be contraindicated. Also, if the patient has major risk factors such as smoking, hypertension, hyperlipidemia, diabetes mellitus, obesity and a family history of coronary artery disease, in conjunction with the aforementioned factors, then that patient should be offered cardiac catheterization.

If a man agrees to undergo a cardiac, catheterization to determine whether or not there is an impending myocardial infarction and/or determines whether the chest pain in question is due to coronary insufficiency because of coronary artery blockage. Then he ought to be given proper informed advice as to why the cardiac catheterization is done and the possible side effects associated with that procedure, along with the risk and benefit of the procedure.

Cardiac catheterization is a procedure done by highly qualified cardiologists who do that procedure as a subspecialty of cardiology. The procedure is done in a special operating room, which is well equipped with all sorts of modern equipment to provide care for the heart under different circumstances.

The procedure is done by a making a large needle-size puncture in the groin, where the femoral artery is located. The area is shaved and properly cleansed with Betadine, and then appropriate local anesthetic is injected in the area. Time is allowed for the anesthetic to take effect, and then a puncture is made with a needle through which a catheter is threaded that goes to the heart, where it can be moved to different parts of its chambers. A dye is injected through the catheter, which is able to display the coronary arteries around the heart. A multitude of very important information is obtained during the cardiac catheterization including the displaying of the coronary arteries. The displaying of the coronary arteries may show evidence of plaques and narrowing in the coronary arteries. If the cardiac catheterization is negative for occlusive coronary disease, it means no gross coronary artery disease is present. Other conditions can cause chest pain that can be seen during cardiac catheterization. Coronary spasm can be seen or induced during cardiac catheterization, and coronary spasm can cause chest pain and when it occurs acutely, it can cut off blood and oxygen flow to the heart muscle, sometimes resulting in acute myocardial infarction. Most recently, a fairly new condition has been described in which men who suffer from long-time hypertension can develop that type of hypertensive cardiovascular disease with enlargement of the left ventricle and increased end diastolic pressure, suggesting that these men have what is called small vessel myocardial disease causing chest pain. Obese men, because of their greater propensity for having hypertension, are quite prone to have that particular condition just described.

After completion of the cardiac catheterization is done, the results are evaluated and the determination is made as to whether the abnormalities found can explain a man's symptoms. In the case of chest pain, the key finding is coronary artery narrowing due to plaques of different degrees.

(Note to layout person) Insert-Normal and abnormal cardiac catheterization photographs.

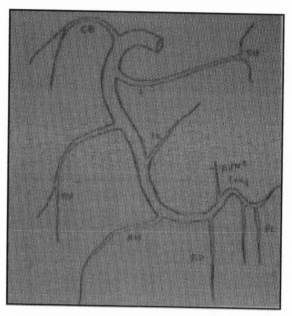

Figure 6.1—A normal right coronary artery.

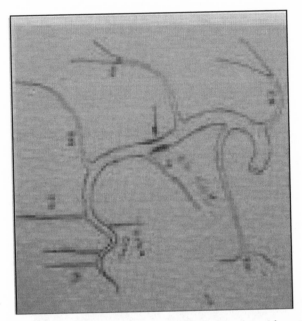

Figure 6.2—*Big arrow shows 50–60% occlusion in the mid-portion of a right coronary artery.*

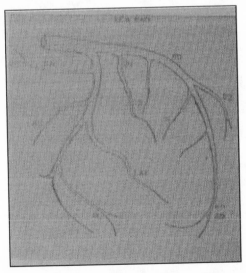

Figure 6.3—*A normal left coronary artery.*

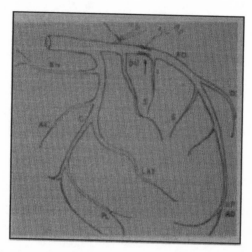

Figure 6.4—*A 50% occlusion of a left anterior descending coronary artery, in a patient with both high cholesterol and hypertension.*

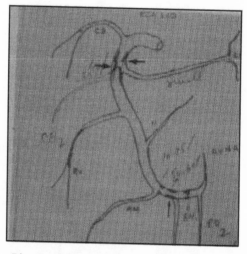

Figure 6.5—*Big arrow showing 40–50% of the proximal portion of the right coronary artery. Small arrow showing 70–75% occlusion of the distal right coronary artery. That right coronary artery has diffused Atherosclerotic changes in other areas.*

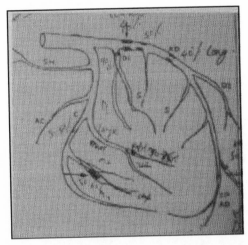

Figure 6.6—Small arrow shows 40% occlusion of the proximal left anterior descending artery. There is a 30% occlusion of the LAD in its proximal portion just before the first major septal artery and there is also a 40% occlusion in the mid-portion of the LAD. Big arrow shows 50–60% occlusion of the epical diagonal branch of the left coronary artery. There are several areas of diffused Atherosclerotic changes involving that left coronary artery. Occlusive changes of coronary arteries in a patient with hypertension and high cholesterol who smoke.

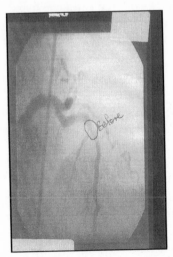

Figure 6.7—Stent placement of narrowed LAD (before)

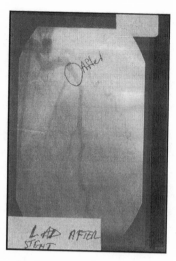

Figure 6.8—Showing how stent placement opens the LAD (after)

Based on the findings of the cardiac catheterization as just mentioned, recommendations are made as to what course of action to follow. If for example, the coronary arteries are found to have plaques in them, then the possibilities are:

1. The patient can be offered angioplasty. (As seen in 6.7& 6.8 above)
2. The patient can be offered cardiac bypass.
3. The patient can be offered medications assuming that the disease cannot be approached surgically and/or the patient refuses to have the angioplasty or cardiac catheterization.

There are contraindications to both angioplasty and cardiac bypass sometimes.

Angioplasty is simpler than coronary bypass, but it also has a higher rate of recurrence of disease. The very fact of going through the vessels to push aside the plaques can damage the inside of the vessels, creating an area for new plaque formation. Sometimes a stent is placed inside a vessel to try to keep it open, which decreases the possibility of new plaque formation.(see Figures 6.7 & 6.8). These men are frequently placed on anti-platelet medications such as Ticlid or Plavix in conjunction with aspirin for several weeks to prevent platelet aggregation and closure of the coronary artery. Angioplasty is done in the cardiac catheterization lab and the same cardiologist who performs the cardiac catheterization usually does it.

On the other hand, coronary bypass requires open-heart surgery which a heart surgeon performs, and it is major surgery and the hospital stay is longer and it costs more money. The success of coronary artery bypass surgery is quite good; though some might say taken together, that coronary bypass relieves symptoms but does not prolong life as compared to medical management on the average. There are reports that some men suffer some degree of dementia after coronary bypass surgery, and it is believed that micro particles that break off from the coronary plaques during surgery lodge into the brain and may be responsible for the dementia.

It is important to stress the point that after angioplasty or coronary bypass, frequently cardiac medication is continued. The list of medications used in cardiovascular disease is very long. The following is a partial list of different cardiac medications that are presently in use:

1. Aspirin.
2. Ticlid.
3. Plavix
4. Nitroglycerin.
5. Beta-blockers
6. Calcium channel blockers.
7. Alpha channel blockers.
8. Digitalis.
9. Diuretics.
    Antiarrhythmic such as Lidocaine, Quinidine, Procainamide, Amiodarone IV Vasotec, IV Verapamil, IV Cardizem, Adenosine, etc.
10. Pacemakers also play a major role in the management of patients with heart disease.
11. Sometimes, a pacemaker is used in the setting of an acute myocardial infarction, and sometimes it is used to treat heart blockage of different types to treat sinus disease, or bundle branch blocks.
12. There are special pacemakers that are used to treat arrhythmias of different types and severity. These pacemakers can on demand shock the heart to eliminate rhythm abnormalities as they occur, without the patient being aware of what is going on. Moreover, these special pacemakers keep a record for the cardiologist to print out and evaluate in his or his management of the patient. It is very important men who are having unexplained cardiac arrhythmias undergo electrophysiological studies to determine both source and the cause of the arrhythmia, so that specific and appropriate anti-arrhythmic treatments can be prescribed for the affected men.

How do these medications work to treat heart disease?

Aspirin, Ticlid, and Plavix work to treat heart disease because these three medications are able to prevent clot formation within the lumen of the vessels around the heart. They do so by preventing platelet clumping, and in so doing they prevent aggregation of platelets, which is necessary for clots to form. Aspirin works both in the prevention of coronary artery disease and also in the acute treatment of coronary artery disease. When a patient presents to the hospital in the process of having a heart attack, if the patient is given two aspirins to chew and swallow, and also, added to that, heparin, that patient frequently can lessen the amount of damage that is done to the heart. On top of that, if tPA is injected into the patient within the first hour or so while the patient is about to have a heart attack, a great deal of heart muscle can be spared.

Beta-blockers are a group of medications that have a great deal of usefulness in the treatment of cardiovascular heart disease of different types. Among the most commonly used beta-blockers are the following:

1. Inderal
2. Lopressor
3. Tenormin
4. Toprol XL
5. Coreg

The beta-blockers work to improve the function of the heart via different mechanisms. Beta-blockers have their main effect on the sympathetic system of the body to decrease stimulation of the heart. They also decrease the forcefulness of the pumping of the heart, thereby sparing the need for greater oxygen delivery. Beta-blockers are also anti-arrhythmic and they prevent arrhythmia from occurring. The long-acting beta-blockers in the Lopressor-type family actually cut down on the amount of adrenalin that the body can secrete, and that decreases the incidence of death from myocardial infarction. That is why long-acting beta blockers are used to protect the heart when a person is sleeping, so that in the early morning hours of the day, when the adrenalin is being secreted in large amounts to prepare the body for the upcoming day's work, protection will continue. By cutting down for adrenalin that is being secreted, the heart is spared the stimulation from the excess adrenalin, thereby cutting down on the incidence of sudden death. The harder the heart pumps, the more blood and oxygen are needed to keep up with the needs of the heart muscle and if plaques, then that demand narrow the vessels around the heart cannot be met. So it is in that manner that beta-blockers are effective in the treatment of angina pectoris, also known as chest pain. Beta-blockers also work in another way in the treatment of heart disease, and that is they slow the heart rate or they make the heart beat in a regular fashion, thereby preventing what are called cardiac arrhythmias from occurring. These arrhythmias are frequently the reason why the heart stops after a heart attack or because of a complex abnormal rhythm which prevents proper pumping activities of the heart that are needed for sustaining life. In fact, using long-acting beta-blockers as just mentioned, especially a dose that has a 24-hour effect on the heart, not only can prevent these abnormalities, but also may in fact prevent heart attacks that frequently as mentioned occur in the early hours of the morning.

Another group of medications that are frequently used in coronary disease are the nitrates. Nitroglycerin, which is a well-known medication, is in the family of the nitrates. The nitrates come in different forms, from sublingual nitroglycerin-to-nitroglycerin capsules, nitroglycerin patches, nitroglycerin paste, to nitroglycerin liquid that can be used intravenously. Nitroglycerin works to relieve symptoms of angina pectoris by dilating the smooth muscles inside the coronary arteries, allowing for better blood and oxygen flow to go around the heart.

Calcium channel blockers are excellent medications that have multiple uses in the treatment of cardiovascular disease. Calcium channel blockers, such as Nifedipine, Cardizem, Verapamil, Norvasc, ACE Inhibitors etc. work to relieve some symptoms associated with coronary artery disease by blocking the effects of calcium to the smooth muscle inside the coronary arteries around the heart. Calcium is needed for muscle contraction to occur at the cellular level. Muscle contraction is associated with vasoconstriction. Vasoconstriction means that the inside of the blood vessel becomes narrowed. The narrowing of the blood vessel prevents proper circulation of blood and thereby prevents proper delivery of oxygen to the heart muscles. When oxygen fails to reach the heart muscle in sufficient amount, the result is chest pain. Another important function of calcium channel blockers is to decrease blood pressure. Increase in blood pressure is a major cause of cardiovascular disease. Calcium channel blockers work to decrease blood pressure by blocking the effect of calcium on the muscle, resulting in relaxation of smooth muscle and that relaxation of smooth muscle causes the blood pressure to come down. In men of color, these medications must be used in combination with diuretics, if a man is not in renal failure, for effective control of blood pressure. The calcium channel blockers are frequently used to treat cardiac arrhythmias and they are very effective. In particular, Verapamil IV or Cardizem IV is used extensively in the emergency room setting to treat different types of ventricular cardiac dysrhythmias.

Diuretics are very important medications in the treatment of cardiovascular disease. When the heart has been damaged, it frequently fails, and heart failure causes fluid to be accumulated in the lungs, the abdomen, the legs, and the ankles. The so-called loop diuretics, such as Lasix, Bumex, etc., are used to remove the fluid from the body, thereby improving heart function and relieving the symptoms of fluid overload from the body. Salt plays a major role in causing fluid accumulation in the body; therefore the intake of salt must be curtailed significantly in the treatment of heart failure. Any man who has chronic congestive heart failure by definition has a total body salt that is elevated.

Heart failure can occur because of acute damage to the heart. Heart failure can complicate heart attack and it frequently does. However, heart failure most frequently occurs because of damage that has occurred to the heart because of longstanding hypertension that was either not properly treated or untreated. Because the muscles of the heart have been stretched to the limit, the heart enlarges and becomes incapable of pumping properly. Once the heart loses its proper pumping ability then fluid backs up in the body, causing the man to be unable to breathe properly and unable to lie down flat. The man must use several pillows to sleep. Heart failure can also occur because of chronic damage that has occurred to the heart because of multiple previous heart attacks, whereby heart muscles have been damaged, and the scarred muscles lose their ability to pump properly. A combination of an enlarged heart, a condition referred to as cardiomegaly, and hypertrophy of the muscles of the heart, can result in heart failure. Men with cardiomyopathy and congestive heart failure, who eat too much salt in their foods, can cause their heart failure to be worse. It is very important to make the point that in the process of using these diuretics to remove fluids from the body, a proper level of potassium must be maintained in order to prevent potassium deficiency, which can cause serious complications to develop. Potassium must be given by mouth for those who are able to take it by mouth in an outpatient setting and it can be given intravenously when necessary for those who are in the hospital and cannot take it by mouth because they are acutely sick. About 550,000 people are diagnosed with heart failure every year. A total of 5 million individuals in the U.S. have heart failure. Some 2,400,000 men have heart failure in the U.S. 2.5% white males have heart failure. 3.1% black males have congestive heart failure. 2.7% Mexican American males have congestive heart failure.

In the year 2001, 19,805 men died of congestive heart failure in the US. During that same period of time, 17,782 white males died of congestive heart failure and 1,802 black males died of congestive heart failure. The yearly cost of congestive heart failure, direct and indirect, is 27.9 billion dollars. (Sources: Heart Disease and Stroke Statistics, 2005 Update, American Heart Association.)

What are the causes of congestive heart failure?

The causes of congestive heart failure are
1. Hypertension
2. Ischemic heart disease
3. Cardiomyopathy
4. Anemia
5. Myocardial infarction
6. Cardiac arrhythmias
7. Valvular heart disease
8. Bacterial endocarditis
9. Myocarditis
10. Hyperthyroidism (Thyrotoxicosis)
11. Pulmonary embolism
12. Acute intracranial hemorrhage with intracranial pressure
13. Infection with high fever, fast heart rate superimposed on a sick heart

What are the symptoms of congestive heart failure?

The symptoms of congestive heart failure are heart failure (CHF)
Shortness of breath (dyspnea and orthopnea) left sided
heart failure

Orthopnea or paroxysmal nocturnal dyspnea right sided heart failure
1. Lassitude
2. Irritability
3. Insomnia
4. Chest pain
5. Head ache
6. Restlessness
7. Tiredness
8. Weakne
9. Abdominal pain due to swollen liver
10. Nausea
11. Anorexia
12. Poor memory due to poor blood flow to the brain
13. Head ache

What are the clinical signs of congestive heart failure?

1. Rapid respiration
2. Labored respiration
3. Rapid pulse rate
4. Bulging neck veins
5. Rapid or irregular heart rate
6. Swollen ankles
7. Swollen legs
8. Swollen abdomen
9. Palpable liver
10. Tender liver to palpation
11. Swollen face
12. Third and fourth heart sounds when listening to the heart with a Stethoscope
13. Rales heard when listening to the lung with the stethoscope
14. Weight gain
15. Using several pillows under the chest to sleep (nocturnal Dyspnea)
16. Raising the head of the bed in order to sleep
17. Jaundice
18. Renal insufficiency (abnormal kidney function)

What is Acute Congestive heart failure? (Pulmonary edema)

Pulmonary edema is an accumulation of fluid in the lungs because of failure of the left side of the heart this happens, more blood entered into the pulmonary circulation than can be removed.

What are the causes of cardiac pulmonary edema?

The causes of pulmonary edema are

1. Acute myocardial infarction (heart attack) resulting in severe muscle damage with heart losing significant pumping ability, thereby causing fluid to back up into the lungs
2. Acute ischemic episode (angina pectoris) superimposed on an already sick heart

3. Decompensated chronic congestive heart failure due too much salt in the diet and or failure to take prescribed diuretic
4. Sinus tachycardia (rapid heart rate)
5. Cardiac arrhythmias
6. Heart blocks
7. Pulmonary embolism
8. Acute bacterial endocarditis
9. Acute rupture of a heart valve
10. Acute intracranial hemorrhage etc.

What are the symptoms of pulmonary edema?

The symptoms of pulmonary edema are
1. Severe dyspnea
2. Severe tachypnea
3. Severe wheezing
4. Diaphoresis (sweating)
5. Tachycardia
6. A feeling of doom
7. Cold feeling of the body etc.

What are the clinical and physical signs of pulmonary edema?

The clinical sings of pulmonary edema are
1. Severe dyspnea (marked shortness of breath)
2. Severe tachypnea (very rapid respiration)
3. Severe diaphoresis (Severe sweating)
4. Marked shivering
5. Distended Neck veins
6. Rapid heart rate or rapid an irregular heart rate
7. Rales and wheezings in both lungs
8. There may be swollen ankles, legs, abdominal walls and scrotum or groins
9. Chest x ray evidence of pulmonary edema involving both lungs with fluid in them
10. There may EKG evidence of acute cardiac abnormality etc.

How to treat pulmonary edema: Give

1. IV Lasix
2. 100% oxygen via re-breather mask
3. IV digitalis if there is bradycardia or significant AV heart block
4. Apply nitro paste to chest wall or give IV nitroglycerin (if the blood pressure is normal)
5. If the patient is hypotensive, give Dobutrex or Dopamine in drip form
6. Give IV Lopressor if the patient's is not too low or there is no significant AV heart block
7. Give IV Vasotec if the blood pressure is not to low
8. Insert a Foley catheter to monitor urine output
9. Monitor oxygen saturation
10. Monitor serial portable chest x-ray
11. Once the acute pulmonary edema is brought under control, continue treatment as per chronic congestive heart failure

How do physicians diagnose congestive heart failure?

To diagnose congestive heart failure

1. History of shortness of breath by the patient
2. History of swollen ankles by the patient
3. History of needing several pillows to sleep
4. History of recurrent coughing when lying down
5. History of difficulty breathing when walking upstairs
6. Enlarged heart seen on chest x-ray with the presence of fluid in the lungs
7. Abnormal left ventricular function seen on Echocardiogram
8. Low Ejection Fraction on Echocardiogram, Rest Muga or Nuclear stress test
9. The presence of S3, S4 galop on listening to heart using the stethoscope
10. Rales heard on listening to the lungs using the stethoscope

How to treat congestive heart failure

1. Lasix IV or by mouth
2. Bumex IV

3. Aldactone
4. Beta Blocker such as Coreg, Lopressor, Toprol XL, Tenormin etc
5. Nitro paste on the chest wall or IV nitroglycerin
6. Digitalis IV or by mouth if the heart is enlarged
7. Nasal oxygen
8. Low salt diet
9. Daily weight when in the hospital
10. BiDil is said to be effective in the treatment of congestive heart failure in blacks

      This a controversial issue because although this medication works to treat congestive heart failure, it is a good medication in all racial groups to treat heart failure.

      The research was to done on this medication only in blacks. No white patients, no Asians patients and no Hispanic patients were treated with BiDil during the research. The two medications in BiDil have been used in the treatment of patients with congestive many years individually and in combination in some settings.

How does BiDil work to treat congestive heart failure?

BiDil works to treat congestive heart failure because

1. Isosorbide one of the two medications in BiDil is a vasodilator which on the venous system causes venous dilation and it also causes the release of nitric oxide which in turn activates guanylyl cyclase resulting in relaxation of the vascular smooth muscle.

   Hydralazine, the other medication in BiDil is an arterial smooth muscle dilator; it also prevents the degradation of nitric oxide. It is said that blacks have lower level of nitric oxide than whites. BiDil works to treat congestive heart failure in all patients with congestive heart failure, without regard to race.

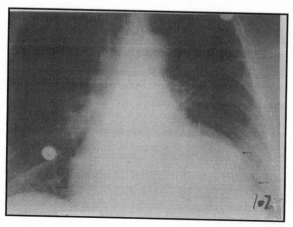

Figure 6.9: Chest x-ray of a man with ischemic myocardial disease with associated congestive heart failure.

Digitalis is a medication that has been around for many years and it still is a very effective medication in the treatment of cardiovascular disease. If the heart is enlarged, the ejection fraction is low and the person has congestive heart failure, digitalis is quite effective in helping the heart to pump well and thereby relieving the symptoms of congestive heart failure. If the rhythm of the heart is irregular, such as in atrial fibrillation, digitalis is the drug of choice. Thus it is used to chronically treat men who have atrial fibrillation to keep the heart rate at normal levels, and sometimes the digitalis itself can normalize the irregular heartbeat. Digitalis has other uses also in the treatment of cardiovascular disease such as in the treatment of paroxysmal atrial tachycardia, and it is quite effective when used for that particular condition. Lidocaine is a very important medication; it is used in the acute setting in individuals who have cardiovascular disease, such as individuals who develop different types of ventricular arrhythmias after more heart attacks. It is very important to realize that frequently when a man has a heart attack; it is often the arrhythmia that causes him to die. If a physician can get to the man, who is having a heart attack promptly and inject Lidocaine into his, quite often his life can be saved. Other antiarrhythmic medications such as Procainamide and Quinidine have been around a long time. Again, they are used for both atrial and ventricular arrhythmias and they are still very effective in the setting for which they are used in men who have these arrhythmias. Quinidine can also be used, at times, as a way to get the rhythm of the heart back to normal in men who have atrial fibrillation.

There is another family of medication called angiotensin-converting enzyme inhibitors; such as Capoten, Zestril and Vasotec, Cozaar, Altace, Aceon are examples of that family of medications. These medications are very important medications and when used in the treatment of congestive heart failure, they can improve the function of the heart These medications can also prevent sudden death in men with coronary artery heart disease Aldactone, when used in the treatment of congestive heart failure, results in markedly improved survival of patients with congestive heart failure. Chronic congestive heart failure causes total body salt retention and increased serum aldosterone. Aldactone works against aldosterone to get rid of salt and water from the body, thereby improving the state of congestive heart failure.

Cardiovascular diseases require a multitude of different medications, frequently used in combination in order to make the heart function properly.

Another common technique that is frequently used to help the heart to function better is the insertion of a pacemaker. Pacemakers are inserted for different reasons. Clinically when a man has sick sinus disease, that is when the area of the heart where the electrical system is located has become degenerated and a man develops heart block, a pacemaker has to be inserted in order to take over the proper electrical functioning of the heart. Heart block occurs usually in the aged or because of an acute myocardial infarction. Pacemakers are used in different sets of circumstances in different age groups for different reasons.

Some of the reasons for which a pace maker may be inserted are
1. Third degree AV black
2. Symptomatic left ventricular block
3. Symptomatic Right ventricular
4. Symptomatic bifascicular block

It is important to realize that the pacemaker, once inserted, must be tested periodically to assure that it is functioning properly. The pacemaker can be tested, even if the man in whose heart the pacemaker is inserted is away in a foreign country. It can be tested using a telephone. It is very important to realize that these things are being modified frequently and the technology has improved remarkably in the last few years. Pacemakers can do wonders to keep people alive who have different types of cardiovascular disease.

An other common problem that individuals with cardiovascular disease have to deal with is cardiac arrhythmias.

Some of the most common cardiac arrhythmias are
1. Sinus tachycardia

2. Atrial fibrillation
3. Atrial flutter
4. Premature ventricular contraction (VPC's)
5. Premature atrial contraction (APC's)
6. Paroxysmal supraventricular tachycardia
7. Ventricular tachycardia (V Tach)
8. Ventricular fibrillation

What are the most common causes of cardiac arrhythmias?
The most common causes of cardiac arrhythmias are
1. Arthrosclerotic heart disease
2. Myocardial infarction
3. Cardiomyopathy
4. Congestive heart failure
5. Ischemic valvular heart disease
6. Congenital heart disease
7. Pulmonary embolism
8. Hyperthyroidism etc.

How to diagnose cardiac arrhythmias?
1. Patient's history of irregular heart beats
2. Examination of the heart using the stethoscope
3. 12 lead EKG
4. 24 hour Holter monitor
5. Monitoring the patient's heart rhythm on telemetry
6. in the hospital
7. Echocardiogram
8. Nuclear cardiac stress test
9. Thyroid blood tests etc,

How to treat cardiac arrhythmias?

Each arrhythmia is treated differently and according to the underline heart disease
The different medications used to treat cardiac arrhythmias are
1. Lidocaine
2. Tocainide
3. Digitalis
4. Quinidine
5. Procaina
6. Amiodarone
7. Beta blockers

8. Adenosine
9. Verapamil
10. Diltiazem
11. Vasotec
12. Aspirin
13. Coumadin
14. Heparin
15. Lovenox

Severe and life threatening ventricular arrhythmias are treated with implantable cardio ventricular defibrillation (ICD)

Atrial fibrillation must be treated with Coumadin, Lovenox or aspirin long term to prevent the development of stroke.

Another aspect of cardiovascular disease, which ought to be mentioned, is valve replacement. The different valves of the heart can be damaged because of infection and because of the aging process. The heart valves can become damaged because of congenital problems. In any event, cardiac valve replacement is being done all over the country and all over the world. Cardiovascular surgeons are using different materials; some of them are prosthetic materials to replace heart valves to make the heart function better. Sometimes, acutely, in the process of a heart attack, a man's heart valve can become damaged and the result can be acute heart failure. The acute heart muscle damage that occurs when a man suffers a heart attack can also cause acute congestive heart failure to develop. Cardiac catheterization can be done to document which coronary artery vessel or vessels is or occluded to have caused the heart attack and which heart valve if any is damaged by the acute myocardial infarction. Following cardiac catheterization, angioplasty, bypass surgery with or without valve replacement may be carried out, depending on the particular clinical situation. The chordae tendineae are little strands—cordlike structures that keep the heart valves together. They can become ischemic and become damaged, they can be damaged because of a heart attack, or they also are damaged because of the aging process. When the chordae tendineae are ruptured, frequently acute heart failure develops.

One of the most common symptoms of sick sinus disease is dizziness, tiredness and a general feeling of UN wellness and, fainting spells. A man may at times, actually lose consciousness. That happens because the person's pulse has become too slow, sometimes less than 30 beats per minute, so that the heart cannot pump enough blood to the brain, resulting in the loss of consciousness or blackout spells. On EKG, different degrees of heart block can be seen to explain the man's symptoms. Third-degree heart block is the heart block most associated with the symptom complex just outlined. In the acute setting, the cardiologist can insert a temporary pacemaker to try to get the patient through the acute period. Sometimes, these patients will need a permanent pacemaker and sometimes they will not. As their hearts recover, the problem that caused the slow pulse may resolve itself and then the pacemaker may not be needed. That usually occurs as part of an acute heart attack. In the setting of sick sinus disease and third degree heart block, a permanent pacemaker is inserted by a chest surgeon. Sometimes, in an acute setting, the so-called bundle branch block can occur, and that bundle branch block can necessitate the insertion of a permanent pacemaker. Be that as it may, if a man has a slow heart rate, a condition referred to as bradycardia, and the heart cannot pump well enough to perfuse the brain, it is very important that a pacemaker be put in, in order to allow for better cardiovascular function.

In 2002, 494,382 men died of cardiovascular disease. During this same period of time, 223,262 white males died of CHD, 24,322 black males died of CHD. In 2002, the prevalence of cardiovascular diseases was 41.1% among black males as compared to 34.3% among white males and 29.2% Mexican-American males. About 2,600 individuals die of cardiovascular heart disease every day in the U.S., nearly a death every 33 seconds. The total direct and indirect cost of cardiovascular disease in the year 2005 was 393.5 billion dollars (Source: Heart Disease and Stroke Statistics—2005 Update, American Heart Association).

A problem that affects the heart quite often is infection:

The different infections that can affect the heart are
1. Infective endocarditis
2. Myocarditis
3. Pericarditis

What is endocarditis?

Endocarditis is when a heart valve becomes infected with a microorganism. There are three different types of infective endocarditis.
1. Native valve endocarditis
2. Prosthetic valve endocarditis
3. Intravenous drug addicts endocarditis

The most bacteria that cause endocarditis in native valve endocarditis are Streptococci, Enterococci Staphylococci and many other gram negative, gram negative bacteria as well different fungi. The different types of native heart valves that that become infected in endocarditis are

1. Normal heart valve
2. Congenital heart valve
3. Degenerative heart valve
4. Rheumatic heart valve

The mechanism through which endocarditis develops is different in different heart valves and in different clinical settings. In an individual with normal heart vale, infective endocarditis can occur, if the individual becomes either bacteremic or septic (bacteria circulating in the blood stream) and the bacteria settle on the heart valve leading to either sub-acute or acute bacterial endocarditis. In congenital bacterial endocarditis the same situation exists as above, except that in this instance, the abnormal valve makes it easier for bacteria that are circulating in the blood to get trapped on causing endocarditis. The same situation occurs in degenerative heart valve and rheumatic heart valve.

Prosthetic valve endocarditis is responsible for about 20% of all caseases of infectious endocarditis. Most of the individuals in this category of patients are men 60 years of age or older.

The different microorganisms that cause prosthetic endocarditis are, Staphylococci epidermidis,

Staphylococcus Aureus, gram negative bacteria and fungi. Prosthetic endocarditis can develop 1 year, 2 years or many years after the prosthetic valves were placed.

Bacterial endocarditis in intravenous drug addicts occurs usually on normal heart valves most of the time and in young men. The skin is the usual site of entry and the valves most frequently affected are tricuspid valve is involved 52% of the time, the aortic is involved 25% of the time, the mitral valved is involved 20% of the time and 3% of the time, multiple valves are involved.

The microorganisms most often involved in causing infectious endocarditis are Staphylococci,

Streptococci, Enterococci, Gram negative bacteria and fungi such as Candida and aspergillus.

The symptoms and clinical signs of endocarditis are:

1. Fever
2. Chills
3. Joints pain
4. Muscle pain
5. Heart murmur
6. Enlarged Spleen
7. Head ache

8. Different types of skin lesions such as Janeway lesions,
9. Roth's spots and Osler's nodes

1. Petechiae
2. Splinter hemorrhages
3. Heart failure
4. The white blood cell count is high there is anemia

Usually there is blood in the urine due to emboli to the kidneys

Because of the blood that is in the urine, there is protein in the urine

The erythrocyte sedimentation rate is quite high

The blood cultures are positive growing the responsible bacteria

The serum BUN and creatinine are usually high due to emboli and immune complexes to the kidneys

The rheumatoid factor is frequently positive

There may be circulating immune complexes

Serum Complement is usually is decreased

Echocardiogram may show vegetation on heart valve or abscesses in the heart muscle

And cardiac arrhythmias may develop

Myocarditis and pericarditis may develop ect.

The cardiology tests that must be done in the diagnosis of endocarditis are:

EKG

24 hour Holter monitor

Cardiac Telemetry monitoring

Echocardiogram

Transesophageal echocardiogram (TEE)

Or transthoracic echocardiogram (TTE)

The following are the different antibiotics that used to treat bacterial endocarditis;

1. Penicillin G
2. Vancomycin
3. Cubicin
4. Ceftriaxone
5. Nafcillin
6. Gentamicin
7. Ceftazidime
8. Piperacillin
9. Cefotaxime

10. Levaquin
11. Ciprofloxacin
12. IV Erythromycin

These different antibiotics are used in different dosages based on the patient's sizes, ages and renal function and clinical settings for 6–8weeks IV

For individuals who are risks to develop endocarditis because of valvular heart diseases or heart murmurs of different types and in individuals who have received prosthetic implants such as heart valves and hip prostheses etc, of one kind or an other, the following antibiotics are used prophylactically when invasive procedures are being done in the body of the affected person.

The invasive procedures that require prophylactic antibiotics are:
1. Intravaginal and intrapelvis surgical procedures
2. Any intraabdominal surgical procedures
3. Intraoral procedures of any kind
4. Any serious skin infection
5. Before colonoscopy etc

Erythromycin by mouth or IV
Amoxicillin by mouth or IV
Ceftriaxone IM or IV
Vancomycin IV
Cleocin by moth or IV

If acute bacterial endocarditis develops, a cardiothoracic surgeon must be brought to take the patient to operating room to replace the damaged heart vale. If vegetation or abscesses are discovered on the heart valve during TEE or TTE, a cardiothoracic surgeon may be brought in to surgically remove the infected part of the heart vale. The patient's life may be saved by this procedure. Infected emboli can be prevented from being thrown to other organs in the body.

Two other significant infectious conditions frequently affect the human heart.
There are;
Infectious myocarditis and
Infectius pericarditis.

Infectious myocarditis develops when a microorganism infects the muscles of the heart.
The most common bacteria are Staphylococcus aureus and Enterococcus.

The most common virus that causes infection of the myocardium is coxsackievirus B.

The AIDS virus can also cause myocarditis. Lyme disease can also affect the myocardium of the heart causing myocarditis etc.

The symptoms of myocarditis are:
1. Chest pain
2. Shortness of breath
3. irregular heart beats
4. Tiredness etc.
5. Although the physical examination is frequently normal, signs of CHF and irregular Cardiac rhythm can be heard
6. Heart murmur

The EKG findings may be similar to that seen when the person is having an acute myocardial infarction. The cardiac enzymes such as the CPK, LDH and SGOT might be elevated as well.

The erythrocytes sedimentation rate is usually elevated.

The tests that used to diagnose myocarditis are:
1. CBC
2. SMA 20 and cardiac enzymes
3. ERS
4. ANA, rheumatoid factor, double stranded DNA to rule out collagen vascular diseases such as Lupus or Rheumatoid arthritis as a possible cause of the myocarditis
5. Blood cultures
6. Urine analysis
7. Viral titers for coxsackievirus B
8. Lyme disease blood tests
9. HIV blood test
10. Chest x-ray
11. EKG
12. 24 hour cardiac monitoring
13. Echocardiogram
14. Myocardial biopsy when appropriate

The treatment of myocarditis is based on the clinical profile and presentation of the affected individual and the best judgment of the treating physician. At presentation, the patient ought to be treated with broad spectrum antibiotics that cover both for gram positive and gram negative bacteria. When bacterial myocarditis is ruled out, then other treatment modality may be considered based on viral titers or collagen vascular test results, such as the ANA, or Rheumatoid factor or other blood tests for Lupus, supportive care with bed rest, nasal oxygen, pain medication and antipyretics to control fever must be provided.

Infectious pericarditis is a condition that occurs when the pericardium becomes infected by micro organism such as bacteria, virus, or a fungus.

Although any microorganism can cause infection in the pericardial sac of the heart if it were to find its way there, the most common bacteria that cause acute infectious pericarditis are:

1. Streptococcus
2. Pneucoccus
3. Staphylococcus
4. Tuberculous etc

The most common viruses that cause acute pericarditis are:

1. Coxsackievirus A Coxsackievirus B
2. Adenovirus
3. Hepatitis viruses
4. HIV etc

The most common fungi that cause acute pericarditis are:

1. Candida
2. Histoplasma
3. Blastoplasma
4. Coccidiomycosis

The most common symptoms of acute infectious peircarditis are:

1. Chest pain that is made worst by coughing
2. Chest pain that is made worst when lying in
3. supine position
4. Chest pain that is made worst by taking a deep breath
5. Chest pain that is relieved by leaning forward
6. Chest pain that is relieved by sitting up

The clinical findings of pericarditis on physical examination are:

1. Distant heart sounds
2. Pericardial friction rub
3. Irregular heart sounds may be heard secondary to different rhythm abnormalities that may develop because of the infection.
4. Many different abnormal findings may be seen on EKG, chest x-ray, in blood tests and echocardiogram in infectious pericarditis.

The most common tests done to diagnose infectious pericarditis are:

1. CBC and blood cultures

2. ESR
3. SMA20
4. Cardiac enzymes
5. Viral titers for Coxsackieviruses A and B
6. Adenovirus titer
7. Hepatitis A, B, and C
8. HIV virus blood test
9. Histoplasma titer
10. Blastoplasma titer
11. Coccidiomycosis titer
12. Blood for Candida culture
13. Pericardial tap and biopsy to obtain specimens for these different cultures including gram stain and AFB stain and culture for mycobacterium tuberculosis
14. Blood test for syphilis (VDRL)
15. EKG
16. Echocardiogram
17. Cardiac Telemetry monitoring
18. Chest x-ray etc.
19. A complete collagen vascular blood profile must always be drawn and sent to the laboratory such as ANA, Rheumatoid factor, double stranded DNA. Blood for Angiotensin-1-Coverting Enzyme ought to be sent to the laboratory as well to rule out the possibility of sarcoidosis as the cause of the pericarditis.

The treatments of infectious pericarditis include:

1. Broad-spectrum antibiotics covering for both gram negative and gram positive bacteria pending the results of blood cultures, pericardia fluid and pericardial biopsy if one was done.
2. Anti fungal IV Amphotericin B if there is a strong suspicion of fungal infection and or if the patient is immunosuppressed.
3. Nasal oxygen
4. Antipyretics to control fever
5. Bed rest and general supportive care
6. In infectious percarditis, pericardial fluid can build up inside the pericardial sac resulting in pericardiac temponade. If pericardial temponade develops in a patient, if it can cause sudden death.
7. The best way to diagnose pericardial is physical examination and echocardiogram;

8. The best way to treat pericardial temponade is surgical intervention by a cardiothoracic surgeon.

Infectious pericarditis can develop into chronic as well as constrictive pericarditis, which can be severely debilitating to affected individuals.

1. Pericarditis can be caused by
2. Trauma
3. Acute myocardial infarction,
4. Lupus,
5. Rheumatoid
6. Arthritis
7. Cancer
8. Kidney failure
9. Hypothyroidism with myxedema and many more.

The following measures can help to lessen the incidence of cardiovascular heart disease in men:

1. Eat a low fat, low-carbohydrate, low salt, and high-protein diet to prevent weight gain.
2. Exercise regularly.
3. Visit the doctor frequently to have the blood pressure checked, so that hypertension can be detected and properly treated.
4. Take chest pain seriously and have it evaluated with an EKG and a stress test.
5. Stop smoking.
6. Do not abuse alcohol.
7. If diabetic, lose weight and control the blood sugar tightly.

If a man has family members who suffer from heart disease, it is very important that he mention that to his physician, so that that fact can be entered into the clinical equation to ensure that he is properly evaluated to detect the existence of heart disease.

The incidence of heart disease in men and the incidence of death from heart disease in men can be brought down significantly, if men understand the gravity of the situation and do the necessary things to try to bring that incidence down.

Another point that needs to be made is that obesity is frequently associated with diabetes and diabetes is a risk factor for cardiovascular disease. Diabetic men frequently have atypical symptoms of coronary heart disease.

Understanding these facts and paying close attention to them will decrease the incidence of death from heart disease in men.

CHAPTER 7

CANCERS IN MEN IN THE US

IN THE YEAR 2007, ABOUT 1,444,920 individuals will be diagnosed with cancer in the United States. 766,860 of that total will be in men. In addition, more than 1 million people developed basal cell carcinoma of the skin yearly. In 2007, according to the American Cancer Society, 559,650 individuals will die of cancer in the United States and of that number, 289. 550 will be men. This means that more than 1,500 individuals die of cancer everyday in the U.S. One in every four deaths in the United States is due to cancer. In a lifetime, a man in the U.S. has a 1-in-3 chance of developing cancer. In 2007, there are 10.5 million cancer survivors in the US. Since 1990, roughly 5 million people have died of cancer of different types in the U.S. The combined five-year survival rate for all cancers diagnosed and treated in the United States is 62%; .the five-year survival rate is higher for some cancers and lower for other cancers.

Overall, according to figures published by the American Cancer Society, Blacks are about 34% more likely to die of cancer than Whites in the United States are. That is an astonishingly great disparity.

Cancer is the second leading cause of death in the United States next to cardiovascular heart disease. Cancer is a very costly disease in monetary terms. The National Institute of Health estimates the total cost of cancer in the year 2004 was 189.8 billion dollars.

What is cancer?

Cancer develops when a cell loses its ability to grow and multiply in a normal growth pattern. A good example of that is contact inhibition. When a normal cell is placed in contact with a hard surface in a Petri dish, the normal cell stops growing. But in the case of an abnormal cell, it continues to grow because it has lost its contact inhibition ability, which allows it to grow uncontrollably, developing into a cancer growth. The cancer cells fail in the process of cell-to-cell interactions. The development of cancer is a multi-step and multi-factorial process. In the multi-step and multi-factorial processes, there is normally a balance between growth-promoting genes (proteins) and growth-suppressive genes (proteins). Once mutation occurs for one reason or another, the growth-promoting genes (oncogenes) stop the suppressive effects of the suppressor genes. The growth-promoting genes take control and promote abnormal cell growth, resulting in the formation of a cancerous clone of cells, resulting in cancer, as it is known. That is an out-of-control process of cell growth whose ultimate goal is to take over the body in which it is growing and destroys it.

The first step in the genesis of cancer is the process of oncogene. Oncogenes can be brought about by a hereditary or familial transmission of a protein from parent or parents to fetus at the time of conception. That protein (oncogene or oncogenes) can then enter over many years into a multi-step process, interactions and reactions that can cause a cell or group of cells to mutate. Once that mutation occurs, then the cell or group of cells loses their ability to grow and multiply normally. The abnormal growth of cells then becomes a cancer mass. Many causative effects can bring about the damage that occurs to the cell or cells that cause that mutation to occur.

All of the following can damage the DNA/RNA materials inside a cell, resulting in a malignant mutant:

1. Transmission of a hereditary cancer oncogene;
2. Exposure to oncogenic viruses such as Epstein bar virus, which can cause nasopharyngeal carcinoma;
3. Exposure to human papilloma virus, causing cervical cancer;
4. Exposure to either hepatitis B or C virus, causing cancer of the liver;
5. Exposure to HTLV-I and HTLV-II, causing T cell leukemia/lymphoma;
6. Sun exposure causing basal cell carcinoma of the skin;
7. Exposure to carcinogens such as tobacco smoking, causing lung cancer, cancer of the mouth, throat, head and neck, etc.;
8. Exposure to ionizing radiation, causing leukemia, lymphoma and other cancers;

9. Exposure to toxic chemicals such as benzene, etc., causing malignancies of different types;

10. Consumption of excessive alcohol, resulting in cancer of the mouth, throat and esophagus;

11. Exposure to estrogen, causing increased incidence of breast cancer and uterine cancer in men;

12. Consumption of too much red meats, resulting in increased incidence of breast, uterine and colon cancer;

13. Alcohol abuse and tobacco smoking, associated with increase incidence of cancer of the esophagus;

14. Long-term exposure to toxic pollutants and chemical solvents in the work place, resulting in the development of different types of cancer;

15. HIV-I and II causing AIDS with its high propensity to cause lymphoma and Kaposi's sarcoma;

16. Non-acquired immunodeficiency and its propensity to cause malignancy of different types etc;

Cancer genetics:

Following are examples of cancers that develop because of oncogene activation:

Multiple endocrine neoplasia (MEN) type 2a and type 2b. MEN 2a include medullary carcinoma of the thyroid, pheochromocytoma and hyperparathyroidism. MEN 2b include medullary carcinoma of the thyroid, pheochromocytoma, mucosal neuromas and bony abnormalities.

Other cancers that occur because of damaged DNA and failure of DNA repair include:

hereditary nonpolyposis colon cancer (HNPCC). That abnormality is responsible for about 10–15% of colon cancers and is associated with ovarian, endometrial and urinary tract cancers.

Other genetically associated cancers include neurofibromatosis 1 and 2, hereditary Wilm's tumor, Li-Fraumeni syndrome, and familial adenomatous polyposis of the colon. The percentage of colon cancer in familial adenomatous polyposis is 100%. Treatment usually requires the affected individual to undergo total removal of the colon by 20 to 30 years of age.

There are many more genes that have been discovered that have association with many other cancers, which in the future will be better clarified. Gene therapy is being actively investigated and the hope is that these investigations will add immeasurably to the treatment of cancer in the future.

In the year 2005, there were 710.040 new cases of cancer in men in the U.S.

The incidence of cancer is higher in black men than men of other racial groups.

The following is a list of the different cancers that men developed in 2005 in the U. S.

1. Prostate cancer: 232,090
2. Lung cancer: 93,010
3. Colorectal cancer: 71,820
4. Urinary bladder: 47,010
5. Melanoma of the skin: 33,580
6. Cancer of mouth and throat: 19,100
7. Non-Hodgkin/lymphomas: 29,070
8. Cancer of the pancreas: 16,100
9. Cancer of Kidney and renal pelvis 22,490
10. Cancer of soft tissue: 5,530
11. Thyroid cancer: 6,500
12. Skin cancer (Non Melanoma) more than 1,000,000
13. Esophagus: 11,220
14. Stomach: 13,510
15. Cancer of the liver: 5.600 in 2003
16. cancer of the brain and nervous system: 10,620
17. Multiple myeloma: 8,600
18. Cancer of the liver and bile duct: 12,130
19. Cancer of the small intestine: 2.840
20. Cancer of the gall bladder: 3.330
21. Hodgkin lymphoma: 3,980
22. Chronic lymphocytic leukemia: 5,780
23. Chronic myelogenous leukemia: 2,640
24. Acute myelogenous leukemia: 6,530
25. Acute Lymphocytic leukemia: 2,100
26. Testicular cancer: 8,010
27. Cancer of the penis: 1,470

Source: American Cancer Society Cancer Facts and Figures, 2005.

The incidence of death from cancer in men in the U.S. all sites during the period of 2005, was 295,280;

Lung and bronchus cancers 90,490;
Colon and rectal cancers 28,540;
Prostate cancer 30,350;
Cancer of the esophagus 10,530;
Urinary bladder cancer 8,970;
Kidney and renal pelvis cancers 8,020;
Liver and gall bladder cancers 10,330;
Chronic lymphocytic leukemia 2,520;
Acute lymphocytic leukemia 850;
Chronic Myelocytic leukemia 430;
Acute Myelocytic leukemia 5.040;
Other forms of leukemias 3,700;
Non-Hodgkin lymphoma 10,150;
Hodgkin lymphoma 780;
Oral cavity/Throat cancers 1,200;
Pancreatic cancer 15,820;
Melanoma 4,910;
Other skin cancers 6,
Testicular cancer 390;
Multiple myeloma 5,660;
Breast cancer 460;

Cancer deaths from all sites in 2005 were:
    245.5 Per 100.000 in white men;
    347.3 Per 100.000 in black men;
    151.2 Per 100.000 in Asian American/Pacific Islander;
    174.0 Per 100.000 in Hispanic/Latino men;
    167.0 Per 100.000 in American Indian/Alaska Native;
The incidence of death from lung and bronchus cancers in the US in 2005 was
    76.6 Per 100.000 in white men;
    104.1 Per 100.000 in black men;
    40.2 Per 100.000 in Asian American/Pacific Islander;
    49.8 Per 100.000 in American Indian/Alaska Native;
    39.6 Per 100.000 in Hispanic/Latino;
The incidence of colon and rectal cancers in the U S was
    24.8 Per 100.000 in white men;
    34.3 Per 100.000 in black men;
    15.8 Per 100.000 in Asian American/Pacific Islander men;

17.1 Per 100.000 in American Indian/Alaska Native;

18.0 Per 100.000 in Hispanic/Latino;

The incidence death from prostate cancer in the US was;

28.8 Per 100.000 in White men;

70.4 Per 100.000 in Black men;

13.0 Per 100.000 in Asian American/Pacific Islander;

20.2 Per 100.000 in American Indian/Alaska Native;

23.5 Per 100.000 in Hispanic/Latino;

The incidence of death from stomach cancer in the US was;

5.8 Per 100.000 in White men;

13.3 Per 100.000 in Black men;

11.9 Per 100.000 in Asian American/Pacific Islander;

7.3 Per 100.000 in American Indian/Alaska Native;

9.7 Per 100.000 in Hispanic/Latino;

The incidence of death from liver and gall bladder cancers in the US was;

6.1 Per 100.000 in White men;

9.3 Per 100.000 in Black men;

15.6 Per 100.000 in the Asian American/Pacific Islander;

8.3 Per 100.000 in American Indian/Alaska Native;

10.6 Per 100.000 in Hispanic/Latino in the US in 2005;

Source: Cancer Facts & Figures 2005 American Cancer Society

1. Heredity plays a role in the causation of different cancers ten to fifteen percent of cancers are hereditary in nature and the rest are due to environmental exposures.

In 2007, 2, 0 30 men will be diagnosed with breast cancer and 450 of these men will die of breast cancer.

How to evaluate a lump in a man's breast

First thing is to take a complete history from the man, including a thorough family history. It is important to determine whether he is taking any estrogen-containing medication. It is also important to find out if he has any pain and how long ago he discovered the lump in his breast. Following the history and examination, a mammogram is to be done and if the breast is very cystic, it is important to do a sonogram of the breast at the same time. The next step is to refer the man to a surgeon for surgical evaluation of the lump. The most up-to-date test to evaluate a man's breast that has a high risk of developing breast cancer because of his family history is to do an MRI of the breast.

In particular, if the man is between 20 and 35 years old, it is very difficult to pick up cancer of the breast because the breast tissue is so dense, and therefore an MRI is most appropriate in that setting.

The clinical approach to the evaluation of a breast mass.

Once a lump is discovered in a man's breast, either by his or his physician, or whether some other abnormalities are found in the breast. The way to proceed to evaluate the breast is to do a mammogram, followed by a sonogram. A biopsy can be carried out or if it is a fluid-filled cyst, an aspiration of the cyst is done and the fluid is sent for cytological evaluation, etc.

There are different methods of doing a breast biopsy:

One type is a needle-guided biopsy (see Figure 7.2).

The second type is a straight needle biopsy of a breast mass under anesthesia.

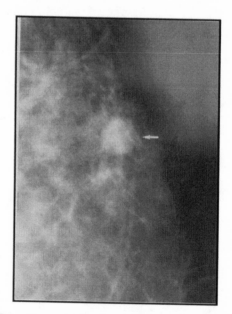

Figure 7.1—X-ray picture of positive mammogram for cancer

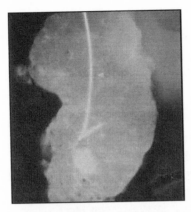

Figure 7.2—Needle biopsy of a breast cancer mass

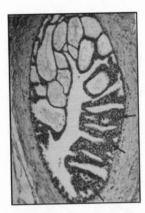

Figure 7.3—Intraductal carcinoma of the breast (arrow)

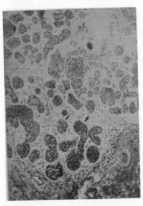

Figure 7.4—Lobular carcinoma of the breast (arrow)

In evaluating the breast cancer, it is important to know the different characteristics of the cancer. These characteristics have major significance in the treatment modalities that are chosen to treat the breast cancer. It is also important to know certain markers that breast cancer may have or may not have, which have major prognostic significance in breast cancer.

These are some of the most important markers used to evaluate and treat breast cancer:

1. Estrogen receptor
2. Progesterone receptor
3. Her-2

As a matter of clinical fact, estrogen receptor-positive breast cancer seems to respond better to such treatments as chemotherapy, radiation therapy or hormonal therapy. The reverse is true in breast cancer that is receptor-negative. It seems to be more aggressive and responds less well to those treatments. More recently, a gene product called Her-2 is found on the surface of 25–30% of breast cancer cells, which, when present, denotes a poorer prognosis for men who are afflicted with that type of breast cancer.

Once it is determined that a man has tissue-proven breast cancer, an evaluation must be undertaken to be sure that the man does not have metastatic disease. A metastatic evaluation for breast cancer includes:

1. Complete blood count, liver function tests (LDH, SGOT, SGPT, bilirubin and alkaline phosphatase). If the alkaline phosphatase is elevated, it may mean that cancer has gotten into the liver or the bone—or it may mean that the patient has some other problem that causes his alkaline phosphatase to be elevated, such as chronic hepatitis, gall bladder disease, or Paget's disease of the bone. To know whether the elevated alkaline phosphatase is coming from the liver or the bone, a test called gamma glutamine transpeptidase (GGTP) is done. If the GGTP is high, it means that the elevated alkaline phosphatase is coming from the liver. If the alkaline GGTP phosphatase is normal, it means that the alkaline phosphatase is coming from the bone, which may mean that the breast cancer has already involved the bones.
2. Bone scan.
3. Abdominal CAT scan or abdominal sonogram to look at the liver.
4. Chest x-ray or chest CAT scan.

If all these tests are normal, indicating that the breast cancer is localized, then a man is now ready for either a lumpectomy with axillary node dissection or a modified radical mastectomy. The decision as to whether a lumpectomy with axillary node dissection or a modified radical mastectomy is done is based on the size of the tumor, the choice of the man or whether the cancer has spread or is localized.

Stages of breast cancer:
Stage 0
Stage I
Stage IIA
Stage IIB
Stage IIIA
Stage IIIB
Stage IV

Stage 0 breast cancer is carcinoma in situ. Intraductal carcinoma. Tubular carcinoma in situ. Or Paget's disease of the nipple with no regional lymph node metastasis or no distant metastasis.

Stage I breast cancer is a breast cancer that is 2 cm or less in greatest dimension with no regional lymph node metastasis and no distant metastasis.

Stage IIA breast is a tumor that is greater than 2 cm and less than 5 cm and has metastasized to the lymph node or nodes in the same side of the breast that has the malignancy.

Stage IIB breast cancer is a tumor that is greater than 2 cm and less than 5 cm and metastasis is found in node or nodes on the side of the malignant breast, or a tumor that is greater than 5 cm in size with no metastasis to regional or distant nodes.

Stage IIIA breast cancer has multiple possible scenarios.
1. Metastasis to node, nodes, or other structures on the same side of the tumor.
2. Tumor no greater than 2 cm with positive lymph node or nodes on the same side of the tumor.
3. Tumor greater than 2 cm with metastasis to node or nodes on the same side of the cancer.
4. Tumor greater than 5 cm with metastasis to node or nodes on the same side of the tumor.

Stage IIIB. A tumor with direct extension to the chest wall with metastasis to the lymph node or on the side of the tumor or metastasis to mammary lymph nodes.

Stage IV is distant metastasis to other parts of the body such as the lungs, liver, bones or brain.

Evaluation and different treatments for breast cancer

The first step in evaluating breast cancer is to examine the breast. The next is to do a mammogram. If there is a suspicion of possible malignant process, because of either suspicious micro-calcification or a suspicious mass in the breast, then a biopsy is done. A needle can aspirate a mass or fluid and the specimen is sent to the histology lab.

A biopsy can also be done via needle-guided technique, or an open biopsy can be done. In either case, the specimen is sent to the pathology lab for histological evaluation. If the pathological report comes back, showing evidence of breast cancer, then a decision has to be made on what type of surgical approach to use to treat the patient. Essentially, there are several approaches. One approach is lumpectomy with axillary node dissection with employment of the sentinel node technique to be sure that nodes that contain cancer are removed during the axillary dissection. Another approach is modified radical mastectomy.

Different stages of breast cancer are treated differently. For patients who choose to have a lumpectomy with axillary node dissection, post-surgical treatment with two cycles of chemotherapy—either with CMF (Cytoxan, Methotrexate and 5FU) or with CAF (Cytoxan, Adriamycin and 5FU)—followed by radiation therapy, then followed by four more cycles of chemotherapy, seems to be the best approach.

Other protocols that are commonly used are CMFVP—Cyclophosphamide, Methotrexate, 5Fluorouracil, Vincristine and Prednisone. Cisplatin, Etoposide, Mitomycin, and Vinblastine are included at times in different protocols to treat more advanced breast cancer.

In metastatic breast cancer, Taxol is also used at a dose of 90 mg/m2 as a continuous IV drip for 96 hours monthly. For men who are Her-2 positive, Herceptin is used to treat them and the results so far have been excellent. The recommended loading dose of Herceptin is 4 mg/Kg IV over 90 minutes followed by a weekly dose of 2 mg/Kg over 30 minutes.

Chemotherapy treatments used in breast cancer and their major side effects: injection, cardiac toxicity, which can lead to heart failure if too much Adriamycin is given over time. It is recommended a test called REST MUGA is done before starting Adriamycin to evaluate the ejection fraction of the heart (what the heart is capable of doing by way of work in any one second). REST MUGA is done periodically during the treatment with Adriamycin and if the ejection fraction is shown to be dropping significantly indicating cardiac malfunction, the Adriamycin is stopped.

Some of the common side effects of chemotherapy are:

Cytoxan: Bone marrow suppression with low white blood cells, low platelets, low red blood cells, (hematuria), alopecia (hair loss), nausea and vomiting.
Methtrexate: Bone marrow suppression with low white blood cells, low red blood cells, low platelets, nausea, vomiting and sores in the mouth.
5-Fluorouracil: Bone marrow suppression with low white blood cells, low red blood cells, low platelets, nausea, vomiting, sores in the mouth, alopecia, darkness of the skin, dakness under nail bed and chest pain.

Adriamycin: Bone marrow suppression with low white blood cells, low red blood cells, low platelets, sores in the mouth, nausea, vomiting and possible cardiac side effects.

Herceptin: The main side effects of Herceptin are cardiac toxicity, anemia and leukopenia. That being the case a REST MUGA and CBC must be done before Herceptin is started and periodically during its usage.

Taxol: The main side effect of Taxol is low white blood cells count; other frequent side effects of Taxol are low platelet count, peripheral neuropathy and loss of hair.

Docetaxel: Is also being used to treat breast cancer. The side effects of Docetaxel are similar to that of Taxol.

Paclitaxel is used in combination Doxorubicin and Cytoxan to treat breast cancer

Paclitaxel is also used in combination with Carboplatin to treat breast cancer

Paclipaxel is also used in combination with Epirubicin to treat breast cancer

Trastuzumab is also used with Docetaxel to treat breast cancer etc.

Amifostine: Can be used in conjunction with these cytotoxic agents to decrease the incidence of peripheral neuropathy.

Neurontin 300 mg. by mouth every 8 hours is also effective in the treatment of chemotherapy-associated peripheral neuropathy.

Lung Cancer

In the year 2007, 114,760 men in the U.S. will be diagnosed with lung cancer and 89, 510 of them will die of this disease.

The most common reason why men develop lung cancer is tobacco smoking.

Some of the symptoms of lung cancer:

1. Chronic cough
2. Coughing with streaks of blood
3. Coughing up blood
4. Chest pain
5. Shortness of breath
6. Weight loss, etc.
7. Recurrent pneumonia and/or pneumonia that fail to respond to treatment over a long period.

Risk factors for lung cancer:

1. Cigarette smoking
2. Cigar smoking
3. Exposure to second-hand smoke
4. Exposures to industrial fumes such as toxic chemicals, arsenic, and air pollution from coal-burning machines, etc.
5. Exposure to asbestos
6. Scar from healed tuberculosis or other inflammatory lung diseases
7. Genetic predisposition to cancer

Sometimes lung cancer is discovered on a chest x-ray without any symptoms. Early detection is crucial in order to increase the chance of curing lung cancer; a chest x-ray is the first test in the diagnosis of lung cancer. The chest x-ray is done either as part of a routine examination or because the patient presents with symptoms such as those described earlier here. Things that can be seen on the chest x-ray or CT when a person has lung cancer include:

1. A mass
2. Effusion (fluid in the lung)
3. An infiltrate and in some cases
4. Calcified mass or calcification seen in the lungs (mesothelioma due to exposure to asbestos)

There are two broad types of lung cancer, large-cell lung cancer and small-cell lung cancer. Large-cell lung cancer may consist of adenocarcinoma of the lung, squamous cell carcinoma of the lung, or scar carcinoma of the lung. Mesothelioma is a form of lung cancer associated with asbestos exposure. Another name for small-cell carcinoma is oat cell carcinoma.

Once cancer of the lung is suspected on chest x-ray, the next test to be done is a CAT scan of the chest, or MRI or PET scan

See CAT scan of the chest lesion in inferior segment of the lower lobe of the lung. Squamous cell carcinoma (cancer) in a smoker (Figure 7.5 [arrows]).

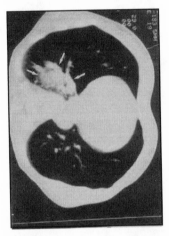

Figure 7.5—See CAT scan of the chest showing lobulated mass (cancer) in the right upper lung in a patient who smokes (Figure 7.6 [arrows]).

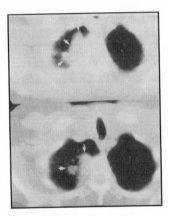

Figure 7.6

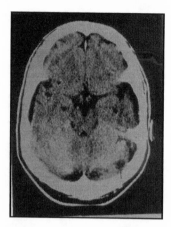

Figure 7.7—CAT scan of brain: Hypodense mass left cerebellar hemisphere—Metastatic cancer to the brain from a lung primary cancer in a smoker (arrow).

Following the CAT scan of the lung, or PET scan, the next step is to refer the patient to a pulmonary specialist for a bronchoscopic examination. Another approach is to refer the patient to a chest surgeon based on the location of the mass. Some masses of the lung are located so peripherally that it cannot be reached via bronchoscopy.

The bronchoscopic examination is a procedure during which a tube is introduced into the lung after spraying the throat with an anesthetic. During the bronchoscopy, either a biopsy or washing is taken from the mass in the lung and sent to the pathology lab for examination. If it is the chest surgeon that takes the patient to the operating room, a piece of tissue is taken from the mass and sent to the pathologist for testing to determine if there is cancer or not (that is called a frozen section). If it is cancer, then a chest surgeon may proceed to remove the segment of the lung that contains the cancer. During the procedure, several lymph nodes are taken out from the surrounding area to check if any of these has cancer or not.

Another method that is frequently used to diagnose lung cancer is CAT-or sonogram-guided needle biopsy to obtain tissue for diagnosis. An invasive radiologist with great precision carries out that procedure and it frequently saves the patient a bronchoscopy or an open-chest surgical procedure. It is always a good idea for a chest surgeon to perform a mediastinoscopy to rule out the presence of cancerous nodes in the mediastinum before proceeding with the resection of a suspicious cancerous mass in the lung.

It is very important to know in advance what cell type lung cancer that the patient has in order to know how to proceed with further treatment. As just stated, there are essentially two different categories of lung cancer, large cells and small cells. The importance of knowing whether a person has small-cell lung cancer, large-cell lung cancer is that small-cell cancer, or oat-cell lung cancer usually has already spread by the time a mass is seen on the chest x-ray regardless of how small the mass is. That being the case, the entire approach to the evaluation and treatment of small-cell cancer is different from any other lung cancer. In fact, it is almost a given that by the time a coin-size lesion is found in the lung of a patient that turns out to be oat cell, the cancer mass probably has already spread to the brain and possibly the liver and other organs as well. Frequently, once the cell type is known to be oat cell because of biopsy, the question as to whether the cancer should or should not be resected becomes a major clinical decision because the prognosis is poor.

On the other hand, once a tissue diagnosis is made that the cancer in the lung is of the large-cell type, and if the cancer is deemed resectable, based on the size, location and overall physical status of the patient, the decision usually is to resect the cancer because the chances of cure are better. Though it must be remembered that 20–25% of people with large-cell-type lung cancer frequently present with metastasis to the brain at the time of diagnosis.

Evaluation of lung cancer includes:
1. History and physical examination
2. Chest x-ray
3. Chest CAT scan
4. Sputum for cytology
5. Lung biopsy
6. Abdominal CAT scan to look at the liver
7. Bone scan to be sure that the cancer has not spread to the bone
8. Brain CAT scan with contrast because a brain CT without contrast will likely miss metastatic disease of the brain
9. PET scan
10. Brain MRI can also be done with contrast

Treatment of lung cancer includes:
1. Surgical resection of the cancerous mass
2. Adjuvant radiation therapy, after surgical resection
3. Adjuvant chemotherapy
4. Or adjuvant radiation followed with chemotherapy

Some frequently used chemotherapeutic agents in large-cell lung cancer include:

Cytoxan
Doxorubicin
Cisplatin
Etoposide
Taxol
Docetaxel
Gemcitabine
Carboplatin
Paclitaxel
Vinorelbine

Tarceva has been approved for use in advanced lung cancer with some encouraging results.

These are used in different combinations.

Some of the commonly used chemotherapeutic agents in small-cell lung cancer care consist of:

Cyclophosphamide
Doxorubicin
Vincristine
Cisplatin
Methotrexate
Carboplatin
Ininotecan
Topotecan

These medications are used in different combinations.

Some of the side effects of these chemotherapeutic agents have been outlined earlier under the treatment of breast cancer. The side effects of Vincristine include double vision, drooping eyelids, headache, jaw pain, tingling of the finger and toes with numbness (peripheral neuropathy), and constipation.

Some of the side effects of Cisplatin include nausea; vomiting; numbness of feet, fingers, and toes; blurry vision; possible kidney damage; and bone marrow suppression, resulting in pancytopenia.

Some of the side effects of Etoposide (VP 16) include bone marrow depression with low white blood cells, low red blood cells, low platelets; sores in the mouth; numbness in feet, finger and toes with tingling; loss of hair; nausea; vomiting; and alopecia.

To decrease the incidence of nausea and vomiting, different anti-emetic medications, such as Zofran or Kytril, in combination with Ativan, Benadryl and Decadron, are used.

Colorectal Cancer

In the year 2007, about 79,130 men will be diagnosed with colorectal cancer in the U.S. and 26,000 of these men will die of this cancer during that same period.

Colorectal cancer is a curable disease when diagnosed early and surgically removed.

Common symptoms and signs of colorectal cancer:

1. Blood in the stools
2. Constipation
3. Diarrhea
4. Abdominal pain
5. Weight loss
6. Poor appetite
7. Hemorrhoids
8. Sudden development of inguinal hernia in a person in the cancer-age group (40 years old and older)
9. Anemia
10. Passing pencil-size stool
11. A combination of these signs and symptoms

How to diagnose colorectal cancer

To diagnose colorectal cancer, a complete history and physical examination needs to be carried out. As part of that examination, a digital rectal examination needs to be done and the stool tested for occult blood. Sometimes, a person goes to the physician and states that he or he sees blood in the stool or on the toilet paper. Sometimes, a man might say that he has had hemorrhoids for a long time and suddenly the hemorrhoids have come out and are now bleeding. At times, a man in his 40s, or older, might come to see the doctor and reports that he has just developed an inguinal hernia with no known precipitating reason.

In all these instances, a complete lower bowel evaluation needs to be done to make sure that these signs and symptoms are not due to colon cancer. Test the stool for occult blood, unless gross blood is seen. It is important that the man being tested stays away from taking aspirin or NSAIDS, for 7–10 days in the case of aspirin and 3–4 days in the case of NSAIDS. It is also important that the man does not eat red meat for three days prior to testing the stool for blood. The man must not take Vitamin C in pill form for one week before the test. In addition, the person must not eat horseradish for several days before testing the stool for blood. Aspirin and NSAIDS will cause the stool hemoccult test to be positive because of the irritating effects on the lining of the stomach. Red meat will cause the stool to be positive for blood because red meats have blood in them. Vitamin C causes the hemoccult test of the stool to be falsely negative for occult blood because Vitamin C is a reducing agent and the chemical reaction that is used in the test is an oxidation reaction. So adding a reducing agent to an oxidation reaction neutralizes the reaction, rendering it falsely negative. Eating horseradish can cause a person's stool to become black when it is exposed to the solution that is used to test the stool for blood. Taking Peptobismol also causes the stool to become black, confusing it with bleeding from the stomach.

The tests most effective in evaluation of colorectal cancer consist of:
1. Digital rectal examination
2. Testing of the stool using the hemoccult test
3. Checking the serum ferritin
4. Checking the red cell distribution width (RDW) during a complete blood count
5. Testing for the soluble serum transferrin receptor level. (If elevated, it proves that the patient has iron deficiency anemia. That test is better than bone marrow iron stain test, the serum ferritin and the RDW.)
6. Barium enema
7. Colonoscopy
8. Flexible sigmoidoscopy
9. Rigid sigmoidoscopy

According to the recent literature, flexible sigmoidoscopy is not very dependable in detecting cancer of the colon. About 34% of colon cancer is missed using flexible sigmoidoscopic examination.

Since the bowel preparation is the same for both colonoscopy and flexible sigmoidoscopy, though there is a difference in price, it would appear that flexible sigmoidoscopy should be abandoned as a technique to evaluate the colon for detecting cancer since it misses more than 1/3 of colon cancer.

Barium enema is an x-ray test during which the bowel is cleansed with cathartics, barium is put in the bowel from the rectum using a tube, and then x-rays are used to visualize the bowel, looking for abnormalities, such as cancerous growth. There are several limitations with the barium enema. Among the limitations:

1. Retained stool in the bowel.
2. Barium enema is not able to diagnose colorectal if the cancer is located between 15 and 30 cm in the lower bowel from the entrance of the anus. That is so because the tube that is used to put the barium in the colon occupies that space, making it impossible to visualize a cancer that may be located in that space.

Cancer is best discovered in that area by sigmoidoscopy or colonoscopy.

In addition, another limitation of the barium enema is that if a mass or polyp is found it cannot be biopsied.

Colonoscopy is the best way to evaluate the colon because not only can the gastroenterologist see the entire lower bowel, but he or she can also biopsy any lesion or polyp that is there. Once a biopsy is taken from either a polyp or mass, the specimen is sent to the pathology laboratory for histological evaluation. Colonoscopy misses about 2–3% cancer in the colon.

It is now recommended that Blacks and Latinos get colonoscopic eaxaminations starting at age 40 because the incidence of colorectal cancer is on the rise in these groups, and the disease is being seen at an earlier age in these 2 groups as well.

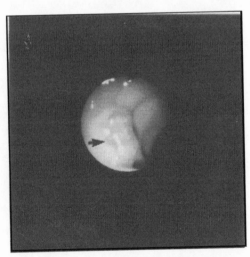

Figure 7.8—Colon cancer: sessile lesion of the colon (arrow)

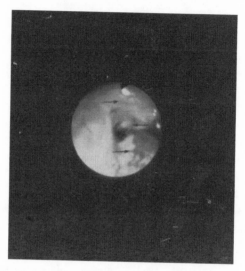

Figure 7.9—Large obstructing colon cancer with bleeding (arrows)

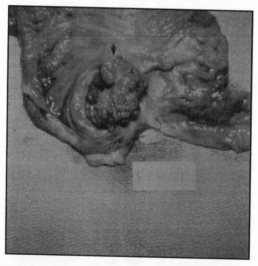

Figure 7.10—Carcinoma in papillary adenoma of cecum (arrow)

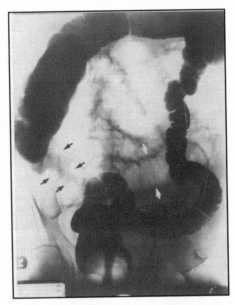

Figure 7.11—Barium enema: Apple core lesion of the cecum (white arrows) with small bowel obstruction (white arrows)

If the pathology report comes, back that the polyp or polyps removed is or are negative for cancer, then in about two years the individual should have another colonoscopic examination. Some people have the propensity to develop polyps in their colon. It takes about 3–5 years for a precancerous polyp to develop into cancer. Some individuals who form a lot of polyps need surveillance colonoscopy every year for 2–3 years so that a polyp that has the potential to become cancerous can be removed before it becomes cancer.

The FDA, to prevent polyp formation in people who are prone to develop too much polyps, has just approved Celebrex, a Cox 2 inhibitor used for arthritis, for use to prevent polyp formation.

It is very important to test frequently the stool of people who have the hereditary predisposition to colon cancer for blood, frequently using the hemoccult. It is also very important to begin to do surveillance colonoscopy for those men starting at age 35 and to clinically monitor them by doing:

1. Digital rectal examination
2. Testing of the stool using the hemoccult test
3. Checking the serum ferritin
4. Checking the red cell distribution width (RDW) during a complete blood count

5.   Testing for the serum transferrin receptor level. (If elevated, it proves that the patient has iron deficiency amenia.)

In a man without hemoglobinopathy, or who is not hemolyzing, who does not have either B12 or folic acid deficiency, who has elevated RDW (15 or greater), that means he is probably losing blood slowly and losing storage iron with it. In the routine setting, the elevated RDW is the earliest sign of slow blood loss. That occurs from the time that the precancerous polyp starts oozing blood, 2–3 years before real cancer develops. So it is crucial that the treating physician understands and knows how to interpret the RDW. The RDW is given as part of the CBC report by most reporting laboratories that do blood counts.

The third very important test that indicates blood loss and iron loss is serum ferritin. The ferritin is the storage iron that humans have in their bone marrow, muscles, liver, spleen, the reticuloendothelial system, the brain and other tissues in the body. A normal-size man has 3.5 grams of iron in his body with 2 grams in the red cells and about 1.5 grams in the store, as ferritin. Keeping in mind that each milliliter of blood has 0.5 mg of iron in it, it is fairly easy to calculate how much iron a man has lost when he becomes anemic by working backwards and calculating how much his serum ferritin is. One unit of blood, which is 500 cc, has 250 mg of iron in it. The normal serum ferritin in men is 22.0–322.0 NG/ML in most laboratories. Note that the serum ferritin is a range and as such it takes several years of slow and chronic bleeding from whatever source to deplete the ferritin down. It is also important and crucial to understand that a man must deplete his serum ferritin totally before he starts using the iron in the circulation. When he is bleeding slowly and chronically—as is the case in cancer of the large bowel, rectum, small bowel, esophagus and stomach—the first iron that is being lost is the iron in the store (the ferritin). Knowing that to be the case then, once it is noted that the range of the serum ferritin is starting to go down (being depleted) it is the crucial time to start evaluating the gastrointestinal tract to look for the reason or reasons for the blood loss. In other words, if an evaluation is undertaken at that juncture, a resectable and curable precancerous polyp can be removed and cancer of the gastrointestinal tract, no matter where it is located, can be cured, in particular, if the cancer is located in the large bowel. The only cancer that may be difficult to cure surgically even if discovered and resected early is cancer of the esophagus.

If a mass is found during colonoscopy and biopsied and the pathology shows cancer, then a metastatic evaluation is carried out to determine if the cancer has or has not spread, before deciding to go ahead with surgical resection of the mass. The metastatic evaluation for colon cancer includes:

1. Complete blood count
2. Liver function tests such as SGOT, SGPT, alkaline phosphatase, LDH
3. CEA (carcinoembryogenic antigen)
4. Abdominal CT to look at the liver and the retroperitoneal area, etc.,
5. Chest x-ray
6. CAT scan of the chest
7. Bone scan.
8. PET scan

If all these tests are normal, then the assumption can be made that the cancer has not spread to these organs; the patient can be scheduled for surgical resection of the cancerous mass.

The resected mass including dissected lymph nodes are sent to the pathology lab department for gross and histological evaluations. To know the extent of the spread of the colon cancer, a system of staging called Duke's staging is adhered to: Duke's A, Duke's B, Duke's C, and Duke's D.

Or

Stage 1

Stage 2

Stage 3

Stage 4

Duke's A is when the cancer penetrates into the wall of the bowel but not through it. Duke's B is when the cancer penetrates through the wall of the bowel. Duke's C is when the cancer penetrates through the wall of the bowel and spreads to the surrounding lymph nodes. There exists more refinement of the Duke's staging, which defines Duke's A, B, BII, Duke's C and Duke's C2. Duke's D is widespread distant metastasis.

The Duke's staging of colon cancer is very important in that it dictates the type of treatment modalities that are provided for the patient with colon cancer. It is also important in outlining the prognosis of the individual who has colon cancer.

Duke's A and B colon cancer are surgically curable cancers. Duke's BII oftentimes requires surgical resection with 6 months of adjuvant 5FU and Leucovorin. Duke's C colon cancer is less likely to be surgically curable.

After surgical resection, the best adjuvant chemotherapeutic treatment for Duke's C colon cancer is Levamisole 150 mg every 8 hours for 3 days every 3 weeks with 5FU 450 mg/m2 weeks for 52 weeks. Or Camptosar 125mg/m2 IV over 90 minutes and 5FU 500mg/m2 IV bolus and Leucovorin 20mg/m2 IV over 2 hours on day 1, 8, 15 and 22 and 1 week off every month for 1 year.

At times surgical resection may be necessary in Duke's D lesion if a large cancer mass is found and is deemed to be potentially about to obstruct the colon. To avoid that problem, the surgeon then may decide to resect the cancer mass. Otherwise, the treatment of Duke's D 5FU 500 mg/m2 IV bolus, Camptosar 125 mg/m2 IV over 90 minutes and Leucovorin 20 mg/m2 IV over 2 hours on day 1, 8, 15 and 22 and 1 week off every month for 1 year. Another frequently used regimen to treat Duke's or Stage 4 colon cancer is Oxaliplatin on Day 1, 85 mg/m2 IV over 2 hours, Leucovorin 200 mg/m2 over 2 hours IV, 5FU 400 mg/m2 IV bolus and 5FU 600 mg/m2 as a continuous infusion over 22 hours. On day 2 Leucovorin 200 mg/m2 IV over 2 hours 5FU 400 mg/m2 IV bolus, and 5FU 600 mg/m2 as a continuous infusion over 22 hours. That is repeated every 2 weeks. There have been good results seen using both these two regimens. Surgical removal of isolated liver mass from colon cancer has been done and is said to be at times successful.

The addition of Avastin to the treatment protocol of patients with metastatic colon-rectal cancer who are epidermal growth factor receptor positive has extended the lives of some of these patients.

The same thing can be said for Erbitux.

Megace is at times added to the 5FU to increase the appetite of the patient with colon cancer and it helps with weight gain. Megace can cause clots to develop in the legs with serious clinical consequences. Oxandrin is also used to improve appetite in men with advanced colon cancer. Some the side effects are similar to that of Megace.

Another form of cancer that oftentimes develops in the large bowel is carcinoid tumor. The preoperative evaluation is the same, except that if the treating physician suspects carcinoid tumor, then serum serotonin or a 24-hour urine for (5HIAA) 5 hydroxyindoleacetic acid can be obtained as a baseline and also to help firm up the diagnosis. These tests are helpful in the subsequent management of the patient with carcinoid tumor.

Non-Hodgkin's lymphoma of the large bowel does occur. The treatment approach is the same. First, surgical resection followed either by radiation therapy or by chemotherapy, depending on the histology and the extent of disease found at surgery.

Colorectal cancer is curable when found early. Therefore, yearly rectal examination and testing of the stool for blood once or twice per year and doing a complete blood count with RDW, serum ferritin and the serum-transferring receptors level together, can prevent colon cancer from ever killing anyone. If the treating physician does these tests and follow up on the results, pre-cancerous lesions of the colon, rectum, small bowel, and stomach can be discovered early and treated appropriately.

Cancer of the Pancreas

Cancer of the pancreas usually develops symptom free until it is too late. In 2007, there will be 18, 830 new cases of cancer of the pancreas in men in the U.S. During that same time, 18,340 men will die of pancreatic cancer.

Signs and symptoms of cancer of the pancreas usually occur when it is too late to do much to save the patient. If the cancer is located near the head of the pancreas, it might cause the common bile duct to become obstructed, causing the patient to become jaundiced with no pain. However, if the cancer is located either at the body or at the tail of the pancreas, jaundice may occur due to metastasis to the liver. Therefore, early development of jaundice due to cancer of the head of the pancreas may in some instances lead to the person seeking medical help. That could result in positive outcomes because of early surgical intervention. Left-sided, mid-abdominal pain in association with weight loss and poor appetite may also be signs of and symptoms of cancer of the pancreas. Risks for cancer of the pancreas consist of:
1. Tobacco smoking
2. Chronic pancreatitis
3. Diabetes mellitus
4. High fat diet
5. Cirrhosis of the liver.

CA19.9 is a blood test marker for pancreatic cancer.

During the ER CP, if a mass is present, it can be seen and material can be obtained for diagnosis. In addition, a stint can be placed to relieve the obstruction of the common bile duct to relieve the jaundice, etc.

Cancer of the pancreas is very difficult to cure, but if found early, surgical resection is the preferred treatment but that cancer is hardly ever found early. There are many gastrointestinal procedures available to relieve the many symptoms and complications of pancreatic cancer but none is curable. The most effective chemotherapeutic agent is Gemzar 600mg/m2 IV days 1, 8, and 15, plus Docetaxel 60mg/m2 day 1. This cycle is repeated every 28 days. The FDA to treat advanced pancreatic cancer has approved Tarceva. The starting dose of Tarceva is 100 mg by mouth daily.

Cancer of the Mouth, Throat and Neck

Cancer of the mouth, throat, and neck is most common in tobacco smokers and heavy alcohol abusers and men who have had radiation to the neck area to treat enlarged tonsils, or men who have been exposed to industrial cancer causing materials etc. In 2007, about 24,180 men will be diagnosed with cancer of head and neck and 5, 180 of these men will die of these cancers.

Some signs and symptoms of mouth, throat and neck cancers include:
1. A sore that bleeds often and easily and fails to heal
2. Persistent hoarseness that is not accompanied by pain
3. Change in voice from normal to a persistent deeper voice
4. Persistent hoarseness that is accompanied with pain
5. Difficulty in swallowing
6. Difficulty in chewing, swallowing and moving the tongue
7. Painful swelling around the neck.

Some risk factors for mouth and throat cancer are smoking cigarettes, cigars or a pipe as well as heavy alcohol consumption and radiation around the neck area during childhood.

The best treatment for head and neck cancers is radiation therapy given 5 days per week for 6 weeks together with Cis-Platinum 100mg/m2 given on day #1, day #22 and day# 43. The response rate for radiation and chemotherapy for stages 1, 2, and 3, head and neck cancers is in the range of 75% worldwide. The response rate for surgical resection of head and neck cancers with adjuvant radiation/chemotherapy parallels the response rate of radiation and chemotherapy without surgical resection. Frequently surgical resection of head and neck cancers requires the removal of the voice box with a permanent tracheostomy.

Most recently, Erbitux has been used with some degree of success in the treatment of head and neck cancer.

In evaluating the throat using the fiberoptic laryngoscope, it is mandatory that the physician doing the scoping passes the laryngoscope through both nasal passages so as not to miss cancer and other lesions that may be located in the upper right or upper left of the nasal anatomy.

One of the most debilitating long term side effects of the radiation treatment given to individuals afflicted with head and neck cancer is xerostomia (dry mouth) no sputum production. It interferes with speech, it interferes with eating, it causes tooth decays and it causes weight loss and general weakness etc. In addition radiation treatment to the head and neck areas causes loss of taste which interferes with proper nutrition etc.

Cancer of the Urinary Bladder

Cancer of the urinary bladder is expected to develop in 50,040 men in the US in 2007 and 9,630 of these men will die of bladder cancer during that same time. Cancer of the urinary bladder is the forth most common cancer in men. This cancer is most common in men over 65 years old. The signs and symptoms of cancer of the bladder are hematuria (blood in the urine) and frequent urination.

Some risk factors associated with cancer of the bladder are:

1. Cigarette smoking
2. Chemicals used in rubber, leather, dye used in industries and materials used in hair coloring
3. Exposure to Cytoxan chemotherapy
4. History of external radiation to the rectum
5. Decrease fluid intake over extended period of time
6. Exposure to schistosoma heamatobium parasite; etc

The best treatments for cancer of the urinary bladder are surgery, chemotherapy plus radiation or chemotherapy alone. BCG is also used to treat bladder cancer.

The most frequently used chemotherapeutic agents employed to treat cancer of the urinary bladder are:

1. Methotrexate 30mg/m2 IV days 1, 15, and 22

Vinblastin 3mg/m2 IV days 2, 15, and 2

Doxorubicin 30mg/m2 IV day 2

Cisplatinum 70mg/m2 IV day 2

Repeat every 4 weeks

Or

Cisplatinum 50mg/m2 IV day 1

Gemcitabine 900mg/m2 IV over 90 minutes on day 1

Ifosfamide 1000mg/m2 IV over 30 minutes on day 1

Repeat every 14 days.

There several more protocol in use to treat metastatic cancer of the urinary bladder.

Cancer of the Kidney:

In 2007, 31,590 men in the US will be diagnosed with cancer of the kidney and during that same period, 8,080 will die of this cancer.

Quite often, cancer of the kidney is discovered incidentally. Early stage cancer of kidney usually presents with no symptoms. Often time blood is found during a routine urinalysis which triggers and evaluation resulting in establishing the diagnosis.

If a man presents

1. With either microscopic hematuria (Red blood cells seen under the microscope) or gross hematuria blood seen by the naked eyes.
2. Low back pain.
3. Flank pain

How to evaluate a patient for possible cancer of the kidney

1. Do a urinalysis
2. Do a urine culture and sensitivity
3. Do a hemoglobin electrophoresis is the man is Black, Hispanic, South Asian, Middle Eastern or Mediterranean, because these men can carry the sickle hemoglobin which can cause both gross as well as microscopic hematuria. (see Chapter 10 for a full explanation).
4. Do renal ultrasound
5. If suspicious mass is seendo Abdominal CAT SCAN
6. MRI may be necessary
7. Chest xray
8. Refer the patient to a urologist for further evaluation

The differential diagnosis of blood in the urine in a man includes in addition the above bladder problems, prostate problems and kidney stones,
Urinary tract infection and prostatitis etc.

The different Stages of kidney cancer are:
Stage 1
Stage II
Stage III
Stage IV

In Stage I kidney cancer, the cancer is 7 cm or less and is contained only inside the kidney.

In stage II kidney cancer, the cancer is larger than 7 cm and is contained only inside the kidney.

In stage III kidney cancer, the cancer is contained inside the kidney plus there is cancer in 1 lymph node.

In stage IV kidney cancer, the cancer is found in at least two lymph nodes in addition to other organs.

The most effective treatment for early cancer of the kidney is surgical resection of the. The 5 year survival of stage I cancer of the kidney is greater than 90%.

Metastatic cancer of the kidney is treated with

1. Interleukin-2 5–7 million IU/m2 SC 5 days per week on weeks 1–4 (premedicate with Tylenol) repeat every 6 weeks

or

2. Interferon 1–5 million IU/m2 SC 5 days per week continuously (premedicate with Tylenol)

or

3. Gemcitabine 600mg/m2 IV on days 1, 8, and 15
5-FU 150mgmg/m2 on day 1 over 24 hours days 1–21 repeat every 28 days.

Testicular Cancer:

In 2007, 7,920 men will be diagnosed with testicular cancer in the US and during that same period, 380 men will die of this cancer.

Early testicular cancer presents with no symptoms. The first sign of testicular cancer is a palpable mass in the testicle. Usually, the mass is felt by the affected man and confirms by an examining physician.

How to evaluate a testicular mass?

Do an ultrasound of the testicle

Do an abdominal Cat scan

Do a chest x-ray

Do a serum pregnancy test on the man serum (in testicular cancer, the serum pregnancy test is positive in man)

Do Alpha feto-protein

6. Refer the man to a urologist

Treatments of Testicular cancer:

> Surgical removal of the affected testicle
>
> Bleomycin 30 units IV (bolus or Continuous infusion over 24 hours) on days 2, 9, and 16
>
> Eptoposide 100mg mg/m2/day on days 1–5
>
> Cisplatinum 20 mg/m2 on days 1–5
>
> Or
>
> Etoposide 100mg/m2/on days 1–5
>
> Cisplatinum 20 mg/m2 on days 1–5

There are several more drug combinations in use to treat Testicular cancer.

Prostate Cancer:

In 2007, 218,890 will be diagnosed with prostate cancer and 30,350 men will die of prostate cancer.

What are the symptom and signs of prostate cancer?

> Difficulty passing urine
>
> Urinary frequency
>
> Burning on urination
>
> Seeing blood in the urine
>
> Urinary tract infection
>
> Elevated prostatic specific antigen (PSA)
>
> An enlarged, hard and irregular prostate gland on digital rectal examination
>
> A palpable prostate nodule on digital rectal examination

Normal PSA is 0–4.0, depending on the man's age.

The PSA can be elevated because of

> Urinary tract infection
>
> Benign prostatic hyper trophy (enlarged prostate)
>
> Ejaculation

How to evaluate a man for prostate cancer

> Do a digital rectal examination
>
> Do a serum PSA
>
> Do an ultrasound of the bladder and prostate gland
>
> Do a prostate biopsy

If the prostate biopsy is positive for cancer

> Do a cat scan of the abdomen
>
> Do a bone scan
>
> Do a CBC

Do an SMA20 chemistry profile

How to treat prostate cancer

Early prostate cancer is treated with
  a. Radical prostatectomy
  b. Radio active Seeds implantation
  c. External beam radiation

Advanced stage prostate cancer is treated with

Radioactive Seeds implantation

External beam radiation

Either Radioactive Seeds implantation or External beam radiation with Hormone

Other treatments that in use to treat prostate cancer are

Paclitaxel 80 mg/m2 IV over 1 hour weekly for 6 weeks

Estramustine 280 mg by mouth 3 times per day Monday-Friday for 6 weeks

Caboplatin AUC 2 weekly for 6 weeks

Taxol IV is also used to treat prostate cancer

Repeat every 8 weeks

There are many more drugs combinations in use to treat advanced prostate cancer.

Intramuscular Lupron is an effective hormonal treatment for advanced prostate cancer.

Leukemias:

In 2007, 24,800 new cases of leukemia will be diagnosed in men and 12,320 men will die of leukemias. during that same period.

There are seven different types of leukemia:
  1. Acute lymphocytic leukemia
  2. Chronic lymphocytic leukemia
  3. Acute myelogenic leukemia
  4. Chronic myelogenic leukemia
  5. Monocystic leukemia
  6. Myelodysplastic syndrome
  7. Acute megakaryocytic leukemia
  8. Acute Promyelocytic Leukemia
  9. T-cell leukemia/lymphoma due to HTLVI and II.
  10. Burkitt's Leukemia
  11. Hairy cell Leukemia

Signs and symptoms of leukemia include weight loss, fatigue, frequent infections, easy bruising, nosebleeds and hemorrhages.

Some of the risk factors include Down's syndrome, AIDS, exposure to ionizing radiation, chemicals like benzene and other toxic chemicals, and viruses.

Different types of leukemias are treated with different chemotherapeutic regimens, including bone marrow transplantation.

Acute Lymphocytic Leukemia is treated with

> Cytoxan
> Mesna
> or
> Vincristine
> Doxorubicin
> Dexamethasone
> or
> Methotrexate
> Cytarabine
> Chronic Lymphocytic Leukemia is treated with
> Cytoxan
> Fludarabine
> Rituximab
> or Leukeran by mouth
>
> Acute Myelogenous Leukemia is treated with
> Cytarabine
> Idarubicin
> or
> Fludarabine
> Cytarabine

These medications are used in different doses based on the patient weight and height per meter square.

> Chronic Myelocytic Leukemia is treated with
> Imatinid (Gleevec) 400mg per day by mouth
>
> Acute promyelocytic Leukemia is treated with
> All-trans-retonoic Acid 45mg/m2/day by mouth in 2 divided doses till the patient enters into remission.
> Idarubicin IV 12mg/m2/day 5–8
> or all-trans-retinoic acid 12 mg/m2/day divided in 2 doses days 1–14 by mouth.

Hairy cell Leukemia is treated with

    Cladribine 4mg/m2/day day 1–7

Burkitt's Leukemia is treated with

    R-hyperCVAD

    Plus Rituximab 375mg/m2 IV on days 1–8 of each cycle.

Recently, Imatinid (Gleevec) has been shown to be very effective as a treatment for chronic myelogenous leukemia.

Lymphoma:

In 2007, a total of 38,670 new non-Hodgkin's lymphoma cases will be diagnosed in men and 10,370 of these men will die of this type of lymphoma. During that same period, 4,470 men will be diagnosed with Hodgkin's lymphoma and 770 of these men will die of Hodgkin's lymphoma.

Some of the signs and symptoms of lymphoma are enlarged lymph nodes, fever, and weight loss, loss of appetite, night sweats, anemia, and sometimes diarrhea. Sometimes a fever can come and go for several weeks—referred to as fever of unknown origin (FUO). Some of the risk factors associated with lymphoma include:

1. Immunodeficiency syndrome (acquired and non-acquired).
2. Men who receive organ transplants (because these men have been made immunosuppressed to prepare them to receive organs to be transplanted).
3. Infection with HTLV I is a high risk for the development of T-cell leukemia/lymphoma. HTLV I can be transmitted sexually, through needle punctures, and via blood transfusions. That disease is frequently seen in the Caribbean, southern islands of Japan, northeastern South America, Central America, and New Guinea. HTLV II is associated with the development of hairy-cell leukemia.
4. AIDS is associated with B-cell lymphoma, 90% of the time, usually of the large-cell category. In 50% of these cases, the Epstein-Barr virus is involved as a causative agent.

Other cancers seen in patients with AIDS are:

1. Kaposi's sarcoma
2. Anorectal cancer.

Herpes virus number 8 is said to be associated with Kaposi's sarcoma as a causative agent.

Other associated risk factors for lymphoma consist of:

Epstein-Barr virus in Burkitt's lymphoma in Africa
Exposure to previous chemotherapy or radiotherapy treatments
Being male (more men are afflicted with Hodgkin's lymphoma than female)
Previous infection with infectious mononucleosis
Higher educational level.

How to evaluate men suspected of lymphoma:
1. Take a complete history
2. Do a physical examination
3. Chest ray
4. Chest CAT scan
5. Abdominal Cat scan
6. PET scan
7. Do biopsy of a palpable lymph node
8. CBC
9. SMA 20
10. Serum LDH
11. ESR
12. Bone marrow aspiration
13. Bone marrow biopsy from both iliac crests

Men who have had infectious mononucleosis due to Epstein-Barr virus are three times more likely to develop Hodgkin's lympoma. (Epstein-Barr virus is said to be associated with some cases of Hodgkin's disease.) Exposure to herbicides and chemicals is also associated with increased incidence of Hodgkin's disease

The most commonly used drugs combinations used to treat Hodgkin's disease are:

ABVD
1. Doxorubicin 25mg/m2 IV on days 1&15
2. Bleomycin 10units/m2 IV on days 1&15
3. Vinblastin 6mg/m2 IV on days 1&15
4. Dacarbazine 375mg/m2 IV on days 1&15
   Repeat every 28 days
       Or

ASHAP
1. Doxorubicin 10 mg/m2/day continuous infusion day 1–4
2. Methylprenisolone 500mg/day IV days 1–5

3. Cisplatinum 25mg/m2/day continuous infusion over 24 hours days 1–4
4. Cytarabine 1.5 g/m2 IV day (when the cisplatimun is finished)
    Repeat every 21 days
    There are several other drug combinations in use to treat Hodgkin's disease.

The most frequently used drug combination used to treat non-Hodgkin's lymphoma is

CHOP-Retuxin
Cytoxin 750 mg/m2 IV day 1
Doxorubicin 50mg/m2 IV day 1
Vincristine 2 mg IV day 1
Prednisone 100mg by mouth day 1–5
Rituxin 375/mg/m2 IV day 1
Repeat every 21 days
Allopurinol 300mg per day by mouth is used daily to prevent urates from clogging up the kidney tubules causing renal failure to develop.
There are several other drug regimens in use to treat non-hodgkin's lymphoma.

Multiple Myeloma

Multiple myeloma is a cancer that comes from plasma cells. Plasma cells are cells that produce antibodies in the body to help fight infections. In 2007, 10,960 men will be diagnosed with multiple myeloma in the US and 5,550 men will die of multiple myeloma during that period. Multiple myeloma is more common in black men than in white men. A rate of 9.0 per 100,000 for black males as compared to a rate of 4.4 per 100,000 for white males. There exist no clear risk factors for multiple myeloma, although exposure to agricultural chemicals, radium, benzene and radioisotopes has been mentioned as being associated with a higher incidence of multiple myeloma.

Some of the symptoms of multiple myeloma are bone pain, weakness, anemia, recurrent infections such as pneumonia, osteoporosis, kidney failure, and high serum calcium and its associated problems such as seizures, etc. It is said that Interleukin 6 (a growth factor) is the causative protein that supports the growth of myeloma cells.

The diagnosis of multiple myeloma is made using bone marrow aspiration and biopsy, along with skeletal survey looking for lytic lesions. Other tests that are used to establish the diagnosis of multiple myeloma include serum protein electrophoresis, serum immunoglobulins levels, and urine immunoglobulins, CBC and SMA20, ESR. serum LDH, and Beta-2-microglobulin.

The most commonly used drug regimens to treat multiple Myeloma are

Thalidomide 100mg by mouth at bed time for 7 days after that 200mg at bed time by mouth Dexamethasone 20mg/m2/day days 1–4, 9–12, and 17–20
Repeat every 28 days
Or
Cytoxan 300mg/m2 IV over 2 hours every 12 hours days 1–4 with mesna
Vincristine 0.4mg/day as a continuous infusion days 1–4
Doxorubicin 9mg/m2/day as a continuous infusion over 24 hours days 1–4
Dexamethasone 20mg/m2/day by mouth days 1–4, 9–12, and 17–20
Repeat every 28 days
Or
Vincristine 0.4mg/day as a continuous infusion days 1–4
Doxorubicin 9 mg/m2/day as a continuous infusion over 24 hour's days 1–4
Dexamethasone 20mg/m2/day by mouth on days 1–4, 9–12, and 17–20
Repeat every 28 days.

Melphalan by mouth with prednisone is also an effective protocol to treat Multiple myeloma.

Radiation therapy is used to treat different bony complications of Multiple myeloma as the clinical situation warrants. Ample doses of pain medication must be used to alleviate the pain that these patients experience, because the intensity can be quite severe.

Basal Cell Carcinoma of the Skin

The most common cancer is basal cell carcinoma (skin cancer) affecting about one million people yearly in the United States. This form of cancer appears most frequently in people of fair skin and also people who are exposed more frequently to the sun.

In 2007, 37,070 men in the USA will be diagnosed with basal cell carcinoma and 7,140 men will die of basal cell carcinoma cancer during that same.

Too much sun exposure is a major risk factor for skin cancer.

The most effective treatments for basal cell cancer include:
1. Surgical resection
2. Radiation therapy
3. Cryosurgery
4. Laser treatments and at times chemotherapy may help.

Melanoma

The most serious and malignant form of skin cancer is melanoma and in 2007, there will be 33,910 cases of melanoma will be diagnosed in men in the US and 5,220 men will die of melanoma during that same time. Melanoma is ten times more common in white males than in men of color.

Signs and symptoms of skin cancer include a mole that has changed in size and color (usually darkly pigmented), a mole that oozes, and a mole that bleeds or changes in appearance. Sometimes there is pain and tenderness, and oftentimes the mole may itch. A dermatologist must quickly and immediately evaluate any skin lesion that causes a person a concern to be sure that it is not cancerous.

Risk factors for the development of melanoma include:
1. Ultraviolet rays (exposure to the sun)
2. Being of fair complexion
3. Exposure to arsenic compounds
4. Exposure to radium
5. Exposure to coal tar
6. Family history of skin cancer
7. History of multiple skin moles

The most effective treatments for melanoma are surgical resection with regional lymph node removal, radiation therapy, immunotherapy and chemotherapy.

Thyroid Cancer

In 2007, 8,070 men will be diagnosed with cancer of the thyroid gland and 630 of them will die of thyroid cancer. Risk factors for thyroid cancer include low-dose radiation given in childhood to treat enlarged tonsils and adenoids. Other causes of thyroid cancer are not clear.

Signs and symptoms of thyroid cancer—see chapter on thyroid disease.

To evaluate a patient for thyroid cancer, a complete history must be taken, including family history as well as work history and child hood history. Any history of pain in the neck or difficulty swallowing is important etc.

The major risks for thyroid cancer are radiation and family history of thyroid cancer.

A complete physical examination must done, paying particular attention to neck looking for possible enlargement of the thyroid gland or a distinct thyroid nodule, or palpable nodes around the neck area.

How to detect thyroid cancer:

1. Do a thyroid scan looking for cold nodules (hot nodules are most likely to be benign) and cold nodules can be cancerous.
2. Do a thyroid ultrasound
3. If a thyroid nodule is suspicious, do a fine needle biopsy of the thyroid under ultrasound guidance
4. Do serum T4, TSH, Free T4, and T3

There are four distinct types of thyroid cancers:

1. Follicular thyroid cancer 10%
2. Papillary thyroid cancer 80%
3. Medullary thyroid cancer 5%
4. Anaplastic thyroid cancer 2%

Many other cancer can metastasize to the thyroid gland, mainly because of the fact that the thyroid gland is very vascular (carries a lot of blood).

How to treat thyroid cancer:

For follicular thyroid cancer the treatments are:

1. Total thyroidectomy (removal of the entire thyroid gland)
2. radioactive ablation
3. Thyroid Stmulating Hormne (TSH) suppression 4. and Survaillance

For papillary thyroid cancer the treatments are:

1. Total thyroidectomy
2. Modified neck dissection
3. Radiotherapy

Anaplastic thyroid cancer has a very poor prognosis and patients live for only a few months following diagnosis.

Treatments for anaplastic thyroid cancer are:

1. Chemoradiothrapy to shrink the size of the fast growing cancer

2. Surgical resection
3. Paclitaxel, Doxorubucin and Gemzar in combination.

Cancer of the Esophagus:

In 2007, 12,130 men will be diagnosed with cancer of the esophagus in the US and 10,900 men will die of this cancer.

Signs and symptoms of esophageal cancer are:

Difficulty swallowing
Chest pain
Weight loss
Anemia
Vomiting
Vomiting blood etc;

Risk factors for cancer of the esophagus are:

Heavy alcohol drinking
Tobacco smoking
Chewing tobacco
Accidental swallowing of corrosive acid;

How to evaluate cancer of the esophagus:

Take a complete history

1. Do a complete physical Examination
2. Do an endoscopic examination
3. Take biopsy of any lesion found
4. Do a CBC
5. Do a serum ferritin
6. Do an SMA20 chemistry profile
7. Do a serum carcino embriogenic antigen (CEA)

How to treat cancer of the esophagus: Early stage

1. Surgical resection
2. Radiation therapy
   5FU 425 mg/m2 IV on days 1–5
3. Leucovorin 20mg/m2 IV on Days 1–5
   Repeat every 28 days

Advanced stage cancer of the esophagus:

1. Radiation therapy
2. Cisplatinum 75 mg/m2 IV on days 1, 29, 50, and 71
   5FU 1,000 mg/m2/day as continuous infusion on days 1–4
   29–32, 50–53, and 71–74

Cancer of the Stomach:

In 2007, 13,000 men will be diagnosed with cancer of the stomach in the US and during that same time, 6,610 men will die of this cancer.

What are the signs and symptoms of cancer of the Stomach?
1. Pain in the stomach
2. Vomiting
3. Indigestion
4. Vomiting blood
5. Black stools
6. Weight loss
7. Anemia
8. The stomach filling up easily

How evaluate cancer of the stomach.
1. Take a complete history from the patient

Do a complete physical examination

Do CBC

Do an SMA 20 chemistry profile

Do a serum ferritin

Test the stools for blood by doing a hemoccult

Do a serum CEA

Do an endoscopic examination of the stomach

Biopsy any lesion that is found

Do a clo test for H pylori

If the biopsy of the stomach is positive for cancer, treat the patient his way:
1. Surgical resection
2. 5FU 425 mg/m2 IV on days 1–5
3. Leucovorin 20 mg/m2 IV on days 1–5
4. Radiation therapy for 5 days per week for 6 week
5. After a 1 month rest period
6. 5FU 425 mg/m2 IV on days 1–5
7. Leucovorin 20 mg/m2 IV on days 1–5
8. Repeat every 28 day x 2 cycles

For metastatic cancer of the stomach treat his way:
1. Docetaxel 75 mg/m2 IV over 1 hour on
Day 1

2. Cisplatinum 75 mg/m2 IV on day 1
3. 5FU 750 mg/m2/day as a continuous
    Infusion on days 1–5
    Or
5FU 1,000 mg/m2IV on days 1–5 as a Continuous
Cisplatinum 100 mg/m2 IV on day 1
Repeat every 28 days
There are several more chemotherapy
Combinations in use to treat metastatic cancer of the stomach.

In 2007, 13,650 men will be diagnosed with cancer of the liver in the US and 11,280 men will die of this cancer during **that** same time.

What are the signs and symptoms of liver cancer?

Abdominal pain

Weight loss

Poor appetite

Fatigue

Fever

Jaundice

Anemia etc.

How to evaluate a patient suspected of having liver cancer.

1. Take a complete history
2. Do a complete physical examination
3. Do an abdominal ultrasound
4. Do an abdominal cat scan
5. Do a PET scan
6. Do a chest x-ray
7. Do CBC
8. Do an SMA 20 chemistry profile
9. Do a Prothrombin time (PT& INR)
10. Do a Partial thromboplastin time (PTT)
11. Do a CEA
12. Do an Alpha Feto protein
13. Do a liver biopsy if a mass is on radiographic studies.

Extreme caution must be under taken in doing the liver biopsy because if the patient, is harboring a hepatoma, it and bleed rather profusely.

If the tissue taken is positive for liver cancer, the following approaches can be taken

1. Surgical resection of the cancerous mass
2. Post radiation radiotherapy

3. Gemzar 1250 mg/m2 IV on days 1, 8, and 15
4. Repeat every 28 days.

Much progress has been made in the detection and treatment of cancer and many cancers are curable when detected and treated early. But much more needs to be done to understand the genetic transmission of cancer, the way cancer cells grow in the human body, so that genetic engineering can be used to prevent the growth of cancer cells in the human body. Society must do more to stop men from being exposed to cancer-causing agents and other toxic materials. Men must stop self-destructive habits such as cigarette smoking and eating too many fat-rich foods; abusing alcohol etc and they must exercise more to lose weight to decrease their incidence of cancer. Both government and the private sector must make available more money for cancer research and cancer treatments.

CHAPTER 8

KIDNEY DISEASE
IN MEN

THE DIFFERENT DISEASES THAT ARE associated with renal (kidney) diseases in men are:

1. Hypertension
2. Diabetes mellitus
3. Acute renal failure because of hypotension resulting from acute myocardial infarction as seen in men who are hypertensive and diabetic or who have had hypotensive episodes during such things like gastrointestinal bleeding, sepsis etc.
4. Chronic pyelonephritis
5. Sickle cell anemia
6. Polycystic kidney disease.
7. Azotemia (renal insufficiency
8. End stage renal disease

Hypertension is one of the leading diseases in men in the United States. 65 millions individuals have hypertension and 70 millions have prehypertension. In 2002, there were 29,400,000 men with hypertension in the US. One out of every four men aged 55 and older is hypertensive. The incidence of end-stage renal disease (ESRD) leading to renal failure is higher in minority men than in white men.

There are roughly 19 million black men in the United States and since three out of four black 55 years and older are hypertensive, it is not difficult to figure out the percentage of these men who stand the chance of getting renal disease from hypertension. Therefore, about 19 million black men who have the potential of developing ESRD if they are not treated properly for hypertension. Twelve percent of adults in the US have chronic renal disease of one degree or an other. If chronic renal failure is not recognized early and treated properly, it can prevent the development of ESRD.

The best way to evaluate the kidneys for chronic kidney disease is to measure the glomerular filtration rate (GFR) and the amount of albumin in the urine. Chronic renal disease has 5 stages, 1–5.

Stage 1. is GFR 90 ml/minute/1.73m2

Stage 2. is GFR 60–89ml/minute/1.73m2

Stage 3. is GFR 30–59ml/minute/1.73m2

Stage 4 is GFR 15–29ml/minute/1.73m2

Stage 5. is GFR less than 15ml/minute/1.73m2

If a man suffers with an underline heart condition such as coronary artery heart disease, stress associated with the job can cause the person to secrete too much adrenalin, which causes the heart to beat too fast, raising the need for more oxygen delivery to the heart muscle, which, in turn, can cause an acute heart attack to occur.

The reason that hypertension causes ESRD that ultimately results in the need for dialysis is that the kidneys have many vital structures within them that are essential for their proper functions. Among those structures are the glomeruli, which are indispensable in the proper functioning of the kidneys. The elevated blood pressure causes plaques to develop inside the small vessels that carry blood and oxygen to the kidneys and the glomeruli within them. Ordinarily, the inside of the blood vessels is smooth, and blood passes through them freely. When the blood pressure is high, as the blood passes through those vessels, the high pressure causes these vessels to lose their smoothness. The high pressure therefore damages the first layer of the vessels within the kidneys, resulting in plaque depositions. The deposition of plaques in turn causes the narrowing of these vessels. The narrowing of the small vessels that is necessary to carry blood and oxygen to the glomeruli of the kidneys results in ischemia of the tissues of the kidney, resulting in the deaths of the glomeruli. The deaths of these glomeruli and other vital structures result ultimately in end-stage renal disease.

All hypertensive men have the potential to develop kidney disease to one degree or another if their blood pressure is poorly treated.

In order to determine if the kidneys are sick and are about to fail from long years of being affected by hypertension, the physician needs to do the followings.

1. Take a complete history

2. Do a physical examination
3. Do an SMA20 chemistry profile
4. Do a urinalysis
5. Do a CBC
6. Do a 24 urine creatinine clearance and protein
7. Do a renal ultrasound
8. Do a chest x-ray
9. Do an EKG

It is very important to do a good examination of the eyes to see if the patient has evidence of hypertensive retinopathy (inside the eyes is the only place a physician can see a naked blood vessel in the human body without cutting the patient open). By examining the fundi of the eyes, the physician can tell if damage has occurred in the vessels inside the eyes because of longstanding of untreated or poorly treated hypertension and the degree of the damage.

The kidneys are referred to as end organs as are the eyes, the heart and the brain. If any of these end organs are damaged by the chronic effect of hypertension, then the examining physician can have a very good idea as to how long the blood pressure has been uncontrolled. Further, the physician, by taking a history and examining the patient, can tell whether or not the patient has entered into the uremic stage.

In uremia, a patient may have sweet breath, may have flaky salty material over his skin, or the patient may have swollen abdomen, swollen legs, the patient may be confused, the patient may also develop seizures and if not treated, may go into coma. etc. On laboratory examination of the patient's urine whose kidneys are failing chronically, the urine may be unconcentrated with a very low specific gravity. Normal specific gravity is about 1.010–1.025. A chronically sick kidney can only concentrate the urine to about 1.002–1.005. The specific gravity is a measure of the ability of the kidneys to concentrate urine. The sicker the kidneys are, the lower the specific gravity.

A chronically sick kidney from hypertension filters out plenty of protein. So by testing the urine during a routine urinalysis for proteins, the physician can be alerted as to how sick the kidneys are. On microscopic examination of the urinary sediment, certain cellular materials such as certain types of casts can be seen. By examining the electrolytes, sodium, potassium and chloride in the urine of a patient with failing kidneys, in particular the sodium, the physician can tell whether the kidneys are failing acutely, a condition called acute tubular necrosis due to some sort of acute event such as heart attack with a drop in the blood, sepsis with shock, acute and heavy bleeding with hypotension, etc., or a slow, progressive chronic disease such as hypertension with damage to the kidneys. The urinary sodium is easy to do. One needs only to get a few milliliters of urine from the patient and send it to the lab for urinary sodium testing.

In acute failure of the kidneys (acute renal failure), the urinary sodium is low 10 mEq/L or less. In chronic renal failure (kidneys that have been failing for a long time), the urine sodium is high 20 mEq/L or greater (different laboratories may have a different scale for what is low urinary sodium or high urinary sodium). That quick and easy test is of paramount importance in the treatment approach of a patient who shows up in the emergency room or the doctor's office with unexplained evidence of renal failure. When the kidneys are failing acutely, they hold sodium in order to hold on to water to maintain the blood pressure to preserve the body and keep it alive.

On the other hand, chronic failing kidneys have lost their ability to hold on to sodium a long time ago, due to chronic damage that has occurred in the kidneys because of the insults of high blood pressure or diabetes to the kidneys; because, a large quantity of sodium is allowed to pass in the urine. Knowing this simple fact, allows the physician to know how to approach both the acute and chronic medical management of the patient with failing kidneys.

Another indispensable crucial test that is done in every patient with failing kidneys who can pass urine is the 24-hour creatinine clearance. That test allows the physician to know the ability of the kidneys to function. It allows the physician to know how much function is left in the kidneys. The normal range of creatinine clearance in men is 125 milliliters per minute down to about 75 milliliters per minute; as a person gets older, these numbers decrease accordingly.

In order to do that test, the serum creatinine must be measured and a complete collection of all urine passed by the patient in 24 hours must be obtained and placed in a plastic bottle and sent to the laboratory to be tested. That urine must be kept refrigerated.

The next series of tests that are essential in evaluating the status of the kidneys are serum electrolytes, which comprise sodium, potassium, chloride, bicarbonate and other renal function tests such as BUN (blood urea nitrogen) and serum creatinine. The reason why these tests are so important is that when the kidney is failing, it is unable to filter waste materials from the bloodstream properly, allowing these substances to accumulate in the body, and a reflection of this problem manifests itself with a rise in the BUN and serum creatinine first. Then as the kidney failure progresses, the serum potassium rises while the serum bicarbonate decreases, resulting in a serious condition called hyperkalemic acidosis. Serum potassium of 6 or greater is a medical emergency that must be dealt with immediately because the high serum potassium can trigger cardiac arrhythmias, which can cause the death of the affected person with kidney failure. Other serum chemistry tests that are important in evaluating a patient with kidney failure include the serum calcium, the serum phosphatase, the serum bilirubin, the LDH (lactic dehydrogenase), the CPK (creatinine phosphokinase), the total protein, and the serum albumin.

What role does an abnormality of each of these blood chemistry tests and CBC play in the evaluation of a patient with kidney failure? The blood tests to obtain in evaluating the kidney failure in patients include:

Serum sodium
Serum potassium
Serum bicarbonate
Serum BUN
Serum creatinine
Serum Phosphate
Serum calcium
Serum bilirubin
Serum protein
Serum protein
Serum albumin
Serum LDH
Serum CPK
CBC with differential
Urine Sodium
Serum GFR (glomorular filtration rate)
24 hour creatinine clearance and protein

If the serum sodium is very high, 150–160, it means that the kidney probably failed because of loss of volume (fluid) due to dehydration and that rehydrating the patient with hypo-osmolar fluid such as water by mouth or water and sugar (D5W) intravenously, the sodium will normalize and, depending on how long the dehydration state existed, the kidney function will probably return to normal.

High serum potassium is quite a bit more complex and complicated than that because there are other conditions that can cause the serum potassium to be high that has nothing to do with renal failure.

Assuming that the high potassium is due to kidney failure, then this occurs because the kidneys are unable to get rid of the breakdown products of proteins, which contain potassium plus potassium ingested as foods or beverages. That also occurs because of electrolyte abnormalities of different types that cause the kidneys either to reabsorb too much potassium or to be unable to excrete enough potassium to maintain good potassium tolerance. The potassium accumulates in the blood, risking severe cardiac arrhythmias with potential lethal consequences if not brought down with either medications or dialysis.

Low serum bicarbonate known as acidosis, though important, is less crucial because the human body is made to tolerate acidosis much better than alkalosis—the reverse of acidosis—meaning the serum bicarbonate is high. When the serum bicarbonate is high, low potassium results which is as serious as high potassium in causing cardiac arrhythmias which can lead to sudden death. Medications and/or dialysis can correct acidosis.

The high serum BUN is a reflection of the inability of the kidneys to function well enough to get rid of the breakdown products of proteins. High BUN and creatinine are some of the indices of kidney failure. Even though high BUN and creatinine are important indices of renal failure, by themselves, they do not represent a threat to the life of a patient. However, when the BUN and creatinine are high, the potassium is at the critical level of 6.5 or greater. If the phosphate is high, the serum calcium is low, the creatinine clearance is 10 ml per minute or less and the patient looks and feels sick, then the time has arrived for dialysis to start.

High phosphatase is a very important abnormality that must be corrected quickly because as the phosphatase goes up, the serum calcium goes down and the low serum calcium is potentially deadly because low calcium can cause cardiac arrhythmias, seizures, tetany with muscle cramps and twitching. Examining the blood for possible elevation of both total and indirect bilirubin is important because in acute and severe hemolysis, the kidney can acutely fail due to the clogging effect of debris from red blood cells, damaging the tubules of the kidneys.

Testing the blood for serum albumin is very important in renal failure because as the kidneys fail they allow protein to pass into the urine, reducing the serum albumin. This, in turn, causes fluid to pass into the extra vascular compartment of the body, resulting in swelling of the abdomen and lower extremities, resulting in anasarca. This set of problems is referred to as "nephrotic syndrome." In nephrotic syndrome, the patient passes three (3) grams of protein or greater in the urine over a 24-hour period. Testing the blood for total protein is very important because there are conditions such as multiple myeloma and other types of plasma cell dyscrasias in which the total protein is elevated and when protein is elevated, many bad things can happen, including a condition called hyperviscosity syndrome. If viscosity syndrome develops, the patient may experience blurred vision, dizziness, unsteady gait, memory loss, etc. The acute treatment for hyperviscosity syndrome is plasma pheresis.

In multiple myeloma, renal failure occurs because light chain proteins filter out of the kidneys, resulting in severe damage to the kidney tubules, which causes renal insufficiency or renal failure to develop. There is a form of myeloma called light chain myeloma in which the total protein is typically low and that is so because the light chains are passing out in the urine in large quantities and not accumulating in the blood to be reflected as elevated total protein. As the light chain proteins pass through the kidneys' tubules, the light chain proteins damage the kidneys. In fact, light chain myeloma is more frequently associated with renal failure than multiple myeloma. Multiple myeloma is much more common in black and Hispanic men than in white and other men. So it stands to reason that more minority men suffer from myeloma kidney than do white men.

It is very important to test the blood for lactic dehydrogenase (LDH). For example, an elevated LDH may be seen in a patient who has an occult cancer that no one knows about yet. Sometimes many routine blood tests and the physical examination are normal but the LDH, BUN and serum creative are elevated. This could be a case of lymphoma, because in lymphoma and other cancers, the cancer cells grow via the anaerobic pathway, meaning that these cells grow in the absence of oxygen. When cells grow in the absence of oxygen, lactic acid is produced as the end product of the anaerobic pathway and lactic acid leads to lactic dehydrogenase (LDH). Therefore, a unilateral elevation of LDH in association with acute renal failure can mean one of several things:

1. Acute lymphoma with rapid cancer cell turnover, resulting in large breakdown products of protein making it difficult for the kidneys to filter them out in the urine, and the result is acute renal failure.

2. When the LHD is unilaterally high, it could be acute hemolysis due to hemolytic anemia or any other number of medical problems that can cause red blood cells to hemolyze.

Once hemolysis occurs, the by-products of the red cells will clog up the kidney tubules, which can result in acute renal failure. Black and Hispanic men as well have the propensity to hemolyze because of sickle cell disease, thalassemia and sickle thalassemia, etc., and if these hemolytic episodes are not handled in a proper clinical way, acute renal failure can be one of the results. Some men of Greek and Italian ethnic background also have the propensity to have hemolytic diseases such as the beta thalassemia.

Elevation of serum creatinine phosphokinase (CPK) can be very important in the development of acute renal failure. There are many medical conditions that cause the CPK to be elevated so high as to be threatening to the health of the kidneys. Among these conditions are rhabdomyolysis, caused by severe muscle trauma, severe seizure with muscle damage, muscle trauma because of a long march with trauma to the feet, trauma to muscle because of marathon bongo drum beating with hands; all these conditions and more can cause damage to the skeletal muscles, resulting in acute damage to the tubules of the kidneys, which, if not treated properly, can cause kidney failure. Therefore, when a patient presents with unexplained acute failure, testing the serum for elevation of CPK is an important thing to do. Any one of the statin anti-cholesterol medications can, at times, cause muscle breakdown, which if not recognized and properly treated, can lead to acute renal failure.

Doing a complete blood count in a patient who presents with acute renal failure is extremely important. There are three parts of the CBC that a physician caring for a patient with acute renal failure must be concerned with:

1. The white blood cell count (WBC)
2. The platelet count
3. The hematocrit

A WBC of greater than 100,000 with lymphocytosis represents evidence of lymphoproliferative disorder out of control. The rapid cell turnover that occurs in that condition results in the production of a large amount of purine, a protein breakdown product that can clog the kidney tubules, resulting in acute renal failure.

If the platelet count is very low, less than 40,000–50,000, in association with acute renal failure, this could mean several things. Low platelets, low hematocrit and acute renal failure could be seen in DIC, TTP, sepsis, Evan's syndrome as seen in SLE, leukemia or lymphoma, red cell transfusion reaction, AIDS, etc. Low hematocrit and acute renal failure could mean acute hemolysis with debris from the break-up of red cells clogging the kidney tubules, resulting in acute renal failure such as what occurs in thrombotic thrombocytopenia purpura (TTP).

To prevent the devastation of the kidneys that leads to kidney failure, hypertensive men have to decrease the salt in their diet by half. Rather than eating an average of 7–8 grams of sodium per day, they ought to eat 3–4 grams of sodium per day. The decrease in sodium will decrease high blood pressure in men, which in turn will decrease their incidence of kidney failure.

African-American men are obese at a rate of 50%, Hispanic men 46%, white males 35% and the incidence of obesity in American Indian men and Pacific/Islanders is significantly higher than among white men. Obesity is highly associated with diabetes mellitus. Diabetes mellitus is the second leading cause of renal failure in men. About 40% of men with chronic renal failure who are on dialysis are in that condition due to end-stage renal failure brought about by diabetes mellitus.

Men ought to exercise, eat a low-fat and low-carbohydrate diet, which will help them to lose weight. That will decrease or delay the onset of diabetes mellitus and hypertension and reduce their susceptibility to kidney disease.

Another common cause of kidney disease in black and Hispanic men is sickle cell anemia. Sickle cell anemia damages the kidneys, because of both the occlusive and its inflammatory nature. Blood and oxygen flow to the glomeruli of the kidneys are both impaired, resulting ultimately in a significant percentage of people suffering with sickle cell disease developing end-stage renal failure requiring dialysis.

Sickle cell trait often causes papillary necrosis, causing bleeding from the kidney, often the right kidney.

When hypertension and diabetes mellitus are seen together in the patient who has sickle cell disease, the incidence of kidney failure increases. A blood pressure of 130/80 is normal in a person not suffering from sickle cell disease but in someone with sickle cell anemia that is hypertension. The blood pressure is usually low in people with sickle cell disease.

1. The most effective treatments for renal failure are a low-salt and low-protein diet.
2. When the renal function deteriorates to the point that the BUN and the creatinine are excessively high, along with high serum potassium, high phosphatase, low calcium and a very low creatinine clearance combined with evidence of uremia, dialysis becomes necessary.

There are two types of dialysis that are in routine use:

1. Peritoneal dialysis
2. Hemodialysis.

Different clinical situations along with the patient's preference will help to determine which type of dialysis will be used to treat the individual patient with end-stage renal failure.

Quite frequently the kidney becomes infected with bacteria because of a lower tract infection that started out in the urinary bladder and migrated upwards into the kidney causing the development of a condition calls pyelonephritis. The symptoms of acute pyelonephritis are:

1. Burning on urination
2. Urinary frequency
3. Low back pain
4. Flank pain

5. Fever
6. Chills
7. Nausea
8. Vomiting
9. Head ache
10. Dizziness
11. Fatigue

The best ways to evaluate a patient for acute pyelonephritis are:
1. Take a complete history
2. Do a complete physical examination
3. Do a urinalysis
4. Do a urine Culture
5. Do blood cultures
6. Do CBC
7. Do SMA20 chemistry profile
8. Do a renal ultrasound
9. Do a Chest x-ray

The best ways to treat acute pyelonephritis are:
1. Start the patient on IV fluid
2. Start the patient on broad spectrum antibiotic to cover for gram negative bacteria
3. Such as Levaquin 500 mg IV every 24 hours for 14 days
4. Or Cipro 400 mg IV every 12 hours for 14 days
5. Or Ceftazidime 1 gram IV every 8 hours for 14 days
6. Once the patient becomes afebrile, the IV antibiotic can be switched to antibiotic by mouth for a total of 14 days.

The most common bacteria that cause urinary tract infection are enteric bacteria from the stools.

Any man, who develops urinary tract infection and pyelonephritis, must be evaluated by a urologist to rule out underline abnormalities in the bladder, kidneys or urological tract to explain the reason for the urinary tract infection.

Some the most common reasons that men have urinary tract infection are:
1. Enlarged prostate
2. Bladder dysfunction resulting in residual of urine in the bladder allowing bacterial growth causing UTI.
3. Kidney stones
4. Foley catheter insertion
5. After urological procedures
6. Congenital malformation of the urological tract

An other common problem that affects the kidney is stone.

The stones are usually made up of urates, oxalates, phosphates and carbonates. Kidney stones are very painful, causing lower back pain and flank pain.

Hematuria (blood in the urine) is frequently seen in individuals who suffer with kidney stones.

1. The best way to evaluate a patient suffering with kidney stones is to do a plain abdominal cat scan
2. Urinalysis
3. Renal ultrasound

The best treatments for kidney stones are:

1. Pain medication
2. IV fluid
3. Diet
4. Thiazide diuretic
5. Strain the urine to find the stone so that it can be sent to the laboratory for chemical examination.

CHAPTER 9

DISEASES OF THE STOMACH AND INTESTINE IN MEN

DISEASES OF THE GASTROINTESTINAL TRACT are among the most common diseases that men suffer from. The most frequent GI symptoms that men go to see the doctor for consist of:

1. Heartburn
2. Bitter taste in the mouth
3. Indigestion
4. Bloating
5. Gaseousness
6. Increased flatus
7. Nausea
8. Vomiting
9. Loss of appetite
10. Easy filling of the stomach when eating (dysphagia)
11. Pain on swallowing food
12. Pain in the stomach area
13. Pain in the abdomen
14. Recurrent diarrhea
15. Rectal bleeding
16. Pain on defecation
17. Hemorrhoids

18. Constipation etc.
19. Diarrhea

The reasons for these symptoms include:

1. *Hiatal hernia*
2. *Reflux esophagitis*
3. Slow motility of the esophagus
4. Esophagitis due to fungal infection of the esophagus
5. Cancer of the esophagus, etc.
6. Gastroesophageal reflux disease (GERD)
7. Peptic ulcer
8. Helicobacter Pylori gastritis
9. Uclcerative Colitis
10. Crohn's disease
11. Diverticulitis
12. Small bowel obstruction
13. Large bowel obstruction
14. Cancer of the stomach
15. Cancer of the large bowel
16. Parasitic infestation of the large bowel
17. Spastic colon or irritable bowel disease
18. Viral gastroenteritis
19. Infectious gastroenteritis etc.

"There are two different types of hiatal hernia: the sliding type and the paraesophageal type" Both types cause significant symptoms such as heartburn, symptoms of regurgitation, and bitter taste in the mouth, acid and chest pain. In hiatal hernia, acid backs up toward the throat, causing the symptoms just outlined. As the acid bathes the part of the esophagus that dips into the stomach, the symptoms develop. Bleeding due to hiatal hernia occurs frequently because of erosion that the acid causes in the wall of the part of the esophagus affected by the acid. More bleeding occurs in paraesophageal hernia than in sliding hernia. The reason why more bleeding occurs in paraesophageal hernia than in the sliding type, is because in the paraesophageal type of hiatal hernia, the part of the esophagus that is involved is stuck in one place, while in the sliding type of hiatal hernia the affected part slides up and down into the area containing the acid, exposing the esophageal tissues much less to acid and thus reducing the incidence of bleeding.

Chronic coughing and throat irritation are frequent symptoms of GERD.

Another important and serious condition that affects the esophagus is *achalasia*. People who have AIDS frequently suffer with *esophagitis* due to fungal infection, viral infection such as cytomegalovirus, or herpes viral infection resulting in severe pain on swallowing. The incidence of smoking and alcohol abuse is quite high among men and, because, their incidence of cancer of the esophagus is higher than among men who do not drink alcohol and do not smoke cigarettes.

One of the most common complaints that the physician sees in his or her office is stomach pain. The reasons for the stomach complaints are many and wide-ranging in characteristics. A frequent contributor to stomach problems is the ingestion of contaminated foods resulting in indigestion and/or acute gastroenteritis with nausea and vomiting. Another common reason for acute gastroenteritis is viral infection affecting the stomach, resulting in stomach pain, stomach cramps, nausea, vomiting and fever. When men eat foods that are contaminated, they frequently become sick and develop infectious gastroenteritis from bacteria such as Staphylococcusylococci bacteria, E. Coli, Salmonella, Shigella, Campylobacter.

Another common and frequent complaint of the stomach in men is stomach pain due to ulcers. Stomach ulcers are more common in men of color, as compared to white men. Men of color face racial discriminations of one type or an other every day. As a person faces racial bigotry, the person first becomes intensely angry, followed with intense fear. Both anger and fear cause the stomach to produce an excessive amount of acid and the increased level of acid in the stomach causes a burning pain, indigestion, and, eventually, ulcer of the stomach. In order to cope with the daily pressure and stress of racial discrimination, some men of color frequently resort to alcohol abuse and cigarette smoking, both of which, via different mechanisms, can cause severe stomach problems including peptic ulcers to develop.

Smoking cigarettes places a large amount of nicotine in the bloodstream, causing marked acid secretion, which increases symptoms of peptic dysfunction and increases the incidence of peptic ulcer disease. Therefore, people who smoke have more ulcers of the stomach.

Peptic dysfunction is one of the common symptoms of alcohol abuse. Some of these symptoms include nausea, vomiting, retching, stomach pain, gastritis, hematemesis (vomiting of blood), and Mallory-Weiss, because of forceful and persistent vomiting due to the adverse effects of alcohol on the stomach and the junction into the stomach. (Mallory-Weiss tear is a tear that occurs at the junction where the esaphogus enters into the stomach-Gastro-Esaphpgeal Junction, that tear can occur because of forceful and prolonged vomiting/retching from any cause, but it is seen most frequently in alcoholics.) A Mallory-Weiss tear causes severe upper gastrointestinal bleeding, occurring because of forceful vomiting and retching, resulting in a tear at the junction where the esophagus meets the stomach. An other type of esaphogeal tear that can occur from forceful vomiting and retching is Boerhaave tear as seen in Boerhaave's syndrome.

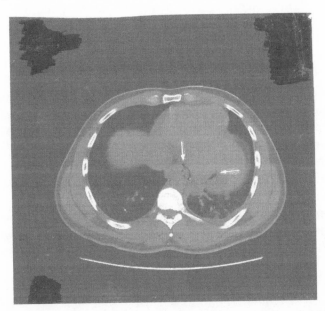

Chest CAT scan (Boerhaave tear in a man who got a piece of chicken stuck in his esophagus)

One of the most serious upper gastrointestinal complications of chronic alcohol abuse is esophageal varices. Varices are small superficial blood vessels that develop on the surface of the esophagus because of portal hypertension, which is the result of occlusion of the small vessels within the liver. The occlusions of these vessels cause the spleen to become enlarged, which in turn causes the development of portal hypertension. Because the esophageal varices are superficial, they bleed easily, frequently and profusely. It is almost impossible to stop bleeding from esophageal varices. All the different treatments that have been tried have very little effectiveness. Bleeding from gastritis is an extremely common occurrence. Alcohol is quite irritating to the lining of the stomach, and because of that irritation, bleeding occurs. That bleeding can be quite profuse at times.

Attached to the lower part of the stomach and to the beginning of the large bowel is the organ called the small intestine. The three common abnormalities that affect the small intestine are:

1. Malabsorption.
2. Inflammatory bowel disease (Crohn's disease).
3. Cancer of the small bowel.

There are many other conditions that affect the small intestine.

Malabsorption can occur because of sprue, parasitic infestations often associated with a disease such as AIDS. Fungal and viral infections of the small intestine, such as candidiasis and cytomegalovirus infection, etc., are seen frequently in patients suffering from AIDS, resulting in severe diarrhea with massive loss of minerals, electrolytes, and vitamins. Malabsorption results in general weakness, overall worsening the patient's condition.

Sprue-tropical type, the cause of which is not known but is probably due to some form of microorganism, which releases a toxin into the small bowel, resulting in malabsorption of iron, folic acid, vitamin B12 and a multitude of minerals and electrolytes. Weight loss, anorexia, diarrhea, and anemia are some consequences of tropical sprue.

Nontropical sprue is another abnormality of the small bowel. That form of sprue is due to intolerance to gluten, which is a protein found in wheat and its products. It is believed that that form of sprue is inherited via a dominant gene of incomplete penetrance. The result of that type of sprue is diarrhea, malabsorption, weight loss and anorexia.

One of the common symptoms of small bowel disease is pain around the umbilicus. Another frequent symptom of small bowel disease is diarrhea. Still another common symptom of small bowel disease is rectal bleeding.

The rectal bleeding can be due to angiodysplasia or AVM, ischemic colitis, Crohn's disease, Meckel's diverticulum, cancer, etc.

The lower part of the small bowel is attached to the large bowel and the large bowel is afflicted with the most devastating disease of the gastrointestinal tract, namely cancer. In the year 2007, it is expected that 72,800 cases of colon rectal cancer will be diagnosed in men in the United States and 27,870 of these men will die of their cancers during that same time.

Another common cause of colon-rectal bleeding is polyps of the colon. Polyps of the colon can bleed, but can also give rise to cancer of the colon. Still another frequent cause of colon and rectal bleeding is diverticulosis of the colon. Diverticular disease of the colon is more common in the men who live in developed countries as compared to the men who live in the third world. Men who live in the third world have more meager diets that contain more roughage, more fibers and less fat, which allow for more regular and more bulky bowel movements. The lack of roughage, the lack of fibers and too much fat lead to constipation, which is associated with increase in the incidence of diverticular disease of the colon and colon cancer. Diverticular bleeding can be both painless and at times painful. Painful diverticular bleeding may be associated with diverticulitis. Diverticulitis is a condition that results from an infected diverticulum. Diverticulum is an outpouching from the inside wall of the bowel. Every now and then erosion occurs in these diverticula due to actions of the stool on them. The result is acute diverticulitis, which causes abdominal pain, fever, chills and malaise. Diverticulitis is a very serious condition, which can cause abscesses and sometimes perforation of the large bowel, resulting in peritonitis and death of the affected person if left untreated.

Another frequent cause of bleeding from the lower GI tract is AVM. Bleeding associated with AVM (arteriovenous malformation) is not only common but, at times, very difficult to diagnose and even more difficult to treat. Ulcerative colitis and Crohn's disease are common in men and the most common problems associated with these conditions are rectal bleeding and anemia. Ischemic colitis is seen most frequently in elderly individuals and people who suffer from diabetes mellitus and atherosclerotic disease. Ischemic colitis is associated with rectal bleeding, abdominal pain, fever and elevated white blood cell count. Bloody diarrhea can be seen frequently in AIDS patients because of enterocolitis due to fungi, viruses, bacteria, protozoa and parasites. Enterocolitis is a serious problem in anyone who is afflicted by it, but it is particularly devastating in AIDS patients because of their already weakened condition.

Constipation is a common problem and one of the reasons men frequently seeks medical advice. Constipation can be due to many different things. Poor dietary habits can lead to constipation. A diet deficient in roughage, fiber and bulk can cause constipation. An underlying condition such as hypothyroidism can cause constipation. Taking medications such as calcium channel blockers to treat hypertension or to treat angina pectoris can cause constipation because the calcium channel blocker relaxes the smooth muscle of the colon, decreasing contraction of smooth muscles, which is necessary for the colon to excrete its contents, namely the stool. Many more medications cause constipation. Taking too much laxatives too frequently is a frequent cause of constipation. When an individual uses laxatives too frequently, the colon becomes lazy, loses its ability to contract properly, and will not work without help to excrete stool. That condition is called cathartic colon. The treatment for that is to retrain the person as to the proper bowel habits to help his or his to refrain from using cathartics to bring about a bowel movement. Constipation must always be brought to the attention of the physician because frequently constipation can be the first sign noticed in cancer of the large bowel. The same can be said of diarrhea as it is related to cancer of the colon. Any significant changes of bowel habits ought to be brought to the attention of a physician because major pathologies can be the reason of the change in bowel habits.

Another frequent ailment is hemorrhoids. Hemorrhoids are found on the very end of the lower GI tract, namely the anus. Hemorrhoids have many causes, but the most frequent ones consist of:

1. Straining at stool due to impatience
2. Constipation causing a person to strain at stool
3. Obesity resulting in too much pressure being placed on the anal area
4. Too much weight gain during pregnancy resulting in too much pressure on the anal area
5. Occupational hazards such as driving long distances over long periods of time
6. Standing for long periods of time over many years
7. Obstructive colonic polyps or cancer of the colon resulting in straining at stool.

If a person suddenly protrudes a hemorrhoid while at the same time passing pencil-thin stool, that usually means there is something obstructing the normal passage of the stool resulting in acute protrusion of a hemorrhoid and that person needs immediate medical attention to evaluate the large bowel by colonoscopic examination to seek out the problem. One of the frequent symptoms associated with the anal area is bleeding. Bleeding from the rectum is always serious and must always be evaluated medically. It is necessary to bring it to the attention of a physician anytime blood is seen coming from the rectum. Self-diagnosis of rectal bleeding, assumed to be due to hemorrhoids, leads frequently to the missing of early diagnosis of colon and rectal cancer.

Men have a tendency to be bashful to seek medical help when they see blood in their stool. That is a most dangerous habit, which can cause a person to delay the diagnosis of serious problems such as colon or rectal cancer.

In addition to hemorrhoids, there are other conditions that cause bleeding in the part of the perirectal area; among these conditions are anal fissures and inflammation-associated colitis, both of which can cause rectal bleeding.

How to evaluate gastrointestinal complaints

The first thing a physician must do is take a careful history. The next step is to carry out a careful physical examination. Having done these two things, the doctor should next try medications along with diet modifications. Depending on the severity of the symptoms and/or the physical findings, intervention by way of blood tests, x-ray tests or endoscopic examination might be carried out in an attempt to establish a diagnosis. If the patient's complaint is inability to swallow liquid or solid foods, then a CBC, SMA 18, and serum ferritin are the necessary and appropriate blood tests to do. Doing an upper GI series, with an esophagram, or doing an endoscopy of the upper GI tract is the appropriate and necessary x-ray or endoscopic examination. These examinations are capable of discovering any abnormality that causes symptoms and diseases of the upper GI tract.

If a patient's complaint is pain in the stomach, heartburn, hyperacidity, vomiting blood or bleeding from the stomach, then doing a CBC, serum ferritin, upper GI series, endoscopic examination and abdominal sonogram are sufficient to discover most of the problems associated with the upper GI tract, the gall bladder and the pancreas.

Frequently, an abdominal CAT scan is needed to help evaluate the pancreas to be certain pancreatic cancer is not causing the patient's abdominal pain. Abdominal sonogram is the choice test to diagnose stones in the gall bladder, while the abdominal CT is good to evaluate cancer of the gall bladder and the liver.

To evaluate the small intestine, one needs to do an upper GI series with a small bowel follow-through. It is not routine to do endoscopic examination of the small bowel. To evaluate the large intestine, one can do a barium enema, which is putting barium in the intestine through the rectum into a rubber tube, and once the barium is in the large bowel then x-ray pictures are taken in different positions.

An instrument called a sigmoidoscope can be used to look inside the lower bowel. There are two different types of sigmoidoscopes, a rigid one and a flexible one. The rigid scope can be passed up to 30 cm, the flexible scope can be passed up to 60 cm. Different complaints, and different circumstances dictate which procedure is done.

There is an instrument called a colonoscope, which is a long, flexible and hollow instrument that allows the gastroenterologist to examine the entire large bowel, looking for abnormalities. Biopsies can be taken during these procedures and lesions such as polyps can be removed entirely, preventing the need for open abdominal surgical procedures to remove polyps in most instances.

According to the recent literature, flexible sigmoidoscopic examination missed up to 34% of cancer of the colon. Therefore, since the bowel preparation is the same for both colonoscopy and flexible sigmoidoscopy, it is preferable to do a colonoscopy instead of flexible sigmoidoscopy.

When necessary, an anoscope can be used to look inside the rectum to evaluate local problems in that part of the bowel.

How can men prevent the development of some of these gastrointestinal ailments?

Starting with the esophagus, men will decrease their incidence of esophageal cancer by stopping cigarette smoking and alcohol abuse. Both of these bad habits cause a predisposition to the development of cancer of the esophagus. Esophageal varices are associated, most frequently, with alcohol abuse and alcoholic liver disease. If men would abstain from alcohol abuse, their incidence of alcohol-associated esophageal problems would likely disappear.

Hiatal hernia is a frequent problem seen in men and it can be quite troublesome, at times resulting in heartburn and sometimes in iron deficiency anemia as because of slow but chronic bleeding from the hiatal hernia. Men can help themselves by losing weight and in so doing they can either prevent and/or decrease the incidence of hiatal hernia. About 50% of men in the United States are obese, and obesity plays a significant role in the development of hiatal hernia and the worsening of its symptoms.

Symptoms associated with diseases of the stomach are more common in men of color as opposed to white men and the reasons are many. To start with, the foods that minority men like to eat have too much fats salt, carbohydrates and spices in them. When a diet is rich in fats, spices, salt and carbohydrates and is combined with cigarette smoking, alcohol abuse is added to the day-to-day stress that poor minority men have to deal with, it is easy to see why the incidence of stomach ailments of all sorts is so much higher in minority men than in the men who eat a better diet and who don't have deal with the daily and constant stresses of racial discrimination and bigotry (His is referred to in part by some one as the "**STATUS SYNDROME**"). JAMA, March 15, 2006-Vol 295, No 11.

About 36% of men in the United States are obese and obesity is very highly connected with gallstones and gall bladder diseases. Further, many Black, Hispanic, Middle Eastern Mediterranean and Asian men suffer with hemolytic diseases such as sickle cell anemia and sickle thalassemia and thalassemias that predispose them to gall bladder stone disease. Men who suffer from these hemolytic anemia produce a substance called bilirubin in excess, which is a pigment that comes from the breakdown products of the hemolyzed red cells. The bilirubin pigment forms bilirubin stones in the gall bladder. Most of the gallstones seen in obese men however are cholesterol stones. Symptoms of gall bladder stones, which include nausea, vomiting, right-sided abdominal pain—which can at times be referred to the left side of the upper abdomen, etc.—can easily be confused with diseases of the stomach such as peptic ulcer or hiatal hernia with reflux. Symptoms of gall bladder disease can also be confused with diseases of the pancreas. Both acute and chronic pancreatitis can have symptoms that are similar to gall bladder disease. Frequently, a person would present to the doctor with jaundice and no pain. Then the question becomes is it due to gallstones occluding the common bile duct, resulting in backing up of bile into the bloodstream, or is it due to a tumor (usually cancer) at the head of the pancreas pressing on the common bile duct, causing the jaundice to occur? That condition is called painless jaundice.

There are many other serious conditions that can affect the gall bladder, such as ascending cholangeitis, cancer of the gall bladder, gangrene of the gall bladder, etc. Another common cause of abdominal pain is disease of the pancreas. In men, the most common disease of the pancreas is acute pancreatitis. The reason why acute pancreatitis is so common in minority men is because 50% of African-American, 46% of Hispanic men and 35% of white men are obese, and obesity increases the incidence of gallstones. Gallstones are the second most common cause of pancreatitis. Gall bladder and gallstones diseases are quite high in incidence in American Indian and Eskimo men.

The bilirubin, once in the blood, turns into bile, which then causes the development of bilirubin gallstones. Gallstones cause pancreatitis by blocking some of the tubes that carry enzymes out of the pancreas, resulting in back flow of enzymes into the pancreas and causing inflammation of the pancreas. That pancreatic inflammation starts the process of acute pancreatitis.

The most common reason why men suffer from pancreatitis is alcoholism, the incidence of alcohol abuse is extremely high among men in the US. Alcohol is very toxic to the pancreas, resulting in acute inflammation causing acute pancreatitis. Acute pancreatitis causes abdominal pain, nausea, vomiting, fever, dehydration, electrolyte imbalance and high serum or urine amylase. When pancreatitis occurs along with other tissue damage, resulting in chronic pancreatitis, pseudocyst of the pancreas and pancreatic abscess can also occur. The symptoms of chronic pancreatitis include the symptoms outlined in acute pancreatitis, plus severe diarrhea, malabsorption, weight loss, and diabetes mellitus, etc.

The reason why malabsorption and diarrhea occur in chronic pancreatitis is that the pancreas, having been destroyed by the effect of alcohol, is not able to produce the different enzymes that are necessary for proper digestion of foods. In particular, fatty foods cannot be digested, resulting in oily diarrhea. The reason that diabetes mellitus occurs in chronic pancreatitis is that the cells that produce insulin are located in the pancreas, and once the pancreas is destroyed then insulin cannot be made. The result is high blood sugar in the blood and all of its consequences.

There are many more conditions that affect the small bowel and large bowel that can cause pain, and among them are ulcerative colitis and Crohn's disease. Both of these conditions are reasonably common in men. Some of the first signs are rectal bleeding, cramps, diarrhea, pain, iron deficiency anemia, etc. No one knows what causes Crohn's disease and ulcerative colitis. To diagnose inflammatory bowel diseases, both barium studies and colonoscopic examinations are used. To diagnose inflammatory bowel of the small bowel, barium study is needed. Diagnosis of inflammatory bowel disease of the large intestine can be made both by barium studies and by colonoscopic examinations. In inflammatory bowel disease, the inner surface of the bowel is swollen and inflamed and bleeds easily. The cause or causes of these changes are not known in spite of many years of research. In addition to abdominal pain, diarrhea, and rectal bleeding, there is an increased incidence of colorectal cancer in people suffering with inflammatory bowel disease.

How to evaluate diseases of the gastrointestinal tract

The beginning of the GI tract is the mouth, and the best way to evaluate the mouth is by the naked eye.

To evaluate the throat, sometimes an instrument like the laryngoscope may be used. To evaluate the esophagus, either barium swallows followed by x-ray or endoscopy can be used.

To evaluate the stomach, the best two ways are upper GI series with barium swallow or endoscopic examination, during which the different parts of the stomach can be directly visualized and, when necessary, biopsies can be done. It is important to understand that if a gastric ulcer is detected during the upper GI series, then endoscopic examination must be carried out so that it can be biopsied to rule out cancer. Gastric ulcers have a high propensity to be cancerous and must always be biopsied when discovered. There are multitudes of other abnormalities that can be found in the upper GI tract during the endoscopic examination. The best way available to evaluate the small bowel is using barium swallow with small bowel follow-through. Some of the diseases found in the small bowel are Crohn's disease, cancer, malabsorption, Meckel's diverticulum, arteriovenous malformation, etc.

To evaluate the large bowel (colon or intestine), barium enema, colonoscopy, rigid or flexible sigmoidoscopic examination is used. Using these examinations, the physician can evaluate the entire large bowel from the anus up to the area where the large bowel is joined with the small bowel. Conditions such as cancer, polyps, diverticula, ulcerative colitis, arteriovenous malformations, hemorrhoids, anal fissures, etc., can be discovered and, when necessary, biopsies can be taken to determine the true nature of some of these diseases, to allow for appropriate treatments," whether surgical or medical treatment".

Ninety per cent of cancer of the colon develops from polyps. Twelve per cent of benign polyps develop in the colon every year. Two per cent of polyps that cause cancer in the colon develop every year. The type of polyps that cause cancer of the colon are usually greater than 1.4 cm in size and are of villous histology.

In order for a polyp to develop, an inflammatory reaction must first begin and this inflammatory reaction is mediated by the enzyme CYCLOOXYGENASE.

Because aspirin and non-steroidal anti-inflammatory drugs block the effects of CYCLOOXYGENASE on inflammation, that is why these drugs help to decrease the development of colonic polyp formation thereby, decreases the incidence of colon cancer and possibly several other solid tumors.

How to best treat the different diseases of the gastrointestinal tract

One of the common complaints that bring patients to the physician's office is heartburn. Heartburn is due to hiatal hernia with reflux esophagitis. Men suffer a lot from that condition because of the fact that a large percentage of men are obese and obesity has a close association with hiatal hernia and heartburn. The best treatments consist of:

1.   Weight loss
2.   Low-fat diet
3.   Decrease of caffeine intake
4.   Decrease of alcohol consumption
5.   Sleeping with head of the bed up, or placing 2–3 pillows under one's head when sleeping, to prevent the free flow of acid to reflux up towards the throat
6.   Raglan 10 mg, 15 minutes before meals, three times a day and at bedtime.

That medication works to propel the foods down the stomach with more ease, preventing too much acid production. When food sits in the stomach too long, too much acid is produced. It backs up toward the upper chest, causing hyperacidity, heartburn, and bad taste in the mouth, bad breath and, frequently, severe chest pain simulating cardiac chest pain and, at times, a chronic cough. Whenever the stomach detects food it sends a signal to the lining of the stomach where the acid-producing cells are located to secrete more acid to digest the food. The idea then is to help move the food along so that less acid is produced, thereby decreasing the symptoms of heartburn. H^2 blockers such as Tagamet, Axid, Zantac, and Pepcid are used also in hiatal hernia with reflux with very good success because these medications block the production of excess acid, preventing the formation of ulcerations around the esophagogastric junction, thereby decreasing the symptoms of heartburn. Protein pump inhibitors such as Prilosec, Prevacid and Nexium are also very effective in medical management of GERD (gastroesophageal reflux disease). There is no definite surgical procedure available to repair hiatal hernia in common use, though there have been some recent claims being made that hiatal hernia can be repaired using laser. However, GERD is being treated laparoscopically using a wraparound surgical technique that seems to be enjoying some degree of success.

Antacids such as Mylanta, Maalox, Rolaids, etc. are also helpful in relieving symptoms of heartburn and hyperacidity associated with hiatal hernia with reflux.

The most common disease of the stomach is ulcer. Other diseases of the stomach that are frequently seen are cancer, lymphoma, gastritis associated with aspirin ingestion or alcohol abuse and H. Pylori infection, etc.

The best treatment available to treat stomach ulcers is the H2 blockers, such as Tagamet, Axid, Zantac, Pepcid and more powerful acid blockers (Protein pump inhibitors) namely Prilosec, Nexium, Prevacid etc. These medications are commonly used for two months to treat ulcers that are proven by upper GI series or endoscopic examination. After two months, a repeat upper GI series or endoscopic examination is done. If the ulcer is healed, then based on symptoms, the physician may choose whether to continue treatment for a few more weeks or not. If the ulcer is only partially healed, then treatment with H2 blockers or PPI can continue for two more months. If the last two months of treatment trial of the ulcer still fails to heal it fully or not at all, then at that point a biopsy via endoscopic examination becomes mandatory to rule out cancer. It is now accepted practice to test for H. pylori at the time of endoscopic examination, using gastric tissue via biopsy to test for the presence or absence of that microorganism. H. pylori is believed to play a major role in the causation of peptic ulcer disease and malignancy of the stomach, such as lymphoma, etc. There are several ways to make the diagnosis of H. pylori. One way is to test the gastric juice for the presence of H. pylori using a color change test (the CLO test). If the color changes from yellow to red when the juice is tested then it means H. pylori is present. Another way is to test the blood of the patient for antibody to H. pylori and if the antibody is found then H. pylori is documented. Still another way to document the presence of H. pylori is to look for the organism in gastric biopsy taken from the stomach at the time of endoscopy. There is a breath test as well as a stool test available to diagnose H. pylori. H. pylori is the most common nosocomial infection in the world. About 50% of the world population is infected with H. pylori. About 70% of the population of New York City is said to carry the H. pylori organism in their stomach because of migration of people from different parts of the world who live there. Countrywide in the U.S., the incidence of H. pylori is 30%. Chronic peptic ulcer disease is associated with H. pylori, the latter being tagged as a causative reason for the development of the ulcer. There are several protocols available to treat H. pylori but Prevpac is a frequently used one. It is used for either 10 days or 14 days. H. pylori get into the body through the" oral/fecal" route. It is important to understand that diagnosing peptic ulcer using the upper GI series is only 65%-70% accurate, while diagnosing peptic ulcer using endoscopy is about 95%-100% accurate.

Surgical treatment is still used for treating ulcers of the stomach under specific circumstances. When an ulcer of the stomach fails to stop bleeding in spite of all medical treatments and in particular, when the patient who is bleeding receives too much blood; a gastrectomy is usually carried out to stop the bleeding and save the patient's life. Another situation that requires gastrectomy is when a biopsy of the stomach reveals the presence of cancer, a gastrectomy is usually undertaken to remove the cancerous part of the stomach. More often than not, other treatments such as chemotherapy and/or radiotherapy are used as additional treatments when cancer of the stomach is surgically removed.

The small intestine is frequently affected by Crohn's disease, and the most frequent treatment for Crohn's disease is steroids with Azulfidine steroid enemas with added folic acid to prevent the folic acid deficiency that the Azulfidine causes. Surgical resection of part of the small intestine is also frequently carried out as part of the treatment for small bowel Crohn's disease.

Another common disease of the small bowel is cancer. The cancer seen in the small bowel can vary from solid tumor like adenocarcinoma, lymphoma, carcinoid tumor and different types of metastatic cancer to the small bowel.

Another frequent disease of the small bowel is sprue, both tropical sprue and non-tropical sprue.

The treatment of choice for tropical sprue is antibiotics such as Tetracycline and the treatment for non-tropical sprue is a gluten-free diet.

Many other serious medical problems can affect the small intestine such as arteriovenous malformation causing severe bleeding, Meckel's diverticulum with severe bleeding and severe malabsorption due to chronic pancreatitis and a multitude of other causes. The different treatments for these different diseases of the small intestine are handled individually as each disease situation warrants.

"The large intestine, and its long list of possible diseases."

The large bowel is the site for a multitude of diseases, some very serious and some less serious, but, nevertheless, many are afflicted by them. Some of the most frequent diseases and conditions of the colon include:

1. Diarrhea
2. Constipation
3. Diarrhea alternating with constipation
4. Abdominal cramps
5. Flatulence
6. Abdominal pain
7. Rectal bleeding
8. Ulcerative colitis
9. Crohn's disease of the colon
10. Diverticulosis
11. Diverticulitis
12. Bacterial overgrowth
13. Lactose intolerance
14. Acute infectious gastroenteritis
15. Parasitism
16. Ischemic colitis
17. Intestinal obstruction
18. Colon cancer
19. Rectal cancer
20. Rectal fissures
21. Hemorrhoids
22. Inguinal hernias
23. Familial polyposis.

Diarrhea occurs for a multitude of reasons in humans, resulting in serious discomfort and inconveniences. Cancer of the colon is frequently presented with diarrhea as an initial complaint. Sometimes the diarrhea occurs because there is a mass obstructing the colon but watery stool is able to pass around it, expressing itself as diarrhea. Sometimes diarrhea occurs because of other cancers such as carcinoid tumor, mucus-producing adenocarcinoma of the colon, etc. Diarrhea is frequently seen in people who are suffering from ulcerative colitis or Crohn's disease of the colon. Diarrhea is seen in both acute and chronic pancreatitis. Diarrhea is frequently seen in individuals suffering from sprue. Diarrhea is seen frequently in people suffering from irritable bowel syndrome. Parasitic infestations such as giardiasis are frequently manifested with diarrhea and there are a multitude of other parasitic infestations which cause diarrhea. Many individuals abuse cathartics and come to the physician with a complaint of chronic diarrhea when in fact the diarrhea is self-afflicted.

Lactose intolerance is quite common in black and Hispanic people. About 60% of individuals of African origin suffer from this condition and develop the disease to one degree or another at some point in their lives. About 35% Caucasians of European extraction suffer from the condition; 45% of Jews and about 40% of Asians, etc. In addition to abdominal cramps, flatulence, nausea, gaseousness, lactose intolerance causes diarrhea. There is an enzyme called lactase, which is produced by certain cells in the lining of the intestine. The role of this enzyme is to break down lactose into glucose and galactose. If a person lacks lactase completely or has a diminished quantity of this enzyme, when that person ingests dairy products such as milk, cheeses, butter, etc., he or she develops symptoms of lactose intolerance as just outlined. The ingested lactose becomes almost like a cathartic, resulting in bowel discomfort. Lactose intolerance is hereditary, but oftentimes it gets worse as a person gets older. Avoiding dairy products is the mainstay of treatment. Some individuals with a mild to moderate form of this condition may benefit from taking a pill called LactAid or drinking milk-containing LactAid.

AIDS is one of the most prevalent diseases of our time and diarrhea is one of the most severe problems that AIDS patients have to deal with. The causes of the diarrhea seen in AIDS patients are due to a multitude of different microbial, viral and parasitic organisms, and in some cases cancer, such as rectal cancer or Kaposi's sarcoma, can also cause rectal bleeding and diarrhea. CMV-associated enterocolitis is quite common in AIDS patients. Herpes simplex gastroenteritis with diarrhea is common in AIDS patients.

In addition, AIDS patients frequently have gastroenteritis with diarrhea due to Giardiasis, amoebiasis, candidiasis, cryptosporidium, Isospora belli, salmonella, shigella, etc. Lymphoma of the GI tract with diarrhea is reasonably common. Another common cause of diarrhea is acute infectious gastroenteritis with diarrhea due to contaminated foods. The foods, water, raw vegetables, poultry and meats can become contaminated with fecal-associated bacteria including salmonella, shigella, E. coli, or typhoid organisms. These foods also can become contaminated with staphylococcusylococci resulting in severe abdominal pain, nausea, vomiting, diarrhea, and fever, sometimes resulting in dehydration, electrolyte imbalance, rectal bleeding and, at times, death of the affected individuals. Poorly cooked meats can be a good source of E coli contamination. In the case of staphylococcus food poisoning, the endotoxin that that organism produces is actually ingested by the individual being contaminated, resulting in symptoms 6–8 hours later. That happens quickly because the bacterial organisms do not have to multiply in the intestine in order to produce the endotoxin that is produced by the staphylococcal organism. In other situations, the bacteria need time to multiply in the colon to bring about the symptoms. Therefore, a person may get sick 1 day, 1 ½ days or 2 days later. Diarrhea is clearly a very common medical problem and must be dealt with seriously when it develops. Self-diagnosis can be very dangerous. It is a good idea to let your physician know if you are troubled with diarrhea so that appropriate steps can be taken to evaluate the cause or causes of the diarrhea and the proper treatments can be prescribed. Other causes of diarrhea include hyperthyroidism, irritable bowel syndrome, lactose intolerance, chronic pancreatitis, short loop syndrome, etc.

Constipation is an extremely common complaint. Constipation is found in all ethnic groups. Blacks and Hispanics living in the third world suffer less with constipation because their diets have more grains and roughage, resulting in more normal bowel movements. Constipation, as a condition, can be due to numerous things, and prominent among these are the following:

1. Stress
2. Poor eating habits
3. Hypothyroidism
4. Taking laxatives too often, resulting in a condition called cathartic colon—that is to say, the colon has lost its ability to contract properly because the individual is compulsively abusing laxatives to bring about daily bowel movements. It is not necessary to have a bowel movement every day. A bowel movement every other day is perfectly fine.
5. Constipation due to medications. Good examples of medications that can cause constipation are the calcium channel blockers. The very reason why these medications work to bring down blood pressure is by relaxing the smooth muscles within the vessel in the people taking them. The intestines have smooth muscles in them and once these smooth muscles are relaxed, the bowel is likely to lose its contractile force, resulting in constipation. Fortunately, these very important medications don't cause that problem in everybody who takes them.

6. Irritable bowel syndrome, a condition associated with spasm of the bowel is frequently associated with abdominal cramps and constipation.

7. The most feared condition sometimes seen in people who are constipated is cancer of the large bowel. Cancer of the large bowel causes constipation by mechanically preventing stool from passing through the area where the cancer is, resulting in pencil-sized stools and straining during defecation.

Before prescribing treatments for any of these conditions, thorough evaluations must be carried out to be sure of the cause or causes of these symptoms. In the case of constipation, it most probably plays a major role in the causation of cancer of the large intestine. That happens because the foods and fluids we consume in the developed world contain a lot of cancer-causing materials. These materials are either outright carcinogens or cancer promoters. Some of these cancer promoters are things produced by the human body itself. For instance, when a person eats a lot of fat containing foods such as red meat, the body via the biliary system produces many bile acids in order to digest fats contained in these red meats. These bile acids are very harsh and irritating to the tissue of the large intestine. The long-term effects of the constant irritation of the tissues of the colon result in the development of colon cancer. Constipation is bad, because not only is it uncomfortable, but it also can predispose the colon to the development of many serious medical conditions, and colon cancer is among them.

Abdominal cramps are a very common complaint and it can be due to things such as constipation, diverticulitis, lactose intolerance, irritable bowel syndrome, acute and chronic infections, parasitic infestation, ulcerative colitis, Crohn's disease, enterocolitis, acute and chronic pancreatitis, cancer of the stomach, cancer of the gall bladder, cancer of the pancreas, cancer of the colon, and stress, etc.

Flatulence is a condition that manifests itself by excessive passing of gas from the rectum. It is a normal biological function to pass gas from the rectum. The gas that is formed and expelled from the rectum is essentially methane. It is, however, abnormal when the gas a person passes is malodorous (smells bad) and when the frequency of passing gas is excessive and when the amount of gas one is passing is excessive. When a person passes large amounts of malodorous gas from the rectum too frequently, that is clearly a situation that requires medical evaluation. There are many conditions that affect the GI tract that can cause a person to produce too much and malodorous gas from the rectum, but the most common reasons are lactose intolerance and eating too much gas-producing foods such as green bananas, cabbage, peas, beans and dairy products when one is lactose intolerant.

Abdominal pain can be due to many things, including acute appendicitis, acute peritonitis due to conditions such as intra-abdominal abscess of different types, ischemic colitis, ulcerative colitis, cancer, peptic ulcer, perforated peptic ulcer, gall bladder disease, acute and chronic pancreatic diverticulitis, kidney stones. Other common causes of abdominal pain are acute gastroenteritis due to viral, bacterial, fungal, and parasitic and protozoal infections.

Rectal bleeding is a frequent complaint for which people seek help from a doctor. Most people think they have hemorrhoids when they see blood in their stools. While hemorrhoids are frequently responsible for rectal bleeding, it is wrong to assume that if blood is coming from one's rectum, it must be due to hemorrhoids that are bleeding. Yes, hemorrhoids can bleed but so can rectal cancer, colon cancer, small bowel cancer, cancer of the stomach, colon polyps, diverticulosis of the colon, ischemic colitis, Meckel's diverticulum, angiodysplasia of the GI tract, and anal fissures, etc. In fact, a person with no previous history of hemorrhoids who suddenly develops hemorrhoids either with or without bleeding would be wise to seek medical help because an obstructing polyp or cancer of the colon or rectum can cause that person to be straining during defecation, resulting in the development of hemorrhoids. That is not to say that every time someone develops a hemorrhoid he or he necessarily has colon or rectal cancer, but that possibility exists if the person is in the cancer age group of 45 years or older. The incidence of colon cancer has increased in recent in Blacks and Hispanic in their 40's. If a person bleeds from the rectum, regardless of age, he or he requires a lower gastrointestinal evaluation by colonoscopy to determine the cause. In point of fact, a person in the cancer age group with known hemorrhoids, which have been quiescent, that suddenly comes out and starts to bleed ought to also seek medical care to be certain that he or he does not have other reason or reasons to explain the sudden aggravation of the heretofore-quiescent hemorrhoids. Poor men seem to have a higher predilection to the development of hemorrhoids because they eat a poor diet with lots of fat, less grain, less vegetables and overall use less bulk, resulting in more constipation, which in turn leads to more hemorrhoids due to more straining during defecation. Another obvious reason that minority men have more hemorrhoids than do white men is that minority men tend to be more obese and obesity places a great deal of stress on the lower end of the GI tract, namely the anal area, resulting in hemorrhoids and their associated pain and bleeding symptoms.

Bleeding from the rectum is always abnormal and ought to be evaluated by a physician. The treatments for hemorrhoids are many and each person's case may be different from another person, because the cause or causes can differ. Conservative treatments, such as anal suppositories containing steroids, along with Sits baths or surgical removal of hemorrhoids, either the conventional way or with laser, are being used. Stool softeners, weight loss, and diet modifications are all approaches that can work for different people. It is best really to see your physician who can evaluate you and tailor a treatment program that is suitable for you.

Inflammatory bowel disease, which represents in the aggregate ulcerative colitis and Crohn's disease, are diseases of unknown cause, which cause different degrees of inflammations of the gastrointestinal tract, resulting in bleeding from the rectum, abdominal pain, and sometimes fever, weight loss, diarrhea, iron deficiency anemia, etc.

Sometimes, people suffering from inflammatory bowel disease can develop acute abdominal pain, megacolon, perforated viscous, intestinal obstruction, intestinal abscess, peritonitis, requiring emergency surgical intervention. Inflammatory bowel disease cuts across racial lines and oftentimes starts in the pediatric age group. Inflammatory bowel disease imposes a major burden on the individuals suffering from it and frequently these individuals develop significant psychological problems such as depression and the like.

No cure has been found for inflammatory bowel disease, but significant progress has been made with different forms of steroid medications either in pill form, intravenously, or in enema form. Medications such as Azulfidine as well as Asocal have made a big difference in the majority of people suffering from inflammatory bowel disease. There is a higher incidence of colon cancer in people suffering from inflammatory bowel disease. The reason is not altogether clear, but certainly the repeated inflammatory reactions and scarring that the bowel is exposed to for sure play a major role in the genesis of the development of bowel cancer in these individuals.

Polyps of the colon are quite common in modern society. It is believed that that is so because those who live in the modern world eat poorly. That is to say, people in the developed world eat poorly because they eat too much fats, carbohydrates and salt and not enough grains, roughage, and vegetables and fruits. Some of the vegetables and fruits that people eat in the developed world are contaminated with insecticides placed there by some food growers to prevent insects from destroying their crops, hence maximizing their profit margins at the expense of the consumers. It is believed that the interplay of all these factors plus genetic predisposition facilitates the development of colonic polyps, which in time—three to five years—may become cancerous. People in the third world develop only a fraction of the colon cancer that people in the modern world suffer from.

Men in Africa and other third world countries suffer only a fraction of the colon cancer that American men suffer from. Dietary habits have a lot to do with minority men health problems. They eat too much red meat, too much bacon, too many eggs, too many sausages and therefore too much fat and too little grains, fruits and vegetables. The "soul food" tastes good but it's not healthy food. The inability to pay for the foods that are healthy is real and remains a serious problem among poor men, and that economic problem is getting worse instead of better. As the economic situation of minority people in his country worsens, the health of minorities will continue to get worse. The incidence of colon cancer is going to get worse as the minority people's diet gets poorer in the United States and the poorer diet is a direct reflection of the poor economic status of minorities as compared to whites.

Another condition that predisposes to the development of colon cancer is familial polyposis. Familial polyposis is a hereditary condition that parents who carry that gene pass it on to their children. The children who inherit that gene develop multiple polyps in their colons and, unfortunately, develop colon cancer arising from these polyps. Once a diagnosis of familial polyposis is established, surgical treatment is advised to remove the colon via total colostomy and prevent colonic cancer from developing.

Diverticulosis of the colon is another common condition seen in the developed world. That is related to the dietary habits of people who live in the developed world. A diet that is deficient in bulk and roughage predisposes to the development of diverticulosis. Diverticula are small outpouchings from the wall of the large bowel. Every so often, the walls of some of these diverticula erode resulting in vascular breakdown, which in turn results in bleeding. Sometimes that bleeding can be severe and life threatening and the bleeding is usually painless and recurrent. Frequently, the only real treatment that is available is surgical removal of the part of the bowel that is bleeding in order to stop the bleeding when all other conservative treatments have failed.

Diverticulitis occurs when a diverticulum or many diverticula become infected and sometimes develop into abscesses. Diverticulitis occurs because the outpouching membrane from the wall of the bowel is bathed with fecal materials and fecal materials contain many bacteria. When the membrane of the diverticulum becomes inflamed and infected, the result is the development of diverticulitis. The symptoms of diverticulitis are abdominal cramps and pain, usually in lower abdominal area, fever, chills; sometimes diarrhea with or without blood and increased white blood cell count (leukocytosis) can occur.

Treatments of diverticulitis include antibiotics by mouth with low-residue diet, for low-grade diverticulitis. For moderate-grade diverticulitis, patients ought to be admitted to the hospital and keep NPO (no foods by mouth); treatment is given through IV fluids and IV antibiotics. Patients with high-grade diverticulitis with possible diverticular abscesses also need to be hospitalized, keep NPO and treated with IV antibiotics. Hyperalimentation may be given to sustain the patient off all foods. Sometimes, if peritonitis is deemed to exist because of perforation of the bowel resulting from diverticulitis, surgical resection of the affected part of the bowel may be necessary.

Bacterial overgrowth or blind-loop syndrome occurs when a situation exists that allows for bacteria to grow in a part or parts of the bowel where a piece of bowel is left in a pouch-like manner due to surgical repair or due to multiple diverticula. One of the consequences of blind loop syndrome is low B12 level and all its consequences. A good indication that blind loop syndrome may exist is a very high folic acid level in the blood in conjunction with a low serum B12 level. The approach to make that diagnosis is to try to correct the problem if possible, by treating the condition with antibiotics to eradicate the bacteria that are causing the overgrowth, and then replenish the B12 level with B12 injections.

The enzyme lactase is found in cells that are located in the walls of the intestine to facilitate breakdown of lactose into glucose and galactose. Both sugars are found in milk. When the amount of lactase is too low or completely absent, that breakdown process (metabolism) is impaired. The result is abdominal cramps, bloating, nausea, flatulence, and, frequently, diarrhea. In children, that is particularly troublesome because infants need the calcium and other nutrients that milk contains for proper growth. In infants the treatment is milk substitutes. In adults, the treatments include abstinence from milk and other dairy products or lactase containing milk or taking Lact-Aid when eating or drinking dairy products.

Acute bacterial gastroenteritis can be very serious and sometimes fatal, as well as moderate-to-mild. That usually occurs because of eating contaminated foods, usually with fecal material from food handlers who don't wash their hands after using the bathroom. The fecal contamination can also occur in the plants where the meat or poultry products are prepared for shipping to supermarkets or a variety of other ways in the chain of events that the foods pass through before they get to the consumer's table. Improperly cooked and contaminated foods in fast food places is a common situation that can result in acute staphylococcus or E. coli gastroenteritis or any number of other causative bacterial gastroenteritis. Microorganisms including E. coli, salmonella, shigella, staphylococcus, Campylobacter cholera and viruses of different types can cause gastroenteritis. Salmonella or shigella gastroenteritis is a common form of gastrointestinal infection that can cause misery for travelers. Acute infectious gastroenteritis causes fever, headache, nausea, abdominal pain, and vomiting, severe diarrhea, which can result in marked dehydration, bacteremia with sepsis and sometimes death if not treated in time and properly. When traveling abroad in certain countries, it is prudent to avoid drinking the water. Use only bottled water even to wash the mouth or to brush one's teeth. Do not eat raw or rare meat. Eat meat or fish that is well cooked. Eat only hard-boiled eggs. Do not eat uncooked vegetables of any kind. Before leaving to go away, make sure you check with your physician to get you a supply of Cipro 750 mg tablets or 500 mg. to be taken one tablet twice per day in the event you get sick with diarrhea. Levaquin 500 mg once per day is just as effective to treat infectious gastroenteritis. Erythromycin 500 mg 4 times per day is the treatment of choice for infectious gastroenteritis that is caused by Campylobacter. Anti-diarrhea medications such as Lomotil, Imodium, and Kaopectate suspension are important to have on hand to treat the diarrhea. Compazine 10 mg tablets to be taken 3 times per day for nausea or vomiting or Zofran 4 mg once per day also are important to treat the symptoms of acute gastroenteritis. Pepto-Bismol taken one tablespoon 4 times per day helps to ease some of the crampy symptoms of acute gastroenteritis. Do not be alarmed if your stool becomes black when taking Pepto-Bismol, it is not blood; it is the bismuth in the Pepto-Bismol that becomes black because of bacterial actions on it. Tarry-black stool, called melena, smells distinctly like old blood and is a terrible smell. Pepto-Bismol associated black stool smells like regular stool, except it is black. When not sure, check with your physician.

Frequently, acute infectious gastroenteritis requires treatment in the hospital with IV fluid, electrolyte replacement IV and IV antibiotics. The IV fluid must contain dextrose with sodium chloride of different concentrations. The purpose of the dextrose is to maintain the affected patients in an anabolic state to hasten recovery. In that setting, even a diabetic patient can be given dextrose with added regular insulin. More commonly, the affected patient can be treated at home with medications by mouth.

Acute gastroenteritis can also be due to viruses. Viral gastroenteritis is quite common and can be very severe if not treated promptly and properly and can lead to a multitude of complications such as electrolyte imbalance, cardiac arrhythmia, renal failure and DIC, depending on different underlying chronic medical problems and the age of the individuals affected, and death can result.

Treatments of viral gastroenteritis are fluid IV or by mouth to prevent dehydration and electrolyte replacement by mouth by ways of soups, sodas, juices or IV. Antipyretics such as Advil and Tylenol are important to bring fevers down. Anti-diarrhea and anti-nausea medications such as just described above are very important in dealing with these conditions.

Differentiating bacterial, viral, fungal or parasitic gastroenteritis is left to the judgment and clinical experience of the examining physician. He or he can usually arrive at the proper diagnosis with a high degree of certainty.

Intestinal parasitism is quite common in people who originate or travel to the tropics or who live in the rural parts of the southern United States. Intestinal parasitism is also commonly seen in people who migrated to the United States from Southeast Asia and other third world countries where poor sanitation and poverty are prevalent. Examples of intestinal parasites are Enactor americanus, Trichuris trichiura, Schistosoma mansoni, Tenia saginata, Tenia solium, Ascaris lumbricoides, pinworm, hookworm, etc. Pinworm is said to infect about 200 million worldwide and about 30 to 40 million of them are in the United States and Canada. It is estimated that hookworms infest about 700 million in the world and the daily blood loss is estimated at 7 million liters. Trichuris trichiura infects about 500 million people in the world. Two million people in the United States are infected with hookworm. Ascaris infestation is a very common parasitic infestation. One quarter of the world's population of 6.5 billion is infected with ascaris and about 4 million Americans are infected with this worm.

The symptoms of intestinal parasitic infection are many and can manifest as nausea, vomiting, constipation, diarrhea, weakness, dizziness, headache, chronic cough, skin rash, generalized itchiness, etc. In recent years, there has been a greater increase in intestinal parasitism brought about by the AIDS epidemic. People who are immunosuppressed are more prone to be infested by parasites of all types including Giardia lamblia, amoeba, etc.

Medications such as Mebendazole, Pyrantel pamoate, Piperazine citrate, and Flagyl can be used to treat different types of parasitic infection. Without any doubt, parasitic infestations afflict more men of color than white men because parasitism is associated with poverty and poor sanitary conditions due to poor housing and overall poor living conditions, which are more common in minority men. Among the conditions that facilitate parasitic infestations are the absence of toilets and lack of running water. Some of these people, due to poverty, walk barefooted, exposing their feet to fecal materials, permitting parasites to enter into their bloodstream and, with no water available to wash hands after bowel movements, hands soiled with parasite-contaminated stool that provides an entry point for intestinal parasitism and all its serious medical complications. Ischemic colitis usually occurs in the elderly with multiple medical problems such as diabetes mellitus, atherosclerotic heart disease, etc.

Ischemia colitis occurs when the blood flow to the affected bowel is impeded either because the patient's blood pressure falls for one reason or another, preventing blood to flow properly to perfuse the bowel. Lack of blood flow causes a segment of the bowel to become ischemic, resulting in abdominal pain. Sometimes, the circulation of blood is occluded by a clot that is thrown to that area from an embolus, usually from the heart, resulting in occlusion of blood causing ischemia of that part of the bowel, which means, if not diagnosed quickly, the affected bowel will die resulting in a multitude of complications with possible death as a final result.

Surgical resection is frequently carried out to treat ischemic colitis. Once ischemic colitis becomes a serious consideration in the differential diagnosis of abdominal pain in an elderly person who presents to the doctor with abdominal pain, a flat plate of the abdomen must be done. A sign called finger printing can sometimes be seen on that x-ray film and if seen, ischemic colitis is highly possibly present. However, even if that is seen or not seen, angiogram is necessary to confirm the presence of ischemic colitis. The most frequently used treatment of ischemia colitis is surgical resection of the ischemic bowel.

Intestinal obstruction is an extremely common medical problem, which brings patients to physicians complaining of nausea, vomiting, and abdominal pain, and feeling generally sick. The list of things that can cause both small and the large intestine to be obstructed is quite long. Things such as:

1. Adhesions resulting from previous abdominal surgical procedures
2. Fecal impaction
3. Tumor of different types
4. In the third world and to some degree in rural south of the United States, where parasitic infestations are common, certain parasites such as ascaris can cause obstruction of the bowel.

There are many inflammatory conditions such as ulcerative colitis or Crohn's disease that can destroy and narrow the lumen of the bowel, causing fistula to develop, resulting in intestinal obstruction. At the other extreme, these inflammatory bowel diseases can at times present with a condition called megacolon, whereby the lumen of the bowel becomes markedly enlarged, representing a surgical emergency. Megacolon is best diagnosed by obtaining a simple x-ray of the abdomen called flat plate of the abdomen. There are many things or conditions that can cause the intestine to become mechanically obstructed or to lose its ability to contract, resulting in the backing up of intestinal contents, resulting in nausea, vomiting, abdominal pain, etc.

Colorectal cancers are common in all groups in the United States. These cancers are more common in minority men as compared to white men. That is due to many reasons, and prominent among these reasons are the fat-rich diet that minority men eat and the fact that 50% of black men, 40% of Mexican-American males and 41% of American Indian men are obese, and the fact that minority men, as a rule, go less frequently to physicians to be examined. By the time a man develops symptoms such as abdominal pain, nausea, vomiting, diarrhea, rectal bleeding because of colorectal cancer, often the cancer is already in an advanced stage. If the man is lucky, the rectal bleeding might be due to a precancerous polyp or some other nonmalignant lesion.

Intestinal obstruction is treated with a Cantor tube that is passed through the nose into the bowel. That tube has a little bag at the end of it filled with mercury to pull it down into the bowel slowly, forcing the area of obstruction to open. Every day an x-ray of the abdomen is obtained to see the progress of the tube and to see if the obstruction has opened up. The tube is attached to a machine called the Gomco machine to suction gastrointestinal contents, relieving the nausea, vomiting and abdominal pain. During that period of time, the patient is fed with intravenous fluid containing saline, glucose and potassium chloride. Suctioning GI contents in that fashion causes the loss of a large amount of potassium chloride and it is crucial that potassium be replaced to prevent severe hypokalemia, which can cause serious cardiac complications.

Rectal fissures are lesions of the rectum, which represent cracks in the rectal tissue. They can bleed and are quite painful. Rectal fissures are treated with Sitz baths and different ointments made specifically for treating superficial rectal ailments.

Hemorrhoids are tissue protrusions that occur immediately inside the rectum (internal hemorrhoids) or immediately outside the rectum (external hemorrhoids). Hemorrhoids may at times be associated with obesity, causing undue pressure to the anal area, and pregnancy, resulting in weight gain and pressure to the anal area. Both pregnancy and obesity occur more frequently in minority men than in white men. That is to say, minority men, as a rule, have more children than white men and with each pregnancy the incidence of developing hemorrhoids increases.

Many other factors are associated with hemorrhoids having nothing to do with obesity or pregnancies.

Conditions such as constipation commonly lead to the development of hemorrhoids. Colorectal cancer can at times result in the development of hemorrhoids or the aggravation of pre-existing hemorrhoids. If pre-existing hemorrhoids suddenly got worse, either by bleeding or by coming out, causing pain that may be the result of an obstructing lesion above in the colon or the rectal area, causing straining at stooling. The high pressure generated during straining causes the development of hemorrhoids and the aggravation of pre-existing hemorrhoids.

It is therefore always necessary to pay close attention to the complaints of rectal bleeding or worsening of pre-existing hemorrhoids by undertaking a lower gastrointestinal evaluation by a skilled gastroenterologist to be certain that no underlying cancerous mass is causing the obstruction.

Inguinal hernia can be associated with colorectal cancer. An obstructing mass within the large bowel inevitably causes the person harboring the mass to generate a great deal of pressure in the muscle of the lower abdomen. That set of interactions can result in tearing of intra-abdominal muscle causing the development of inguinal hernia. It is therefore very important to investigate a man who is in the cancer age group, age 45 and older, who spontaneously develops an inguinal hernia. Any man who fits that profile ought to have a lower GI evaluation with either a barium enema or a colonoscopy before he undergoes an inguinal hernia repair.

Other conditions that can cause abdominal pain include:

1. Gall bladder disease
2. Cholecystis (inflammation of the gall bladder)
3. Pancreatitis
4. Appendicitis

Gall bladder disease occurs because of stones that form inside the gall bladder. Chronic hemolytic diseases such as sickle cell anemia, beta-thalassemia, alpha-thalassemia, hereditary spherocytosis, etc, can cause bilirubin stones to form in the gall bladder. Other stones that are frequently formed in the gall bladder include cholesterol stones and a mixture of bilirubin and cholesterol stones. Obesity is also associated with an increase incidence of gall stone disease. After gastric by-pass surgery, gallstones frequently develop. Other predisposing factors for gallstones formation include being Eskimo and Native American Indians. Both these racial groups have a high incidence of gall stone disease. The most common symptoms of gall bladder disease are:

1. Nausea
2. Vomiting
3. Right upper abdominal pain

4. Poor appetite
5. Fever
6. Chills

The best way to evaluate a patient for the symptoms of gall bladder disease is to

1. Take a complete history
2. Do a complete physical examination
3. Do a CBC
4. Do an SMA20 chemistry profile
5. Do Serum amylase and Lipase
6. Do a flat and upright of the abdomen to look for free air under the diaphragm
7. Do an abdominal sonogram

The best way to treat gall bladder disease if the patient has no pain and fever or chills is with a low fat diet. If the patient is symptomatic, is to refer the patient to a surgeon for Cholecystectomy.

Pancreatitis (inflammation of the pancreas) is commonly seen in alcohol abusers (alcoholics) or in individuals with gall stone disease. Gall bladder disease is the second most common cause of pancreatitis.

The symptoms of pancreatitis are:

1. Nausea
2. Vomiting
3. Left upper abdominal pain
4. Sometime fever and chills can develop

The best way to evaluate a patient for pancreatitis is to do:

1. Take a complete history
2. Do a complete physical examination
3. Do a CBC
4. DO an SMA20 chemistry profile
5. Do serum amylase and Lipase
6. Do a serum alcohol level
7. Do a flat and upright of the abdomen (X-ray) to look for free air under the diaphragm
8. Do an abdominal sonogram
9. Admit the patient to the hospital
10. Keep the patient NPO (food or water by mouth)
11. Start the patient on IV fluid of D5 Normal saline at 150 or 200cc per hour

12. Give the patient anti nausea and anti vomiting medication either IV or IM
13. Give the Tylenol suppository if he is febrile
14. Give patient pain medication either IV or IM
15. Do daily serum amylase, Lipase, CBC and SMA 20 chemistry profile
16. Replace potassium IV as necessary
17. When the situation quiets down, start the patient on low fat, clear liquid diet and advance the diet as necessary.
18. Place patient the on alcohol withdrawal protocol to prevent delirium tremens (DT's)

Frequently, acute pancreatitis that occurs because of alcoholism goes on to develop chronic pancreatitis if the person continues to drink alcohol. Chronic pancreatitis can lead to a multitudes of serious problems such as:
1. Chronic relapsing pancreatitis
2. Chronic abdominal pain
3. Weight loss
4. Poor appetite
5. Chronic diarrhea
6. Chronic nausea
7. Recurrent hospitalizations
8. Abuse of pain medication

In addition, the chronic pancreatitis can lead to pseudo cyst formation with secondary infection of these cysts, which may have to be drained surgically and treated with antibiotics. Sometimes, the pancreas fails altogether causing constant greasy diarrhea containing undigested foods. When his happens, secondary diabetes mellitus often develops requiring the use of insulin.

Viral hepatitis occurs quite commonly in some men. There are three major types of viral hepatitis.
1. Hepatitis A
2. Hepatitis B
3. Hepatitis C

Viral hepatitis occurs predominantly via the oral fecal route although. There are several reports in the literature showing that it can be transmitted as a blood born infection in rare occasions.

The incubation period for hepatitis A is 4 weeks. (the time period

The Symptoms of hepatitis A are when the virus enters into a person's system and the development of symptoms).
1. Malaise
2. Anorexia

3. Nausea
4. Vomiting
5. Joints pain
6. Body aches
7. Head ache
8. Fever
9. Chills
10. Sore throat
11. Runny nose

Take a complete history from the patient including a detailed travel history and any restaurant that he may have gone to and ask if the patient ate raw seafoods recently.

Physical examination usually reveals:

1. Jaundice of the skin
2. Scleral icterus (yellowish in the white part of the eyes)
3. Enlarged and tender liver
4. Sometime an enlarged spleen
5. Elevated temperature
6. Rapid pulse rate

What blood tests to do evaluate a person for hepatitis A:

1. Do a CBC
2. Do a SMA 20 chemistry profile
3. Do a Prothrombin time
4. Do a Hepatitis A, B, and C profile
5. Do an abdominal ultrasound

The treatments for hepatitis include:

Bed rest
Control fever with low dose Tylenol
Control nausea and vomiting with Zofran
Monitor Prothrombin time
Monitor CBC
Monitor SMA 20 chemistry profile
If the patient cannot keep foods and water down
Admit the patient to the hospital for in hospital care
If the prothrombin time is elevated, monitor the patient for possible liver failure.

Most patients with hepatitis A recover. Hepatitis A has no chronic sequalea.

There is a vaccine in use to prevent hepatitis A. It is called VAQTA. It is recommended for individuals who are at high risk of contracting hepatitis A and for those people who are infected with hepatitis B and C.

Hepatitis B is a blood born viral illness that is contracted usually through blood, semen, urine and other body fluid. Intravenous drug abusers are frequently infected with hepatitis B. Hemophiliacs are frequently infected with hepatitis B. People who receive blood and blood products are sometime infected with hepatitis B. People who get tattoos placed on their skins can get infected with hepatitis B and the hepatitis B virus can be transmitted through sexual intercourse. Worldwide, the incidence of hepatitis B is about 200 millions.

The incubation period for hepatitis B is 4–12 weeks.

The symptoms of hepatitis B include:
1. Fatigue
2. Head ache
3. Lassitude
4. Nausea
5. Runny nose
6. Fever
7. Chills
8. Vomiting
9. Abdominal pain
10. Poor appetite
11. Body aches and pain
12. Joints aches and pain

How to evaluate a patient with hepatitis B infection:
1. Take a complete history
2. Do a complete physical examination

On physical examination, the following might be found:
1. sign of weight loss
2. Jaundice of the skin
3. Jaundice of the white part of the eyes
4. Elevated temperature
5. Tender abdomen
6. Enlarged liver
7. Enlarged spleen

What laboratory tests to order in a patient with hepatitis B
1. Do a CBC
2. Do an SMA 20 chemistry profile and serum LDH

3. Do hepatitis B surface antigen and antibody, HBe antigen and antibody
4. Do PT, INR and PTT
5. Do RNA, CPR Viral load
6. Do hepatitis B genotype

What radiology tests to do:

1. Do and abdominal ultrasound
2. Do a chest x-ray

Do a baseline EKG on the patient

How to treat a patient with Hepatitis B:

If the PT and INR are normal and the patient can eat and drink fluid, and is not toxic looking, the patient is best kept at home on best rest and fever control with low dose Tylenol. If the PT and INR are elevated and or the patient looks toxic, then, the patient ought to be admitted to the hospital for in hospital care.

In the hospital, the patient must be kept in isolation with needles and body fluid precautions to avoid infecting the treating medical, nursing and other treating staffs.

Hepatitis infection has different clinical manifestations and different stages.

1. It may be subclinical
2. It may become subacute
3. It may become chronic persistent
4. It may become chronic active
5. It may become fulminant
6. It may entered into the carrier stage

At the appropriate time, a liver biopsy must be done to determined stages 3, 4 and 5. of hepatitis B.

The medications available to treat hepatis Be are

1. Lamividine
2. Adefovir
3. Entecovir

The hepatitis B virus while showing good response to Amividine and Adefovir, resistance to these two medications frequently develop. So far there has bee no evidence of resistance to Entecovir, making it the best medication to treat hepatitis B.

Response to these medications prevents persistent elevation of the hepatitis B organism decreasing the possibility of cirrhosis of the liver and cancer of the liver.

These medications must be used continuously or else the viral load will go back up resulting, in all the chronic problems associated with hepatitis B.

There is a vaccination in use to prevent hepatitis B; it is sold under the name Recombivax HB.

The other most common virus that can cause hepatitis in the US is hepatitis C virus.

There are 4 million individuals with hepatitis C in the US and every year, 10,000 people die as result of hepatitis C in the US.

Hepatitis C has an incubation period of 30 to 180 days.

Hepatitis C is a blood borne infection. All body fluids such as sperm, saliva, urine and vaginal secretion contain the hepatitis C and can transmit if contact is made with them in an infected individual. Hepatitis C infection is very common in intravenous elicit drug users. Other individuals commonly infected with hepatitis C are hemophiliacs, people who are on dialysis, people who receive blood and blood products and hepatitis C can also be transmitted sexually.

The Symptoms of hepatitis C are:

1. Fatigue
2. Loss of appetite
3. Head ache
4. Runny nose
5. Muscle pain
6. Joints pain
7. Nausea
8. Vomiting
9. Abdominal pain
10. Fever
11. Chills
12. Etc

The physical findings in hepatitis C are:

Jaundice of the eyes
Jaundice of the skin
Enlarged liver
Enlarged spleen

The laboratory findings in hepatitis C are:

Low white blood cells count
Sometimes high white blood cells count
Low platelets counts
Low red cells count

Elevated liver functions tests SGOT, SGPT, Alkaline phosphate, LDH, and total bilirubin) The prothrombin time may be elevated On radiographic examinations such as abdominal ultrasound and CAT scan, both the liver and the spleen can be enlarged.

How to evaluate a patient for hepatitis C:

1. Take a complete history
2. Do a complete physical examination
3. Do a hepatitis C blood profile
4. Do hepatitis C genotype
5. Do hepatitis C viral load if the blood test for hepatitis C is positive
6. Do a CBC
7. Do an SMA20 chemistry profile
8. Do PT INR and PTT
9. Do abdominal ultrasound
10. Do abdominal CAT scan when appropriate
11. Do a base line Alpha feto protein blood test

There are 6 genotypes of hepatitis C and some of these genotypes are more responsive to treatments than others.

How to treat patients who have hepatitis C:

Acute hepatitis C is treated with

1. Bed rest
2. Fever control with low dose NSAID'S
3. Anti-emetic to control nausea and vomiting
4. Plenty of fluid and foods as tolerated
5. If the patient cannot keep foods and water down, the patient ought to be hospitalized and intra hospital treatments such as IV fluid administered etc.
6. If the prothrombin time is elevated and the patient looks very sick, he should be admitted into the hospital for close monitoring because of the possibility of liver failure and disseminated intravascular coagulopaty.

Many patients, recovered from hepatitis C with no long term sequalea.

On the other hand, many individuals develop a chronic stage of hepatitis that if not treated leads to cirrhosis of the liver. The cirrhosis associated with chronic hepatic frequently leads to hepato cellular carcinoma of the liver. (Cancer of the liver).

The medications in use to treat chronic hepatitis C are:

1. Pegelated Alpha interferon SQ
2. Ribiviran by mouth

There are 4 millions individuals with hepatitis C in the US and 10,000 individuals die yearly from hepatitis C.

Many other gastrointestinal diseases are seen commonly in men; therefore, it is crucial that men pay close attention to the multitude of factors outlined in his chapter to help them from falling victims of these diseases.

CHAPTER 10

ANEMIAS IN MEN

Anemia is common problem in men.
The most common reasons for anemia in men are:
1. Bleeding
2. Abnormal hemoglobin
3. Autoimmune hemolytic anemia
4. AIDS
5. Starvation
6. Chronic infection
7. Chronic diseases
8. Cancer
9. Chemotherapy
10. B12 deficiency
11. Folic acid deficiency
12. Iron deficiency
13. Chronic kidney failure
14. Arthritis
15. Collagen vascular diseases
16. Alcoholism
17. Malaria
18. Parasitic infestation
19. Iron overload diseases etc;

Bleeding causes anemia in men due to
1. Trauma
2. Gastrointestinal bleeding

3. Bleeding from the kidneys
4. Bleeding from the urinary bladder
5. Bleeding from the kidneys

What is anemia?

Anemia is a condition in which the human body has too little blood. In other for anemia to occur, the following criteria have to be met.

1. A person is bleeding out red blood cells
2. A person is hemolyzing red blood cells
3. A person is not making enough red blood cells
4. Or a combination of the above

Why is too little blood bad for the body?

Too little blood is bad for the body because blood is needed to carry oxygen to all the organs in the body for proper body functions.

When an individual is anemic, the different organs in the body are deprived of the proper amount of oxygen, resulting in the condition referred to as anoxia. An anoxic organ can become sick because of oxygen deficiency. Red blood cells contain a substance called hemoglobin. Hemoglobin has as its function to bind with oxygen in order to carry it to the different places in the human body where it is needed. There exists an invisible man-conceived curve in the human body called the Oxygen Dissociation Curve. When the right amount of oxygen is present in the blood, that curve is well balanced in the middle and is shifted to the right to deliver oxygen to the tissues. When something happens that causes anemia to develop, the result is that the red blood cells hold onto oxygen, and the curve is shifted to the left, resulting in the inability of the red cells to discharge their content of oxygen to the different tissues in the body, resulting in improper perfusion of the tissues with oxygen. The Oxygen Dissociation Curve is also influenced by the pH of the blood.

What are some of the symptoms of anemia?

To answer that question one must know how long the person has been anemic and how severe the anemia is. A normal hemoglobin and hematocrit in a man is 42–50% hematocrit and 14–16 grams of hemoglobin The more acute the blood loss or hemolysis or inability to produce red blood cells results in lower red blood cell count, which results in anemia—the less able an individual is to tolerate it. The younger the man who is losing blood is, the better he is able to tolerate the anemia. The older the man is who is acutely losing blood due to bleeding or hemolysis, the less well he is able to tolerate the anemia. Older men are more likely to have underlying medical problems, such as heart disease, kidney disease, hardening of the arteries in the brain, etc., making it easier for the anemia to complicate these already precarious conditions.

Men who have had anemia for a long time are better able to tolerate their anemia, because they have had enough time for their bodies to adjust to the effects of the anemia. In time, many of these chronically anemic men's vital organs, such as the heart, the brain, the kidneys and many other organs would be affected by the anemic state but it would happen gradually. The most common symptoms of anemia are:

5. Weakness
6. Malaise
7. Headaches
8. Shortness of breath
9. Tiredness
10. Irritability
11. Depression
12. Chest pain
13. Insomnia etc.

What conditions must exist in the human body before anemia can occur?

1. A person must be bleeding or must have bled.
2. A person must be hemolyzing red blood cells (that is, breaking up red blood cells in the body).
3. A person's bone marrow must have stopped producing red blood cells because of bone marrow failure, such as occurs in pure red cells aplasia or aplastic anemia
4. The bone marrow cavity have been replaced by other cells, such as cancer cells etc., leaving little or no room for red blood cells to be made, or
5. The bone marrow may also be replaced by fibrous tissues such as occurs in a condition known as myelofibrosis.

6.   When any combination of the aforementioned conditions develops at the same time anemia can also develops.

What are the physical signs of anemia?

The signs of anemia are many and frequently coincide with the type of anemia the person is suffering from.

If a man presents to the emergency room or to the doctor's office and is acutely bleeding, from the or the rectum, vomiting blood from an upper gastrointestinal tract or from the urinary tract, his pulse rate will be fast, his blood pressure might be low and he may be having pain.

Severe and acute bleeding from any of these sites resulting in about 1800 cc of blood loss or more will likely cause a drop in the blood pressure.

Another frequent sign of acute blood loss anemia is rapid heart rate.

The reason for the rapid heart rate is that, it is the heart's way of trying to make up the difference by increasing the cardiac output in an attempt to help deliver enough oxygen for proper body functions. If the anemia persists for many years, the heart may fail because of what is called high output failure.

Other physical signs of anemia include

1.   Paleness of the skin
2.   Pale nail beds
3.   Pale conjunctivae, in the entire human body the only place where naked vessels can be seen is in the eyes. By looking at the conjunctivae (the white of the eye) the examining physician can see blood vessels with the naked eyes and can tell if these vessels are pale, indicating anemia.
4.   In addition, if the patient is hemolyzing, different the examining physician in the person's eyes can observe degrees of icterus (yellowishness). (There are many other conditions having nothing to do with hemolytic anemia that can cause sclera icterus).
5.   Rapid breathing
     A flow heart murmur, which is a function of the thinness of the blood as it passes through the heart valves, can be heard.
6.   Sometimes the spleen can be palpated depending on the underlying disease causing the anemia
7.   Sometimes the liver can be palpated depending on the underlying disease causing the anemia
8.   Bronze looking skin as seen in individuals with thalassemia major etc.

What are the most common anemias seen in men?

The most common anemia seen in men includes:

1. Iron deficiency anemia
2. The second most common anemia seen in many black men, many Hispanic men, many Asian men, many Greek men, many Italian men, many Indian men and many men of Arabic descent are anemias such as sickle cell anemia (SS), sickle cell C (SC), sickle cell thalassemia, homozygous hemoglobin C, Alpha thalassemia and Beta thalassemia.
3. Another common anemia seen more frequently in men of color is lead poisoning-associated anemia. These men are exposed to lead as youngsters, and never realizing that they had that problem, therefore, they sought no treatment and as adults, they continue to suffer with that anemia.
4. Still another common anemia seen in many poor men is nutritional deficiency anemia. Many poor men are forced by virtue of their impoverished conditions not to eat nutritious foods because these foods are, for the most part, expensive. Moreover, that state of poor nutrition begins at an early age, as many poor young boys go to school with no breakfast and eat only the food that is provided as part of the school lunch program. The quality and quantity of these foods vary from communities to community in many instances; these foods are prototypes of fast foods, which are neither healthy nor nutritious. Frequently, a combination of these different anemias coexists in minority men, making their anemic state much more difficult to diagnose and treat. According to recent reports, 34 million American citizens live below the poverty line and 24.1% blacks in the U.S. live below the poverty line. It has also been reported that some 14 million children in the U.S. go to bed at night hungry and altogether 38 million individuals suffer from hunger in the US. In addition there are more than 100 hundred thousands homeless individuals in the US.
5. Alpha thalassemia is quite common in men of Southeast Asian, Mediterranean and Middle Eastern descent.
6. Beta thalassemia is quite common in men of Italian, Greek and Arabic descent.
7. Sickle cell disease-associated anemia is also seen in some subgroup of men from Italy, India and the Middle East.

8. Autoimmune hemolytic anemia is quite common in men and is frequently seen in association with lupus (SLE).
9. Pernicious anemia is also common in men.
10. B12 deficiency anemia is also quite common in men.
11. Folic acid deficiency anemia is quite common in men of all ethnic backgrounds, but more so in men who abuse alcohol.
12. Anemia of acute blood loss is also common in men and can occur for a variety of reasons.
13. Another common anemia frequently seen in men is anemia of chronic disease or anemia of inflammatory diseases.

The chronic diseases that cause anemia in men are:

1. Chronic renal failure
2. Diabetes mellitus
3. Cancers
4. Rheumatoid arthritis
5. Osteoarthritis
6. Alcoholism
7. Chronic hepatitis B
8. Chronic hepatitis C
9. Cirrhosis of the liver
10. Hemoglobinopathy
11. Hemochromatosis/iron overload
12. Chronic osteomyelitis
13. AIDS
14. Tuberculosis
15. Malaria
16. Parasitic infestation
17. Hemophilia A &B
18. VON Willebrand disease
19. Chronic diverticular bleeding
20. AV malformation with recurrent GI bleeding
21. Rendu-Osler-Weber disease with recurrent bleeding
22. Myelodysplastic syndrome
23. Myelofibrosis
24. Sideroblastic anemia
25. Chronic starvation
26. Pica for clay, starch etc.

What are the mechanisms of the different anemia seen in men?

Men have iron deficiency anemia because of blood loss because of gastrointestinal bleeding from different diseases of the GI tract, Pica, and eating foods that are poor in iron.

Men who migrated to the United States from regions of the world, such as South America, Latin America, Central America, the Caribbean, Africa and other tropical countries where the incidence of parasitic infestation is high, also suffer from iron deficiency anemia because of blood loss due to worms sucking blood from their intestines. Therefore, blood is lost in the stool. Parasitic infestation is quite a problem for these men, many of whom are surviving on a meager diet to begin with, while at the same time they are losing a significant percentage of their intake of nutrients to parasites that afford them no symbiosis in return. That is clearly an unfair deal.

Many men abuse alcohol significantly and an alcohol abuse is associated with many conditions that can cause iron deficiency anemia. For instance, alcohol abuse frequently causes gastritis. The blood that is lost because of gastritis can lead to iron deficiency anemia when the gastritis occurs recurrently, as is often the case. Alcohol abuse frequency causes esophageal varices with recurrent bleeding, and that too can cause iron deficiency anemia. Alcohol abuse frequently causes damage to the liver resulting in alcoholic liver disease (cirrhosis of the liver) which is the cause of esophageal varices. The incidence of colon cancer is quite high in men in the U.S., and one of the most common signs of colon cancer is iron deficiency anemia.

Many men suffer from a condition called Pica and all the different Picas are associated with iron deficiency anemia. The most common Picas are eating starch, clay, and ice.

Drinking tea with food in the stomach can cause a person not to be able to absorb iron that is contained in the food, making iron deficiency anemia worse. The reason why drinking too much tea can contribute to low iron level in the blood is because tea contains tannic acid, and tannic acid binds the iron that is in the food, preventing its absorption from the stomach. So men ought to be aware that drinking tea is okay but it is best to drink tea on an empty stomach.

Iron deficiency anemia can also occur as because of malabsorption. Some time the malabsorption is the result of a malabsorption disease such as sprue but some time it is due to the fact the individual is aged and is not able to produce sufficient acid in the stomach to allow for absorption of the iron the duodenum, which is the part of stomach where iron is absorbed.

The so-called anemia of chronic disease/anemia of inflammatory disease are in fact a form of iron deficiency anemia. Because in this form of anemia, there is plenty of iron in the body, but the iron is located in reticuloendothelial cells in the parts of the body where iron is stored. The iron cannot be carried to the early red blood cells to be incorporated within the early red blood cells to produce hemoglobin.

There are a series of phase II reacting proteins that develop in the body because of the chronic infectious/inflammatory state which prevent the transport protein (Transferrin) from being able to transport iron and deliver it to the erythroblasts in the bone marrow resulting in the anemia. The iron piles up in the tissues causing a form of secondary hemochromatosis/iron over load with damages to tissues because as the iron degrades, it releases free radicals and free radicals are damaging to human tissues creating all sort of problems such as

1. Iron deficiency state
2. Osteoarthritis
3. Erectile dysfunction
4. Cirrhosis of the liver
5. Type II diabetes mellitus
6. Anemia
7. Hypothyroidism
8. Adrenal deficiency
9. Gonadal hypofunction etc;

Because ferritin is a phase II reacting protein, it becomes elevated in the presence of all infections and inflammations. Serum ferritin equals serum iron and therefore, the higher the serum ferritin the higher the serum iron. Sometime the serum ferritin is high and yet a person may be iron deficient because as stated above, the iron cannot be transferred to early red cells or a person may be iron deficient because a person has lost blood chronically and lost iron as result. A person may have lost blood, becomes iron deficient and still has a high serum ferritin in many medical conditions.

Among these conditions are:

1. Sickle cell disease
2. Thalassemia
3. Hemochromatosis/Iron over load both primary and secondary
4. Hemochromatosis type 1,2,3 and 4
5. Chronic Hepatitis B and C
6. End stage renal failure
7. Rheumatoid Arthritis
8. Chronic osteomyelitis

9. Systemic Lupus Erythematosus
10. Mixed collagen vascular diseases
11. AIDS
12. Lymphoma etc:
13. Cancer
14. Other abnormal hemoglobin diseases etc;

To properly diagnosed iron deficiency anemia in face of a high serum ferritin, the best to do is Soluble Serum Transferrin Receptor Level. This test is elevated when true iron deficiency anemia exists and is not affected by inflammation or infection.

The different types of hemochromatosis/iron over laod:

The gene in the human body that controls the amount of iron
Which a person absorbed from foods is known as HFE.
This gene has two common mutations, C282Y and H63D.
The causative gene for type 1 hemochromatosis came out of Northern Europe.
1 in 10 individuals in Northern Europe caries this abnormal gene.
In other for a person to inherit homozygous type 1 hemochromatosis, he or she has to inherit one each of the C282Y gene from each parent.
The C282Y gene is located on position 6 of the HLA locus.
5 out 1000 individuals or 0.5 per cent in the US carry two copies of the C282Y genes making them susceptible to developing type 1 hemochromatosis.
Type 1 hemochromatosis is very rare in Blacks, Asians, Hispanics and American Indians.

Type 2 Hemochromatosis is the result of a genetic abnormality found
On the long arm of chromosome q1 and in many cases the abnormal gene is G320V. More recently, however a subtype has been discovered involving the hepcidin ferroportin axis.

Type 3 Hemocromatosis is limited to the liver and the mutation is due to TRF2 receptor.

Type 4 is very common in Southern European countries such Greece.
The abnormality is in the gene encoding for ferroportin.

Type 5 Hemochromatosis/African iron overload syndrome does not in reality occurs as originally described because many

Blacks who never been to Africa and therefore have never drank beer from iron contaminated drums have iron primary iron over load. Recent reports have shown that the so-called African iron over load is due to other genetic reasons i,e Source: Prevelance of Iron Overload in African-Americans:

A primary care Experience.

Prestige Medical News Feb, 7th, 2003

Valiere Alcena M.D.F.A.C.P.

The prevalent view now is that primary Hemochromatosis/iron overload is due to decrease Hepcidin level which allows perroportin to remain unchecked, resulting in the over absorption of iron. This condition is seen many whites, Asians, Latinos and people of other ethnic groups.

It is extremely rare to find the C282Y/H63D mutations in blacks and for that reason it makes no clinical sense to screen them routinely for for these mutations.

Hemochromatosis-primary/secondary/Iron overload is very serious medical condition.

It can affect people of all racial groups and all sexes. When present in a person as evidence by an elevate serum ferritin of 300 and over, it affects the following organs and can cause the following problems:

1. The hematopoeitic system causing anemia
2. Osteoarthritis
3. Cirrhosis of the liver
4. Hepatocellular cancer of the liver
5. Hepatomegaly (large spleen)
6. Cardiomegaly (enlarge heart)
7. Congestive heart failure
8. Cardiac arrhythmias
9. Gonadal deficiency
10. Erectal dysfunction (male sexual impotency)
11. Diabetes mellitus type II etc.

Hemochromatosis/Iron overload is frequently treated by 1.

1. Phlebotomy
2. Desferal SQ
3. Exjade by mouth for transfusion induced iron over load
4. Epogen/Procrit when there is anemia

Men who have hemochromatosis/iron overload from any cause, when they are anemic and therefore cannot have blood taking away from as a form of treatment, can be treated with Procrit/Epogen 10,000–20,000 units SQ every week or every 2 weeks.

This modality of treatment achieves two things:

1. It forces the iron across the threshold where transferring could not and places it into the early red blood cells to allow for the production of new red blood cells and hemoglobin thereby, correcting the anemia.

2. It mobilizes the iron from the tissues, preventing it from causing damage to them and uses it productively for the benefit of the affected person to treat the anemia.

There are no reports in the literature that Procrit/Epogen when used to treat anemia and iron over load causes side effects to patients.

Other medical conditions in which Procrit/Epogen is used:

1. Sickle cell anemia
2. Patients being treated with chemotherapy./Radiation for malignant diseases
3. Rheumatoid Arthritis to get patients ready for different types of surgical Procedures
4. Prior to major GYN surgical procedures to raise the HCT (oral iron is usually given at the same time)
5. End stage kidney failure
6. Chronic hepatic B and C
7. AIDS
8. Chronic Osteomyelitis
9. Osteoarthritis with anemia
10. Any chronic inflammatory/infectious disease conditions ect, that have anemia associated with them will respond to Procrit/Epogen by raising the HCT.
11. Sideroblastic anemia
12. Thalassemia
13. Autoimmune hemolytic anemia
14. Myolodysplastic Syndrome
15. Aplastic anemia etc;

This treatment eliminates the need for blood transfusion in many instances and its associated side effects, such as the possibility of contracting:

1. HIV
2. Hepatitis
3. Malaria
4. Syphilis

5. HTLVIII
6. Blood transfusion reactions etc, etc.

Treating patients with iron overload/secondary hemochromatosis who are anemic and therefore cannot be phlebotomized, with Procrit/Epogen 10,000–20,000 units SQ is the best treatment available. It is safe and effective and it has no known side effects and is highly recommended.

This treatment achieves two things:

1. It decreases the iron load thereby preventing it from damaging the tissues
2. It raises the hemoglobin/hematocrit thereby correcting the iron deficiency anemia making the affected men feel better and stronger.

When treating individuals who have end stage renal disease and sickle cell anemia with Epogen/Procrit, the hemoglobin ought not to be raised above 13 grams to prevent stroke or heart attacks. These individuals have very poor vessels and as such cannot tolerate the viscosity of a hemoglobin above 13 grams or a hematocrit above 36 %.

How to evaluate iron deficiency anemia in men

The first thing to do in evaluating men for iron deficiency state is to do a CBC, reticulocytes count, RDW, and serum ferritin. Iron deficiency has several stages. Stage 1 is called prelatent iron deficiency state. Stage 2 is called latent iron deficiency state or iron deficient erythropoiesis and Stage 3 is late latent or frank iron deficiency anemia.

Each millimeter of blood contains 0.5 mg of iron. It is said, according to the World Health Organization, that 1.6 billion people of the 5.6 billion people in the world suffer from iron deficiency anemia.

Iron deficiency is most probably much more common than the 1.3 billion reported by the World Health Organization. Iron deficiency state is defined as total body iron store depletion that leads ultimately to iron deficiency anemia. Long before iron deficiency anemia comes about, the loss of blood, and the iron it contains, had already begun. The first iron a man loses when he is bleeding slowly is the iron from the store, as reflected by the serum ferritin. Iron is stored as ferritin in the bone marrow, the muscles, the spleen, and other tissues of the body, including the iron that is located in the cytochrome system of the brain, which is needed for proper uses of oxygen by the brain to make the brain function well to carry the daily activities.

When the iron stored is depleted, even before evidence of anemia appears, men whose iron store is absent feel tired all the time, can't concentrate well, yawn a lot, become irritable easily, and feel overall unwell. An adult man usually has about 2 grams of iron in his iron store, which is the equivalent of eight units of blood. About 1.5 grams of iron is located in his circulating blood, which is the equivalent of six units of blood. Once he loses the entire iron store, as reflected by a serum ferritin of less than 10 to 15, then he begins to use up the circulating iron for the production of red cells. As the level of the circulating iron decreases, iron deficiency anemia starts to set in, which gets worse and worse over time, resulting in low hematocrit, low MCV and low red cells per million and high RDW. At that juncture, he looks pale and feels very tired. The numbers of men who suffer from iron deficiency state and iron deficiency anemia are in the billions.

It is important for a treating physician to understand iron kinetics to enable his to determine very early, whether that patient is slowly bleeding and losing iron. When an individual is bleeding slowly and occultly, the very first blood test to become abnormal is the RDW (red cells distribution width). The RDW becomes elevated when an individual begins to lose blood slowly. The RDW is elevated in all diseases that cause microcytosis, such as thalassemias, iron deficiency anemia and macrocytic anemias such as B12 deficiency, folic acid deficiency, and hemolytic anemias.

The next blood test that becomes abnormal when a person is bleeding slowly and chronically is the serum ferritin. Ferritin is a phase 2 reacting protein and therefore can be falsely high in inflammation and infection. It is therefore prudent to always interpret the serum ferritin with that fact in mind. Serum ferritin ought to be looked at as a scale, in that if the level of ferritin is going down, that represents blood and iron loss and the patient must be evaluated accordingly.

In men, the most common sources of blood loss are:

1. Gastrointestinal tract bleeding and
2. Bleeding from the urinary tract.
3. Rendu-Osler-Weber disease

In the case of cancer of the GI tract, the decreased level of serum ferritin can be detected very early, sometimes as much as four years prior to the person becoming anemic or prior to the person having any symptoms that might make his suspect that he may have colon cancer. It is, therefore, important to test the stool for occult blood, which is mixed with the rest of the stool, making it difficult for the eye to see. It takes 25 cc of blood in the gut to cause the stool hemoccult to become positive. The RDW comes with the CBC and, as just mentioned, is elevated in slow chronic bleeding. The serum ferritin test costs only about $56.00 in most clinical laboratories. When it is interpreted properly, the serum ferritin can help to save thousands of men from dying because of GI cancer, because, by evaluating these men early the doctor can remove the precancerous or cancerous lesion either endoscopically via biopsy or via colonoscopic biopsy.

A new test is now clinically available called the **Soluble Serum Transferrin Receptor Level**, which is much more sensitive to diagnosed iron deficiency anemia. This test is not affected by either infection or by inflammation. An elevated soluble serum ferritin level is firm evidence of iron deficiency anemia, even if the serum ferritin is normal or high. Iron is attached to the receptors in the transferrin protein to be carried to the early red blood cells in the bone marrow to produce new red blood cells. When there is no iron, these receptor sites remain unoccupied and, as such, their level is elevated, hence the value of that test.

Starting at age 40 men who are iron deficient ought to have a complete GI work up, involving both the lower and the upper GI tract with colonoscopy and endoscopy, to make sure that no precancerous or cancerous lesions are contributing to the iron deficiency before being started on iron therapy. In general, at age 40 Black men and Latino men should a colonoscopy. White males should have their first colonoscopy at age 50 unless they have GI symptoms or have, familial polyposis or have family history of colon cancer.

Other conditions that can cause iron deficiency consist of:

1. Gastroesophageal reflux disease
2. Peptic ulcer
3. Chronic gastritis associated with ingestion of aspirin or nonsteroidal anti-inflammatory drugs or alcohol abuse
4. Diverticulosis
5. Inflammatory bowel diseases, such as ulcerative colitis, Crohn's disease
6. Bleeding esophageal varices
7. Anemia of chronic diseases/Chronic inflammatory diseases (such as Rheumatoid Arthritis, Systemic Lupus erythematosus, Chronic Hepatitis B,C, Osteomylitis, Cirrhosis of the liver, Hemochromatosis, Chronic renal failure, Chronic hemolytic diseases, Osteoarthritis etc;

What can men do to prevent iron deficiency anemia and what are the best ways to treat it?

A simple bleeding test from the tip of a finger done of aspirin for two weeks and of NSAIDS for 12 hours can help to determine if a man has Von Willebrand's disease or not. The normal bleeding time is up to 7 minutes. Von Willebrand's disease consists of qualitative platelet abnormalities which prevent platelets from aggregating properly, resulting in prolonged bleeding. It is the most common bleeding abnormality in the world, affecting several million individuals to one degree or another. Making the diagnosis can in most instances be quite complicated, so when that diagnosis is being considered, it is a good idea to refer the man to a hematologist for both evaluation and treatment. A Von Willebran's profile can be done to establish this diagnosis.

Excessive bleeding due to Von Willebrand's disease is treated with 20 micrograms of Desmopressin (DDAVP) in 50 cc of normal saline IV over half an hour. The second treatment available for Von Willebrand's disease is fresh frozen plasma. The third treatment for Von Willerbrand disease is platelet infusion.

1. Men from third world countries and African-American men who reside in the rural South must have their stool tested for parasites, which, if found, can be in part responsible for chronic blood loss due to parasites attaching themselves to the wall of the bowel, sucking up blood, resulting in iron deficiency. Men who because of their living condition which place them at high risk for parasitic infestation and also because of menstrual blood loss and childbirth, associated blood loss, suffer from iron deficiency anemia more than their white counterparts. It is advisable for men with iron deficiency anemia, who either lived in the third world before at one point in the past or in the rural South of the U.S. or who visited countries where they could have been infested with parasites, to have their stool checked by the parasitology laboratory for the possibility that parasitism may be partly responsible for their iron deficiency.

2. Another common problem that some men are afflicted with that causes iron deficiency anemia is a habitual condition called pica. There are different types of pica—eating clay or other types of dirt, eating starch, or eating ice. In the United States, some men are afflicted with PICA and in particular those who reside in the South. Eating clay or starch binds iron as it goes to the stomach, preventing its absorption. PICA is a psychological problem that is developed

into a habit and it is very hard to stop. It is ingrained in part of some cultures in certain parts of the minority community and has been going on for hundreds of years and is very difficult to eradicate, but it must be dealt with because it adds to the degree of iron deficiency anemia that these men suffer from.

3. Still another contributing factor to iron deficiency anemia is drinking tea with one's meal. It is a small contributing factor to iron deficiency, but it is one, nevertheless. Tea contains tannic acid, which binds iron in the stomach, preventing its absorption. The best way for a man to drink tea is on an empty stomach or three or four hours after eating iron-containing foods to allow the stomach a chance to absorb the iron.

If the iron deficiency anemia is severe, sometimes, blood transfusion is necessary. Otherwise, iron deficiency is best treated with iron tablets by mouth. There are several iron preparations on the market such as Ferrous Sulfate, Ferrous Gluconate, Ferrous Fumarate, Slow Fe, Chromagen Forte, etc. Chromagen Forte is the best iron preparation on the market. It contains 151 mg of elemental iron, 60 mg of vitamin C, 1 mg of folic acid and 10 mcg of B12. The dose is one capsule per day. It is, though, quite a bit more expensive than the other iron preparations.

In order to treat iron deficiency properly, patients must take one 325 mg tablet daily for one week with foods, then one tablet twice per day for one week, then one tablet three times per day.

Other of anemia frequently seen in many men is hereditary hemolytic anemia.

The genetic abnormalities that cause this different anemia are quite different and, because, the severity varies. The severest of these anemias is sickle cell anemia. 8.5% of the Black-American population carries the sickle cell gene (sickle cell trait). That number is the same between Hispanics and Caribbean Blacks.

According to the most recent U.S. Census Bureau, there are 304 million people in the U.S. There are 40.2 million Blacks (13.8% of the total U.S. population). There are 44.3 million Hispanics (14.8% of the total U.S. population) .70, 000 Black-Americans actually have sickle cell anemia, the homozygous type (full-blown sickle cell disease) and 2,500,000 of them have sickle cells trait. At birth, 1:625 Black-American babies born are expected to develop sickle cell disease. Worldwide there are 10 millions people with sickle cell anemia. In Nigeria there are 4 million people with sickle cell anemia. Sickle cell disease has an important historical background. It was the research done in sickle cell anemia that gave birth to the entire field of molecular biology. The discovery that the substitution of valine for glutamic acid in position 6 of the beta globulin chain is responsible for the basic abnormality that causes red blood cells to sickle in people who carry the sickle cell gene.

A cardiologist from Chicago first discovered sickle cell disease, the clinical entity, in the U.S. in 1910. He made the discovery in a young black dental student from the island of Grenada in the Caribbean. That molecular abnormality causes the red blood cell of the sickle cell patient to become sticky and deformed and develop into a half-moon or banana-shaped cell.

The normal red cell is disc-shaped.

These abnormalities in the red cell membranes cause the red cells to develop a great deal of difficulty passing through small vessels to deliver oxygen to tissues of the heart, the brain, the kidneys, the liver, the bone, the eyes, the spleen, the skin, the muscle and the rest of the tissues of the body. The lack of oxygen delivery to these different organs is responsible for many of the problems associated with sickle cell disease.

Historically, the sickle cell gene can be traced to three main areas of Africa. The most prevalent sickle cell gene came from Benin near Nigeria in Central Africa. Another gene came from Senegal on the West Coast of Africa. The third gene came from the Bantu-speaking area of Central Africa.

The same three genes can be found within North American Blacks and in the Caribbean. The African slaves who were brought here against their will to work the fields and to do forced labor brought these sickle cell genes to the North American continent during the slave trade. Over the close to 500 years since slavery started, the sickle cell gene has had ample time to penetrate the North American Black race causing much devastation and leaving a lot of pain, suffering, despair and death in its wake. As early as 1670, there is evidence that clinical sickle cell disease existed in a Ghanaian family. Sickle cell disease does not only affect Blacks. Sickle cell disease affects some Indians, Italians, and Arabs, and the same percentage of Hispanics throughout the Americas is affected by sickle cell disease as are Blacks, which is 8.5%.

Sickle cell disease is a preventable disease, if individuals who carry the gene for that deadly disease would learn the pros and cons of how the disease is inherited. If a man who is not carrying the sickle cell trait gene marries with a woman who is carrying the gene for sickle cell trait and they decide to have children, 50% of the children will be born without the sickle cell gene and 50% will carry it. If both individuals are carrying the sickle cell trait, 25% of their children will be born normal, 25% will be born with the full-blown sickle cell disease and 50% will be born carrying the sickle cell trait. If one of them has the full-blown sickle cell disease and the other is normal, 100% of the children will be born carrying the sickle cell trait. If one of these two individuals is carrying the sickle cell trait (AS) and one has the full-blown sickle cell disease (SS), 50% of the children will be born with the sickle cell trait (AS) and 50% will be born with the full-blown sickle cell disease (SS). If both of these individuals have full-blown sickle cell disease (SS), 100% of their children will be born with full-blown sickle cell disease (SS).

Once a person is carrying either the sickle cell trait (AS) or sickle cell disease (SS), many factors interplay to make that person sick and suffer from sickle cell disease.

What makes sickle cell anemia so deadly as a disease is the inability of the hemoglobin S to carry oxygen to the different tissues and organs of the body for proper body functions. The basic defect of the hemoglobin molecule is the substitution of Valine for Glutamic acid in the beta globulin chain at position 6, as mentioned earlier, which causes sickle cell hemoglobin to gel where there is lack of oxygen. That process is called polymerization. This basic abnormality is responsible for most of what is wrong in sickle cell disease. Because of polymerization, the red cells become stiff and sticky and therefore are unable to pass freely through small vessels such as venules, arterioles, capillaries and other medium-sized vessels, resulting in vascular occlusion. Vascular occlusion occurs because of these sticky, misshaped, half-moon or banana-shaped red cells prevents red cells from delivering oxygen normally to tissues in the body of men affected by sickle cell disease.

White blood cells also contribute to the occlusive processes that occur in sickle cell disease. White cells secrete a series of adhesive proteins that result in an inflammatory reaction within the vessels of the individuals with sickle cell disease. That inflammatory reaction participates in the vascular occlusion that occurs in painful sickle cell crisis. Platelets may also contribute to the vascular occlusion processes by secreting abnormal proteins within the vessels of these individuals as well.

Sickle cell disease is a multi-system disease and, as such, affects all major and minor organs in the human body, starting with the skin, which is the largest organ in the human body. The lower extremities can develop ulcers due to skin breakdown. The brain of a sickle cell patient is damaged early in life and can become severely damaged, resulting frequently in stroke at an early age, from 4 to 6 years old.

Men with sickle cell disease frequently present acutely with one or several of the following crises:

1. Painful sickle cell crisis
2. Hemolytic crisis
3. Hypoplastic crisis
4. Acute chest syndrome
5. A combination of all the aforementioned crises occurring in tandem
6. Splenic sequestration in sickle thalassemia or sickle cell C disease
7. Priapism

Painful sickle cell crisis

Painful sickle cell crisis occurs as because of occlusion of the small vessels in the body due to the misshaped, sticky red cells making it difficult for them to pass through these vessels to carry oxygen for proper perfusion of tissues. The lack of oxygen delivery to these tissues results in tissue anoxia. The anoxic tissues secrete kinins, mentioned earlier, which cause the burning pain in different parts of the body. That pain can at times be quite severe. The basis of the painful crisis is that when the body of the sickle cell patient is under stress, such as infection, which raises the pulse rate, causing the need for more oxygen delivery to tissues to be more severe, and when that need cannot be met, that further aggravates the anoxia, causing a painful crisis to be triggered and made worse.

Another frequent predisposing factor in the development of painful crises is cold weather, which causes vasoconstriction, preventing oxygen delivery to tissues in sufficient amounts, causing ischemia to occur in these tissues, and the result is pain.

Most recently, new information has come out in the literature outlining some of the mechanisms responsible for the occlusive nature of sickle cell disease. The sickled red cells cause damage to the inner lining of blood vessels. The damaged inner lining of blood vessels produces a series of adhesion proteins. These adhesion proteins are said to play a major role in causing occlusion of red blood cells, resulting in painful sickle cell crises. It is believed that both white blood cells and platelets produce proteins that play a role in the vascular occlusive nature of sickle cell disease (Ref.: *American Society of Hematology Education Program Book, 1998*).

Treatment of painful sickle cell crisis

The painful sickle cell crisis is best treated with pain medication such as Dilaudid IM or by mouth, morphine sulfate IM, IV or by mouth, Percocet, by mouth, Toradol by mouth or IM, and IV fluids. Some men with sickle cell disease, by virtue of the fact that they have an enlarged heart due to repeated assault to the heart by the sickle cell disease over a long period of time, may be in heart failure chronically, so giving them IV fluids may be detrimental. It is important that men with sickle cell disease who come with painful crisis be evaluated thoroughly by physical examination and by chest x-ray to be certain that they do not have congestive heart failure before being given large amounts of fluid. Giving too much fluid to a sickler can throw the patient into pulmonary edema, which, if not understood quickly, can result in the death of the patient. It is important to do a blood test called Beta Natriuretic Peptide (BNP) which if elevated indicates the presence of congestive heart failure.

Pain medication, oxygen, and transfusion of fresh blood are indicated in the treatment of patients with sickle cell disease who are in pain.

It must be clearly understood that the vast majority of patients with sickle cell disease who suffer with recurrent painful crises are, by necessity, addicted to the pain medications that they have been receiving over the years. In spite of that fact, however, these patients must be given ample amount of pain medication when they are in pain, for that is the only way to help them ease their suffering. If it can be determined that an infection triggers the painful crisis, then that infection must be identified and treated with appropriate antibiotics to help alleviate the crisis. Tests, such as chest x-ray, blood culture, urine cultures, etc. and CBC with reticulocytes count must be done before starting antibiotic treatment. Trying to treat a patient with painful sickle cell crisis with an underlying infection, without treating the infection, is just not going to work. The infection must be treated simultaneously, while the pain is being treated in order to handle the situation in its totality.

The most effective pain medication to treat sickle cell painful crisis is morphine sulfate. Demerol (meperidine) is frequently used to treat patients with painful sickle cell crisis, but it is a bad medication for that purpose. The reason that Meperidine (Demerol) is a bad pain medication to use in the treatment of painful sickle cell crisis is because Meperidine breaks down in the body into Normeperidine, which accumulates in the body because of its very long half-life. Normeperidine has no significant pain-relieving effect. Normeperidine, however, causes insomnia, anxiety, agitation and seizure, all of which are very bad for men suffering with pain due to sickle cell disease. Morphine sulfate therefore is the recommended pain medication to treat sickle cell patients suffering with pain.

Hemolytic crisis

Men with sickle cell disease hemolyze a certain percentage of their red blood cells at all times, and that is the nature of their disease. It is, however, not clear as to the reason or reasons why suddenly patients with that disease begin to hemolyze grossly. When men with sickle cell disease develop the hemolytic crisis, they drop their hematocrit abruptly, resulting in shortness of breath, joint pains, general weakness, and sometimes-acute congestive heart failure. The hemolysis can be so brisk, causing the patients to suddenly develop dark looking urine, then their eyes become as yellow as an orange, when, the day before, the situation was not like that at all, and they need to be quickly brought into the hospital and treated appropriately. Other evidence of the hemolytic crisis is a markedly elevated LDH, total and indirect bilirubin and elevated reticulocyte count.

Treatments of the hemolytic crisis

Once it is recognized that a patient is in acute hemolytic crisis, the patient must be admitted to the hospital and oxygen, nasally or by mask, administered along with fresh packed red blood cells. If the patient shows signs of congestive heart failure, Lasix IV must be given to prevent worsening of the CHF. Folic acid, by either mouth or IV, must also be given to the patient.

Treatments of acute hemolytic crisis

Men with sickle cell disease hemolyze their red blood cells all the time, which is part of the disease process. The half-life of their red blood cells is extremely short, maybe 10 to 20 days, as compared to 120 days in a normal person. However, under the stress of an infection or some other circumstances, some of them known, some of them unknown, these men can acutely begin to hemolyze, resulting in a rapid drop in their hematocrit. When that happens, a number of things can develop such as acute shortness of breath, chest pain, drop in blood pressure with shock, and an acute heart attack can occur because of that severe drop in hematocrit. That occurs because of the inability of the heart to pump sufficient blood to carry oxygen to the myocardium.

Acute hemolytic crises must be discovered quickly and treated carefully with fresh packed red cells under the cover of IV Lasix or other loop diuretics to prevent acute pulmonary edema from occurring. In addition to a very low hematocrit, high bilirubin, high LDH, and high reticulocyte count also occur in acute hemolytic crisis.

In addition to replacing blood with fresh packed cells, a high dose of folic acid must also be given when the patient is acutely hemolyzing. The recommended dose of folic acid in patients with chronic hemolytic disease such as sickle cell is as much as 25 mg of folic acid per day and not the usual 1 mg per day of folic acid, which is given for nutritional deficiency. One milligram of folic acid is inadequate in people who are chronically hemolyzing. Failure to understand that fact can result in the inability of the patient who is chronically hemolyzing to make sufficient red cells. As an individual hemolyzes, the body attempts to make new red cells to meet the demand created by the hemolytic state and uses all available folic acid to make new red cells. Everybody who is hemolyzing chronically is, by definition, folic acid deficient.

The need to give fresh packed red cells to chronically anemic patients has been mentioned earlier. That is a very important concept to understand because when a severely anemic patient needs a blood transfusion, the anemia can be made worse if he is transfused with old packed red cells that have been sitting in the blood bank for a long time. As blood sits in the blood bank, the level of 2–3 Diphosphoglycerate (2–3 DPG) constantly decreases. Blood that is depleted in 2–3 DPG, when infused in an already anemic person, shifts the oxygen dissociation curve further to the left, making it much more difficult for that person to deliver oxygen to the tissues. What needs to be done do is to give fresh packed cells, less than a week old, so that a sufficient amount of 2–3 DPG can be delivered in that blood to shift the oxygen dissociation curve to the right, allowing for better delivery of oxygen to the tissues. If a man has underlying ischemic myocardial disease, as is frequently the case in men with sickle cell disease, then the ischemic myocardial disease can be made acutely worse, resulting in either worsening of underlying congestive heart failure or can even lead to an acute heart attack or can cause serious cardiac arrhythmias to occur because of the worsening myocardial ischemia.

Hypoplastic crisis

The hypoplastic crisis usually occurs as because of an infection that suppresses the bone marrow or because of folic acid deficiency or some other insult to the bone marrow that causes it to fail. Evidence that a patient has developed hypoplastic crisis is an acute drop in the hematocrit and a low reticulocyte count.

Treatment of hypoplastic crisis includes oxygen, blood transfusion, folic acid administration and treatment of any underling infection if any exists.

Acute chest syndrome

Acute chest syndrome is the most serious and potentially lethal of all the sickle cell crises. Next to painful crisis, acute chest syndrome is the second most common reason patients with sickle cell disease are admitted to hospitals, and acute chest syndrome is the cause of death in 25% of all deaths of sickle cell disease patients. Surgery is a major risk factor for the development of acute chest syndrome. Some 25% of patients with sickle cell disease who undergo elective surgery develop acute chest syndrome. In acute chest syndrome, the sickle cell patient usually presents with chest pain, tachycardia, fever, cough, shortness of breath, low oxygen saturation, high white blood cell count, high baseline hemoglobin, low platelet count, together with infiltrates on the chest x-ray. The nature of the acute chest syndrome appears to be multifactor and is associated with inflammatory cytokines causing vascular endothelium damage with fat embolism and pulmonary infarction. Secretory phospholipase A2 is an inflammatory substance that is produced in the lungs in ACS and liberates free fatty acids, which in turn cause acute pulmonary fat embolism to occur. The level of secretory phospholipase A2 is quite high in the blood of patients with ACS and is elevated before the onset of ACS and when detected confirms the diagnosis of ACS. Infection plays a major role in ACS. In patients with ACS, when bronchoscoped, a multitude of different microorganisms was found, and included in the list of microorganisms were different bacteria and viruses. The most common bacteria found were Chlamydia pnuemoniae, Mycoplasma pneumoniae, respiratory syncytial virus, Parvovirus, Rhinoviruses.

Treatments of acute chest syndrome

1. Patients who are having pain should be given pain medication such as morphine sulfate to relieve their pain.
2. Oxygen must be given.
3. Incentive spirometry every 3–4 hours while awake is crucial to prevent atelectasis and eventual pneumonia.

4. Transfusion of fresh packed red blood cells must be given and if necessary exchange transfusion ought to be given.

5. Broad-spectrum IV antibiotics must be given because microorganisms are felt to play a major role both in genesis of ACS and in its complications.

6. Blood for secretory phospholipase A2 should be obtained and the level ought to be used to monitor the activity of the syndrome.

7. Daily chest X-ray is necessary to monitor lung infiltrates if there are any.

8. Frequent arterial blood gas is needed to monitor the lung functions of these patients.

9. It is very important to avoid giving too much IV fluid to patients with ACS to prevent the development of pulmonary edema and other complications such as adult respiratory distress syndrome (ARDS), etc and beta-natriuretic peptide (BNP) blood test must be done.

Other common abnormal hemoglobin seen in men of immediate African ancestry and to some degree men of other ancestral descents is hemoglobin C. Homozygous hemoglobin C can cause a chronic hemolytic disease with large spleen, joints pain, chest pain and abdominal pain. Frequently, the hemoglobin C gene is inherited along with the sickle cell gene resulting in sickle C disease. SC disease causes the same type of symptoms as SS disease. The complications of SC disease are similar to SS disease except that individuals with SC disease have the propensity of having more frequent sickle cell retinopathy and all its associated problems such as retinal detachment. In addition, people with SC disease can have infarction of the spleen as well as splenic sequestration, which often present with left sided abdominal pain.

The treatments of sickle cell C disease are the same as that for sickle cell SS disease.

Laser is used to treat most eye problems that sickle cell disease causes.

Splenic sequestration

Splenic sequestration as a sickle crisis is seen most frequently in infants but can also be seen in adults who have either sickle C disease or sickle thalassemia.

The reason why patients with SC or sickle thalassemia can have that form of sickle crisis is because frequently the spleens these individuals have spleens are enlarged.

Therefore, when patients in that category present with acute left-sided midabdominal pain, splenic sequestration with impending rupture of the spleen must be considered and an abdominal CAT scan and a surgical consult must be obtained immediately.

Oftentimes, people who carry the sickle cell trait (AS) do not realize that the AS state carries its own list of medical problems. These problems include prominently:

1. Hematuria with occasional severe gross bleeding from the kidney because of papillary necrosis of the left kidney more often than the right kidney, as mentioned earlier.
2. Arthritis of the hips, knees and spine.
3. Inability to concentrate the urine properly, although general kidney function is normal.
4. Anemia, more severe in menstruating men because of concomitant iron deficiency due to iron loss as part of the menstruation cycle. About 35% to 40% of the red cells are sickle in AS trait as compared to 60% to 70% in people with SS disease.
5. Infraction of the spleen can occur in situations where ambient oxygen pressure is too low in people with sickle cell trait. But, people with sickle cell trait are able to tolerate
6. Simulated high altitude with no problem. People with the sickle cell trait have been engaging in strenuous physical activities, including professional sports, with no difficulty. Usual medical management with analgesics, with IV fluids, blood transfusions, when necessary and high-dose folic acid, up to 25 mg per day, is the mainstay in the everyday treatment of patients with sickle cell disease. The usual 1 mg dose of folic acid given daily is grossly inadequate as outlined earlier.

Other major complications of sickle cell disease include:

1. Gross hematuria due to papillarym necrosis of the kidney
2. Pulmonary embolism
3. Acute myocardial infacrtion
4. Congestive heart failure, due to cardiomyopathy associated with secondary hemochromatosis and myocardial ischemia
5. Acute gouty arthritis, due to rapid red cell turn over associated the secondary hemolytic state
6. Stroke
7. Chronic renal failure
8. Acute multi organs damaged syndrome (which can occur when the hematocric rises above 36%

9.   Sickle cell disease hemolytic transfusion syndrome
10. Priaprism

The thalassemias as well as the major sickling diseases are in great measure responsible for the evolution of the new world from the old world because these diseases allowed some people who lived in the old world to survive the ravages of malaria, mainly because the malarial organism could not flourish inside these abnormal red blood cells.

Other acute complications of sickle cell disease include:

There are several more recently described complications of sickle cell disease, such as the effect of increased viscosity due to high hematocrit in a person with sickle cell anemia. A hematocrit of 30%-35% or higher interferes with oxygen delivery to the tissues, resulting in hypoxia and can be associated with thrombosis (clot formation). As part of that increased viscosity scenario another syndrome, called acute multi-organs damage syndrome, can occur. Because of the hypoxia associated with increased hematocrit, several organs can become damaged at the same time, resulting in an acute medical emergency. These are the most frequently damaged organs during that syndrome: 1. the kidneys causing hematuria (blood) in the urine, or the kidneys can fail (acute renal failure); two. Necrosis of the liver can occur; 3. The bone marrow may become necrotic, resulting in the propagation of fat emboli; 4. Acute pancreatitis can occur; and 5. Acute stroke as well as acute myocardial infarction can occur.

To prevent the acute multi-organs damaged syndrome, the hematocrit of the sickle cell patients ought to be kept between 27%-29% (Ref: *American Society of Hematology Education Program Book,* Dec. 2000).

Still another serious complication of sickle cell disease is a hemolytic transfusion reaction that can occur in patients being transfused with red blood cells to treat anemia associated with sickle cell disease. This problem is called sickle cell transfusion reaction syndrome. Some of the indications that a patient with sickle cell may be experiencing sickle cell transfusion reaction syndrome include: 1. Worsening of the painful crisis while receiving blood transfusion; 2. A marked drop in the patient's hematocrit and acute inability to make new red blood cells, as manifested with a low reticulocytes count; 3. A rapid drop in the hematocrit after receiving blood transfusion (the hematocrit drops to a lower percentage than before the transfusion of red cells were given); 4. Subsequent transfusions of red blood cells may make the anemia worse and, at times, that situation can be severe enough to cost the affected man his life. That problem must be recognized quickly and when and if it occurs, to avoid transfusing a patient who is suffering from that problem. The treatment of sickle cell hemolytic transfusion reaction is administration of corticosteroid intravenously. A rising reticulocytes count and hematocrit is an indication that the patient is getting better (Ref: *American Society of Hematology Education Program Book,* 2000).

The heart is always affected in a rather severe way in patients with sickle cell disease. The mechanism through which the heart gets affected in sickle cell disease is similar to all the other affected organs, through a vascular occlusive mechanism. The vessels carrying blood to the heart to deliver oxygen are of all different sizes. The smaller they are, the easier it is for them to get occluded by the very nature of the sickle red cells. Sickled red cells just cannot pass through these small vessels easily, and there lies the basis of the ischemia that occurs in the muscle of the heart in men suffering with sickle cell disease. The ischemia causes the release of substances called kinins, which are chemicals that tissues of all types release once they become ischemic (starved for oxygen).

Once the kinins are released they cause a burning pain, and that burning pain is responsible not only for chest pain but also is, in fact, the basis of the painful sickle cell crisis, which is most common of the sickle cell crises. The myocardial ischemia that occurs in patients with sickle cell disease is just as detrimental as any other ischemia that affects the heart. It leads to muscle scarring and if one or more of the coronary arteries were to become occluded then acute myocardial infarction can occur. However, more commonly, what happens is that the small vessels that carry blood to the heart muscle is occluded, causing myocardial ischemic disease to occur. Along with the ischemia of the myocardial muscle that occurs in men with sickle cell disease, the red blood cells of these men constantly hemolyze. The homolysis causes lots of iron to be deposited in the bloodstream, resulting in a serious condition called hemochromatosis. That secondary hemochromatosis results in elevated serum ferritin. That storage iron gets deposited in many organs in the body, in particular the heart muscles, the liver, the pancreas, the joints, the testicles, etc. The iron, once it accumulates in the heart muscles, causes the heart to become enlarged (a condition called cardiomyopathy). When the iron breaks down, it releases free radicals, which damage myocardial tissues, as well as many other tissues.

The enlargement of the heart in turn makes blood pumping very difficult, resulting in congestive heart failure. Cardiac arrhythmias of different types can also occur in that situation. The pumping of the heart becomes so sluggish at times that blood within its chambers becomes stagnated, which can cause a clot to form, and that clot can be carried to different organs as emboli. An organ that is particularly vulnerable to that situation is the brain. If a clot gets loose and becomes lodged in the brain, then an acute stroke can occur. To prevent such a problem from arising, these patients with cardiomyopathy are frequently treated with Coumadin (a blood thinner) to thin the blood to prevent the development of emboli.

As just mentioned, these individuals frequently develop different rhythm irregularities of the heart and one of the most common rhythm disturbances seen in that situation is a condition known as atrial fibrillation. The reason why that particular rhythm abnormality is so serious is that in the acute setting it can make the affected man quite sick. Atrial fibrillation can cause the heart to decompensate and it can cause a stroke to develop. Digitalis is used to control the rate of the heart and Coumadin is used to prevent a clot from forming.

Hemochromatosis (too much iron in the body) in men with sickle cell disease is quite serious because of what it can do to the liver, pancreas, heart, and the joints, etc.

The two most effective treatments are phlebotomy (removing one unit of blood—500 cc—from the body at a time) and Desferal (a chelating agent). Desferal, when used in the proper fashion, chelates the iron, removing it from the body and passing the iron out in the urine, thereby decreasing the level of iron in the body.

In addition to the problems just outlined, people who suffer from sickle cell disease (SS), sickle thalassemia, or sickle cell C disease, commonly have a spectrum of clinical manifestations of disease that causes them to be frequently quite sick.

What is the mechanism through which sickle cell disease causes stroke to occur?

Stroke occurs in sickle cell disease patients because the misshaped and sticky red cells clog the small vessels within the brain, preventing oxygen from getting to vital parts of the brain. This lack of oxygen results in ischemia, which in turn causes ischemic stroke to occur, and, depending on the extent and location of the stroke, paralysis may result.

Other major problems that arise because of stroke induced by sickle cell disease, even in a child, are inability to control bowel and urinary functions, and aphasia may occur (the inability to speak), sometimes permanently. The stroke frequently causes difficulty in swallowing, which is quite common, and that can sometimes result in recurrent aspiration pneumonia, which may lead to lung abscesses, bronchiectasis, and, sometimes, pulmonary death is the result.

Other frequent complications are seizures. These seizures can be quite troublesome even when anti-seizure medications are used. Pulmonary problems are also quite common in sickle cell patients such as pneumonia, pulmonary embolism, congestive heart failure, causing marked difficulty in breathing with severe hypoxia (lack of oxygen).

Along with these new concepts and mechanisms in sickle cell disease are the proposed newer treatments of sickle cell disease. Hydroxyurea works in sickle cell disease by not only raising hemoglobin F, but also the fact that it decreases the level of white blood cells and platelets and helps to improve the symptoms of sickle cell disease. So sickle cell patients on hydroxyurea, even if their hemoglobin F level does not go up, benefit because of the lowering of white cells and platelets (Ref: *American Society of Hematology Education Program Book*, 1998).

Other proposed treatment modalities include inhalation of nitric oxide gas to dilate blood vessels, allowing for better tissue perfusion. Another proposed new modality of treatment for sickle cell disease is low-dose aspirin, which works as an anti-inflammatory medication against the effects of the adhesion proteins. Aspirin also works to prevent platelet aggregation, resulting in better blood flow through blood vessels and decreasing the incidence of sickle cell painful crises (Ref:. *American Society of Hematology Education Program Book*, 1998).

Another common problem that frequently occurs in men who suffer from sickle cell disease is gall bladder disease. If gall bladder disease is allowed to go un-diagnosed, it can cause severe problems for the patient. It usually presents with acute abdominal pain, nausea, and vomiting. This constellation of symptoms is usually due to acute cholecystitis. Because men with sickle disease and other chronic hemolytic diseases hemolyze constantly, they dump large amounts of bilirubin pigments into their bloodstream. These bilirubin pigments in turn form bilirubin-containing gall bladder stones. Over time, these gall bladder stones cause the gall bladder to become inflamed and sometimes infected, resulting in a spectrum of acute and chronic gallbladder diseases.

The diagnosis and treatment of gallbladder disease is described elsewhere in that book.

Other frequent problems that men with sickle cell disease have to cope with are things such as:

1. Sickle cell retinopathy (bleeding into the eyes) seen more frequently in SC disease than in SS disease.
2. Leg ulcers
3. Aseptic necrosis of different bones, such as the shoulder joints, the elbow joints, the hip joints, and the knee joints.

4. Microscopic or gross hematuria due to papillary necrosis is quite common. It is seen more often from the left kidney than the right kidney. The reason why papillary necrosis is seen more frequently from the left kidney is that the anatomical position of the two kidneys is different. The left kidney is located higher than the right kidney. The position of the left kidney places it in a situation where it is less able to receive appropriate amount of oxygen as compared to the right kidney. In normal men that does not matter but in men who have sickle cell disease, that becomes a major problem and in the left kidney where that situation occurs, papillary necrosis occurs frequently, resulting in gross hematuria.

5. Men with sickle cell disease have the propensity of getting infected with capsular bacterial organisms such as pneumococci and Haemophilus influenzae. It has been said that patients with sickle cell disease are infected in the bone frequently with salmonella bacteria, resulting in osteomyelitis.

6. The spleens of men with sickle cell anemia (SS) get destroyed by the time these men become teenagers, due to the recurrent insults of the sickling phenomena to the splenic circulation. The hypo splenic state that results causes these men to become immunoincompetent, thus causing them to be infected much more easily. It is therefore recommended that these men get vaccinated with pneumococcal vaccine about every three years or so. The pneumococcal vaccine is protective against 23 subtypes of the pneumococci bacteria. It is also recommended that these men get treated with penicillin 250 mg daily as a prophylaxis against pneumococcal organisms for life. These organisms are exquisitely sensitive to penicillin. If the patient is allergic to penicillin, Erythromycin 250 mg daily or twice a day can be used as a substitute.

7. Men with sickle thalassemia or sickle C disease tend to have large spleens.

8. Men with sickle cell disease are prone to develop sickle hepatopathy (sickle cell liver disease), with large engorgement of the liver, which frequently causes right upper abdominal pain.

9. Another common problem that men with sickle cell disease suffer from is disease of the kidneys. At first, the manifestation of the kidney disease appears as different degrees of renal insufficiency in the blood chemistry tests that evaluate kidney function. As the sickle cell disease progresses chronic renal failure develops, forcing these indi-

viduals to be placed frequently on chronic hemodialysis. Before the kidneys fail completely, hypertension frequently develops, complicating the picture even more because the hypertension can cause strokes or congestive heart failure. As outlined earlier in that chapter, men with sickle cell disease have the propensity to develop strokes and cardiomyopathy. When the blood pressure becomes elevated, it is superimposed on an already sick heart and sick brain, risking decompensation of these and other organs that are frequently affected by elevated blood pressure.

There are no definite treatments available to cure sickle cell disease presently. However, there are several medications and methods available to treat the disease. Hydroxyurea is being used to treat patients with sickle disease to improve the symptoms of the disease. Hydroxyurea works to improve the symptoms of sickle cell disease in some patients by raising the level of hemoglobin F. Hemoglobin F is an excellent carrier of oxygen and in that way the increased hemoglobin F enables oxygen to be carried to tissues much more easily, thereby preventing ischemia from occurring; the result is less pain and improvement in the overall symptoms of the affected patients. Sodium butyrate has been shown in a recent setting to be able to increase hemoglobin F level as well. Recombinant human erythropoietin (Epogen or Procrit) is being used in combination with hydroxyurea to increase hemoglobin F level, use up the excess iron and raise the hematocrit in the process. When Epogen/Procrit is used in a person with sickle cell anemia, the hematocrit must be maintained between 29%-32%. A hematocrit above 36% in this setting can cause a stroke, a heart attack, DVT or pulmonary embolism to occur because the blood is too viscous to pass through these people poor blood vessels.

The same thing applies to individuals with end stage kidney disease. When people with sickle cell anemia is over transfused with packed red cells or given too much procrit to raise the hematocrit above 36% the possibility of acute multiple organs infarction can occur resulting in medical catastrophy.

In spite of all the many millions of dollars that have been spent looking for a cure for sickle cell disease, no cure has been found as of that date. Bone marrow transplantation is being tried as a curative measure for sickle cell disease but it is in its infancy and the results so far have been few although some reports appear to be quite encouraging. As for the future, it is hoped that gene therapy might hold promise in helping people with sickle cell disease.

Genetic counseling remains the most worthwhile approach for those who are affected with sickle cell disease.

Alpha Thalassemia

In alpha thalassemia, the in the individual who is a silent carrier is missing one alpha globin haplotype. In alpha thalassemia trait, the individual is missing two alpha globin haplotypes. In

Hemoglobin H, the individual is missing three alpha globin halotypes and in hemoglobin Bart's, the fetus is missing four alpha globin halotypes and hemoglobin Bart's is not compatible with life. Taken together alpha thalassemia is the most common genetic disorder in the world. About 32% of black Americans carry the alpha thalassemia genetic abnormality. Of this figure, 30% are missing one alpha globin haplotype and 2% are missing two alpha globin haplotypes. The prevalence of the alpha thalassemia gene is also quite high among Hispanics.

Black and Hispanic men do not have any symptoms from that abnormality. Those who are missing two alpha globin haplotypes from opposite sides of the alpha globin haplotype may have a mild microcytic anemia and are said to have alpha thalassemia trait. People of color with immediate African ancestral genes always miss the two alpha globin haplotypes from opposite sides of the alpha globin haplotype. On the other hand, Asian people and others, when they are missing two alpha globin haplotypes, they always miss the chains from the same side of the alpha globin haplotype, creating an unbalanced alpha globin chain situation. That is what happens in hemoglobin constant spring, which causes anemia and symptoms in individuals who are afflicted with it. Individuals who are missing three alpha globin haplotypes have hemoglobin H and are severely anemic. Hines bodies are seen in the red blood cells of these individuals on blood smears.

How to diagnose alpha thalassemia

The best way to diagnose alpha thalassemia is to do a CBC and a quantitative hemoglobin electrophoresis. In alpha thalassemia, the CBC shows microcytosis, low MCV, erythrocytosis and high RDW. The erythrocytosis (elevated red blood cell count) differentiates thalassemia from iron deficiency. For every 10% of the hematocrit there is 1 million of red blood cells and where there is a discordance of about 400,000 or more greater than red blood cells per million, there exists a thalassemia syndrome in the patient. If all the aforementioned conditions exist and hemoglobin A2 and hemoglobin F are normal on the hemoglobin electrophoresis, then the patient has alpha thalassemia of one degree or another.

The treatments for alpha thalassemia are:
1. Folic Acid
2. Blood transfusion
3. Iron chelation with Desferal
4. Bone marrow transplantation

Beta thalassemia

Beta thalassemia affects about 3% of the world population and its distribution is worldwide.

The people who are most affected by beta thalassemia are those of Greek, Italian, Turkish, Iranian, Syrian, Arabic, Pakistani, Indian, Southeast Asians, South Asians, Kurdish Jews, and in North America, Blacks and Hispanics. Beta thalassemia has been reported in some Northern European individuals as well.

Beta thalassemia has three clinical categories:

Beta thalassemia minor

Beta thalassemia intermedia

Beta thalassemia major.

Beta thalassemia minor causes no clinical manifestation or disease. Beta thalassemia intermedia can cause a hypochromic microcytic anemia with moderate degree of iron overload, but growth is normal and life span is also not affected.

Beta thalassemia major causes a severe anemia, serious symptoms with high iron overload, growth retardation, large spleen, large liver, large heart, congestive heart failure along with cardiac arrhythmias. Without early, effective and aggressive treatment, individuals with thalassemia major die before reaching adulthood.

How to diagnose beta thalassemia

The CBC in beta thalassemia major shows low hemoglobin and hematocrit, low MCV, high red blood cell count, high RDW and the blood smear shows many target cells. The quantitative hemoglobin electrophoresis shows elevated hemoglobin A2 or F or both.

How to treat beta thalassemia major

The most effective treatments for beta thalassemia major consist of:

1. Blood transfusion
2. Chelation therapy using Desferal or EXJADE 20 mg/kg body per day
3. Folic acid
4. Bone marrow transplantation
5. Prenatal diagnosis during the first 9–10 gestation can be done, using chorionic villus sampling for DNA fetal analysis. That procedure allows the parents of the unborn fetus to know whether the fetus is homozygous or heterozygous for beta thalassemia major.

Sometime, the Alpha thalassenia gene is carried together with the sickle cell disease gene in the same individual. When this happens, the Alpha thalassemia gene renders the sickle disease to be much less severe and. On the other hand, when the Beta thalassemia gene is carried together with the sickle cell gene in the same individual, the disease sickle thalassemia results that is a bad disease and it behaves in the same way as does sickle anemia most of the time.

Megaloblastic anemias

B12 deficiency:

B12 deficiency is a very common entity.
The different things that cause B12 deficiency are the following:
1. Nutritional deficiency
2. Parasitic infestation
3. Blind loop syndrome
4. Atrophic gastritis
5. Gastrectomy
6. Malabsorption
7. Pernicious anemia
8. Inhalation of nitrous oxide
9. Abnormal secretion of salivary glands
10. Chronic use of H2 Blockers and proton pump inhibitors (such as Tagamet, Zantac, Axid, Pepcid and Nexium, Prevacid, Prilosec etc). Individuals, who are taking these medications on a chronic basis, ought to be taking B12 in pill form to avoid becoming B12 deficient.

How do these different things cause B12 deficiency?

The total store in the body is about 5000 micrograms. The body loses about 1–4 micrograms of B12 per day and the daily requirement for B12 is in the range of 5 micrograms per day. B12 is found in liver, milk, eggs, cheese and meats.

Nutritional B12 deficiency is usually found in strict vegetarians and in people who don't have access to the food products just mentioned.

Diphyllobothrium latum is the fish tapeworm most commonly associated with B12 deficiency.

This worm causes malabsorption of B12 to occur. The tapeworm also takes up the B12; thereby preventing its absorption from the ileum, and the result is B12 deficiency.

Small bowel blind loops/bacterial overgrowth, small bowel diverticulosis, and other pouches and fistulae cause B12 deficiency because the bacteria eat the B12, making it unavailable for absorption. In that condition, the level of folic acid is quite high.

Atrophic gastritis causes B12 deficiency because as individual ages, the stomach is less able to produce acid and an acidic milieu is necessary in order for intrinsic factor to properly work to allow B12 to be absorbed. Along the same line, the elderly are prone to develop B12 deficiency because of a deficiency that occurs in the mouth due to a lack of certain salivary enzymes that are necessary to begin the process of B12 digestion. There are several millions elderly individuals (about 5 million in the US) who, though they do not yet have macrocytic anemia, have B12 deficiency that can cause severe medical problems, including dementia. B12 deficiency state does not always mean B12 deficiency anemia. It takes years before B12 deficiency state becomes B12 deficiency anemia. Anemia is the last stage of the multiple stages of B12 deficiency disease. A person can be very sick from B12 deficiency and not yet develop macrocytic anemia. A good example of that is B12 associated dementia.

Gastrectomy can cause B12 deficiency 5–10 years post gastrectomy because the bulk of the intrinsic factor-producing surface was removed during the gastrectomy, leaving very little or no intrinsic factor behind, so B12 cannot be absorbed, resulting in B12 deficiency. It would take that long to deplete the B12 store of about 5000 micrograms. Therefore patients who have undergone hemigastrectomy ought to receive B12 injection monthly for life about 5 years after the procedure. Individuals who had gastric by-pass surgery must also get injection of B12 post op for life to prevent B12 deficiency.

Malabsorption of B12 occurs in chronic pancreatitis because of exocrine enzyme insufficiency. It also occurs in Zollinger-Ellison syndrome because of low pH in the ileum; it occurs as well in regional enteritis involving the terminal ileum in Crohn's disease. Chronic hemodialysis can also cause of B12 deficiency. Therefore, individuals who are affected by these conditions ought to receive B12 injection on a regular basis.

Pernicious anemia is an autoimmune condition involving an interaction between the stomach and intrinsic factor. This antigen-antibody reaction prevents intrinsic factor from attaching itself to B12 to allow it to be absorbed from the terminal ileum into the bloodstream, where it is taken to the bone marrow to be incorporated in the early red cells for the production of red blood cells.

Pernicious anemia can be seen in association with hyperthyroidism, hypothyroidism, vitiligo, diabetes mellitus, Addison's disease, and sometimes cancer of the colon.

The previous standard way of making the diagnosis of pernicious anemia, which was by doing the Schilling test, is no longer practical because the radioactive B12 that used to be employed to carry out that test is no longer routinely available in that country. Using the patient's symptoms, the low serum B12, the high MCV, the megaloblastic features on the bone marrow smear and the positive intrinsic factor antibody, will suffice to establish the diagnosis of pernicious anemia. If the diagnosis of pernicious anemia is established, then ANA, T4, TSH, fasting blood sugar, serum electrolytes and colonoscopic evaluation of the patient in question ought to be done, for the reasons previously described.

Nitrous oxide interferes in the biochemical pathway of B12 in a way that leads to B12 deficiency and megaloblastic anemia. People who chronically inhaled nitrous oxide are likely to develop that form of anemia and all its medical complications if left untreated.

How to diagnose B12 deficiency

The first thing to do is to take a good history and do a good physical examination.

The next thing to do is to order CBC, serum B12, serum homocysteine, and if the serum B12 is borderline or normal and the diagnosis is still suspected, then serum methylmalonic acid ought to be done. The serum methylmalonic acid is much more accurate in making the diagnosis of B12 deficiency than the serum B12. Methylmalonic acid is elevated in true B12 deficiency. In B12 deficiency both, the methylmalonic acid and the homocysteine are elevated but in folic acid deficiency, only the homocysteine is elevated.

How to treat B12 deficiency in men who are B12 deficient

The first thing to do to treat the underlying problem or problems responsible for the B12 deficiency:

1. In the case of nutritional deficiency, B12 can be given IM at first then added to the diet.
2. In the case of fish tapeworm infestation, treat with anti-tapeworm medication and replace B12 by injection at first, then by mouth until the macrocytic anemia is corrected and the store of B12 is replenished.
3. In the case of blind loops, treat the problem surgically if possible, give B12 by injection, give tetracycline by mouth (if the men are not pregnant), document by tests, physical examination and history that the malabsorption has resolved and add B12 by mouth till the store has been replenished.

As for atrophic gastritis, give injection of B12 monthly for life.

As for post-gastrectomy, give injection of B12 monthly for life.

As for malabsorption, treat the same as for blind loops.

As for pernicious anemia, give 1 mg of B12 IM daily for 7 days, and then give 1 mg of B12 IM three times per week for three weeks and then give 1 mg of B12 monthly thereafter, for life.

It is prudent when treating truly B12-deficient patients with B12 injection to do the following in the beginning of the treatment.

1. Take the patient's baseline weight.
2. Weigh the patient weekly.
3. Listen to the patient's lungs carefully for evidence of heart failure (rales).
4. Listen to patient's heart for evidence of heart failure (S3or s4 gallop).
5. Check the patient's serum potassium weekly for the first 4 weeks.

Patients with true B12 deficiency who receive B12 injection are likely to respond quickly by increasing their blood volume markedly, as though they have just been given 2–3 units of blood, which can throw them into acute congestive heart failure and death.

Acute weight gain would be an indication of water retention and congestive heart failure.

In order to make new red blood cells, potassium is needed to be incorporated into RNA; that process can cause an acute depletion of body potassium, resulting in chest muscle weakness with inability to breathe, as well as acute cardiac arrhythmia and death. Therefore, treating men for true B12 deficiency is serious business and to be carried out by physicians experienced in dealing with that disease.

As for nitrous oxide, those who are exposed to it ought to find ways to decrease their exposure and those who use it as an addicting drug ought to seek help to resolve their addiction and stop using it.

B12 injection at first, followed by B12 by mouth, is the treatment of that form of B12 deficiency.

If a man who is B12 deficient remains untreated, he can develop severe megaloblastic anemia, combined system disease with severe neurological problems, dementia and psychosis.

The neurological problems associated with B12 deficiency are not reversible after going untreated for 5 years.

Folic acid deficiency

The other common cause of macrocytic/megaloblastic anemia is folic acid deficiency.

Folic acid deficiency occurs in
1. Nutritional deficiency
2. Alcoholism
3. Hemolytic anemia
4. Drug-associated folic acid deficiency
5. Tropical sprue
6. Non-tropical sprue
7. Hemodialysis.
8. Dilantin treatment
9. Phenobarbitol treatment etc;

How folic acid deficiency occurs

Nutritional deficiency causes folic acid deficiency as because of poor intake of folic acid.

The total body folic acid store is about 5000 micrograms and in 2–4 months, the body can become depleted of folic acid. The daily requirement for folic acid in an adult is about 400 micrograms. In fact, the body is incapable in a normal individual to absorb more than 400 mcg of folic acid per day. The foods that are richest in folic acid are vegetables.

Poor nutrition causes folic acid deficiency if a person stays on a folic acid-free diet for about 2–4 months.

Alcoholism causes folic acid deficiency via three main mechanisms:

1. Alcoholics as a rule eat a diet that is poor in folic acid.
2. Alcohol as a substance, when consumed in excess, poisons the folic acid biochemical pathway.
3. When the alcoholic develops cirrhosis of the liver, portal hypertension develops, which in turn causes hypersplenism with secondary hemolysis, making folic acid deficiency worst.

Medications such as Dilantin, Phenobarbital, Mysoline, and Methotrexate, to name a few, are known to cause folic acid deficiency.

Tropical sprue is known to cause folic acid deficiency because of the malabsorption that it causes.

How to diagnose folic acid deficiency

To diagnose folic acid deficiency, do a serum folic acid, CBC and a reticulocyte count.

In folic acid deficiency, the serum folic acid is low, the hematocrit is low, the MCV is high and the reticulocyte count is low. Sometime the folic acid level may be in the range even though the patient is folic acid deficient. That may happen because the folic acid level reflects the last folic acid-containing meal that the patient ate before the blood was drawn.

The most accurate test to do to measure folic acid level is red blood cells folic acid level, but that test is not routinely available and is therefore not practical. The bone marrow aspirate in folic acid deficiency shows megaloblastic changes in the red blood cells and a left shift in the early white blood cells white.

How to treat folic acid deficiency

The best treatments for folic acid deficiency are folic acid by either mouth or IV/IM. If the patient is very anemic, then blood transfusion can be given. To treat tropical sprue, in addition to folic acid 5 mg per day, tetracycline 250 mg 4 times per day ought to be given.

Chronic hemolytic anemia is treated with high doses of folic acid, up to 25 mg per day in order to keep up with constant destruction of red blood cells that is taking place.

Anemia of chronic disease/inflammatory disease

Anemia of chronic disease is mediated by cytokines IL1 and TNFa (Interleukin 1 and Tumor Necrosis Factor alpha), these substances cause an inflammatory reaction to occur, which then result in the production of nitric oxide, which in turn suppresses the ability of erythroid blood progenitors (early red blood cells) from being able to make red cells. In that setting iron moves from the blood into to the tissues where it is stored and not made available for red blood cell production. Apparently, this is the body's way of protecting itself from invading microorganisms, such as bacteria, viruses and fungi, by depriving them of iron for their growth. In addition, the body seeks to protect itself from cancer by depriving the cancer cells of iron, which is necessary for their growth. The second apparent advantage of anemia of chronic disease is to deprive cancer cells and microorganisms of sufficient oxygen needed for their growth and their proliferation by not making enough red cells to carry oxygen to them. The third proposed advantage of anemia chronic disease is that that the lack of circulating iron strengthens the cell-mediated immune system. The third advantage mentioned seems to make sense, since having cancer in the human body, by itself, creates an immune deficiency-type state (Source: *American Society of Hematology Education Program Book,* pages 42–45, 2000).

BLOOD SMEAR IN IRON DEFICIENCY ANEMIA

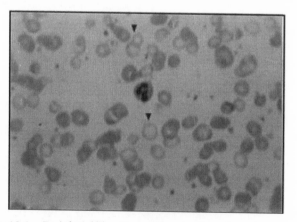

Figure 10.1—Peripheral blood smear showing hypochromic pale red cell showing lack of hemoglobin (arrow head). Arrow showing microcytic red cell (small red cell) due to lack of hemoglobin.

BLOOD SMEAR SHOWING SICKLE CELLS

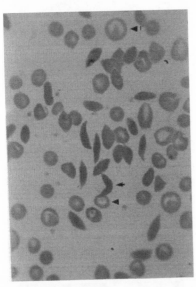

Figure 10.2—Arrow showing sickle cell (banana-shaped cell). Arrow head showing a target cell in a patient with sickle cell anemia, with thalassemia combined (sickle thalassemia).

Other types of anemia seen in men are folic acid deficiency, B-12 deficiency and autoimmune hemolytic anemia.

Sickle cell disease frequently affects the bone and brain of individuals suffering from it.

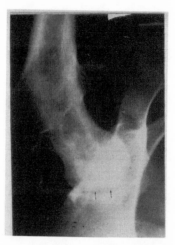

Figure 10.3—*Arrows showing avascular necrosis (lack of blood flow to bone) of femoral head with flattening necrosis of head bone in a patient with sickle cell disease.*

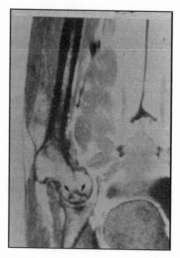

Figure 10.4—*MRI of femoral head of hip of patient with sickle cell disease. Arrows showing avascular necrosis.*

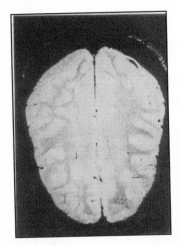

Figure 10.5—*Arrows showing multiple infarcts (stroke) in the brain of a patient with sickle cell disease as documented by brain MRI.*

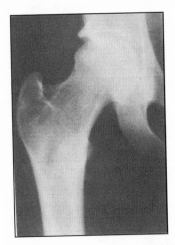

Figure 10.6—*X-ray of a normal hip*

Table 10.7

An example of what a CBC, serum ferritin and Hemoglobin electrophoresis of a person with beta thalassemia trait looks like. this person has the increased HGB A2 variant of beta thalassemia with normal HGB F level.

Normal

WBC	8.6	(4.0–10.5)	TH/MM3
RBC	6.37	(4.2–5.8)	MIL/MM3
HGB	13.4	(13.0–17.0)	G/DL
HCT	42.1	(38.0–50.0)	%
MCV	66.1	(80–96)	FL
MCH	21.0	(27–32)	UUG
MCHC	31.8	(33–35.5)	%
RDW	15.4	(11.0–14.5)	%
PLT	21.9	(130–400)	TH/MM3
MPV	9.0	(6.8–11.0)	FL
NEU	69.6	(43–75)	%
LYMPH	21.4	(15–45)	%
MONO	7.5	(3–12)	%
EOS	1.0	(0–5.5)	%
BASO	0.5	(0–2.0)	%
NEU#	6.0	(1.7–7.9)	TH/MM3
FERRITIN	673	(12–282)	NG/ML
hemoglobin A	93.4	(94.7–98.2)	%
hemoglobin a2	5.80	(1.8–3.3)	%
hemoglobin f	0.80	(0.0–2.0)	%

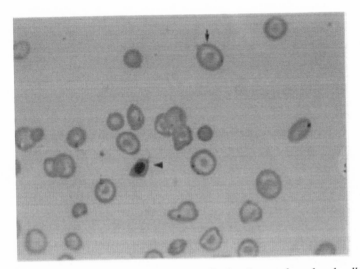

Figure 10.8—Thalassemia *(arrow head) showing nucleated red cell, small arrow showing Howel jolly body. Big arrow shows target cell.*

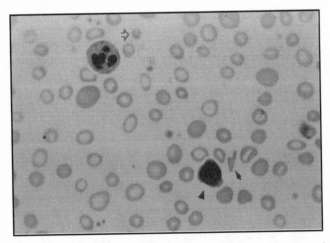

Figure 10.9—Hemolytic anemia *(arrow head) showing nucleated red cell. Arrow showing a schistocyte (fragment of red blood cell). Open arrow showing spherocyte (very small red cell full with hemoglobin).*

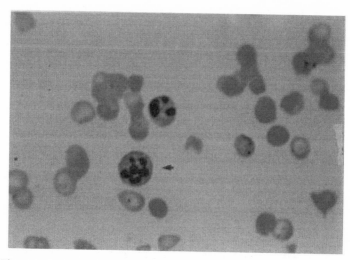

Figure 10.10—Folic acid deficiency and alcoholism (big arrow showing segmented polynucleated white cell with 7 lobes, typical of macrocytic anemia). Small arrow showing a macrocytes (large immature red blood cell).

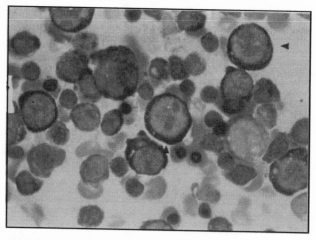

Figure 10.11—Bone marrow aspiration smear (arrow heads) showing megaloblastic red cells (very large immature red cell and pernicious anemia due to B-12 deficiency).

A very serious complication of chronic hemolytic diseases is iron overload, known as hemochromatosis, which was discussed earlier in the section on sickle cell disease. The hemochromatosis seen in the individual who suffers from hemoglobinopathies is the secondary type as compared to the idiopathic type or primary hemochromatosis. About 5% of the U.S. population carries the gene for primary hemochromatosis, and in certain sub groups, as much as 1:200 or 1:2000 have hemochromatosis. Primary hemochromatosis-affected people over-absorb iron because of a genetic defect that forces them to absorb too much iron. New informations have come out that show that most of the individuals who have C 282Y negative primary iron overload; have elevated serum ferritin because of Hepcidin deficiency. A normal level of hepcidin is needed to control the action of Ferroportin. Ferroportin is needed to facilitate the absorption of iron from the intestine and it allows the body to reuse iron that is in macrophages. The low level of hepcidin, allows ferroportin to go unchecked resulting in over absorbption and over production of iron in the body. It is through these two mechanisms that these individuals develop primary iron over load which has the same clinical manifestation as the HFE associated hemocromatosis. In secondary hemochromatosis, which is the result of hemoglobinopathies, the iron gets dumped into the bloodstream because of shortened red cell survivals, resulting in hemolysis. In the full-blown thalassemia, these children classically have bronze skins due to iron deposits under the skin. The iron gets deposited in different tissues and organs in the body of these children who are suffering from thalassemia and sickle cell disease a or any other chronic hemolytic anemia. The organs that are most affected by iron deposits are the heart, the liver, the endocrine organs such as the adrenal glands, the pituitary, the gonads and the pancreas. Iron deposits also affect the joints. Iron deposits cause damage to tissues and organs because as iron particles lie in the tissues they break down, releasing free radicals. These free radicals are extremely toxic to human tissues, damaging the tissues, resulting in diseases such as cardiomyopathy with resulting heart failure. As the free radicals are released, they damage the liver, resulting in cirrhosis, which results in scarring of the liver, which can result in hepatocellular carcinoma of the liver. One of the most sensitive ways to diagnose iron deposits in the liver is by doing an MRI of the liver, which, if positive with iron deposits, shows a starry sky-type picture.

Damage caused by iron deposits in the gonads can result in sexual dysfunction and sexual underdevelopment. Damage of iron deposits into the pancreas often result in diabetes mellitus Type II, because the beta cells within the pancreas get damaged and destroyed. It is these beta cells that are responsible for the production of insulin, and without insulin, sugar cannot be broken down to be used as fuel for proper body functions. Osteoarthritis is a common disease in people who are affected by hemochromatosis, and men are particularly afflicted by that because men, because of their lower economic status, are forced to do heavier work to earn a living, which places their bone structure at most stress and also their musculoskeletal structures at most stress, causing osteoarthritis. When iron deposits are superimposed on that condition, osteoarthritis is made worse.

The free radicals that are released from the breakdown products of iron deposits in the joint spaces cause an inflammatory reaction to occur, which results ultimately in destruction of the joints, causing severe arthritis in these joints and chronic pain. Many men do not know that they have hemochromatosis and that is really a major issue. The worst-case scenario is that oftentimes they are carrying an abnormal hemoglobin which predisposes them to constantly smoldering hemolysis with secondary iron being dumped in their body while, at the same time, they may be carrying the gene for hemochromatosis, which is also causing them to over-absorb iron, having, therefore, two problems affecting them simultaneously, resulting in more frequent problems associated with iron overload.

Primary hemochromatosis is believed by some to be a disease that is found usually in Caucasians of Scandinavian and European descent. This in fact turns out not to be so. While the disease is more common in whites, it does occur with significant frequency in black men, Hispanic men, Asian men and men of other races. The gene that is responsible for hemochromatosis is located in the short arm of chromosome 6 and is on the HLA locus.

Many non-white males with no abnormal hemoglobin frequently have high serum ferritin consistent with heterozygous hemochromatosis/iron overload state with clinical features of primary hemochromatosis." The author was the first in the world to discover the C282Y gene in a black man, in the year 2000, documenting that, this gene, which is responsible for primary hemochromatosis, can also in rare instances found in Blacks. The so-called African Iron Overload Syndrome probably does not exist at all. There are probably other yet-to-be-identified genes in the human body that may be responsible for the primary hemochromatosis seen in Blacks, Hispanics Asians and some Whites frequently in day-to-day clinical practice.

There are in fact many whites who have primary hemochromatosis and are treated for it and yet the C282Y gene is absent in them and they are said to have primary hemochromatosis. However when Blacks have clear and unquestionable primary hemochromatosis, many physicians would say that they have "African Iron Overload Syndrome." This is nothing more than an attempt to say that Blacks cannot possibly have the same disease that Whites have, which is total racial nonsense because the human race began in Africa and all human beings are the same from a DNA standpoint, except for a few minor differences, and since skin color happens to be one of these minor differences, some choose to make a big deal of it for their own social and economic advantages.

"Prevalence of Iron Overload in African-Americans A Primary Care Experience—Revised" *Prestige Medical News*, February 2003, Vol 5 No 3 pp 1–22 Le Negre Publishing
37 Davis Avenue
White Plains N.Y. 10605

Recent reports have shown that many cases of iron overload/hemochromatosis is due to Hecidin deficiency which allows over activity of Ferroportin, resulting in over absorption of iron from the stomach. Still further evidence exists to show that there are several other groups of hereditary iron overload/hemochromatosis different from HFE gene mutation that causes C282Y primary hemochromatosis. (see page 184 above)

The C282Y test to diagnose primary hemochromatosis of different degrees is available in several commercial clinical laboratories.

The best way to determine if someone has hemochromatosis is to do a serum ferritin. A serum ferritin costs about $56.00 to do and it is immensely important. The serum ferritin gives an evaluation of the total body iron. A serum ferritin of 500 or greater points to a possible diagnosis of hemochromatosis. Once he stops menstruating and is not losing iron through his menstrual period, then the iron level will gradually go higher.

Another organ that is frequently affected by hemochromatosis is the skin, which, in fact, is the largest organ in the human body. In primary hemochromatosis the skin has a bronze color to it. The easiest and best treatment for hemochromatosis is phlebotomy, which is removing blood from the body if the person is not anemic. During that procedure 500 ml of blood is removed. Each time 500 ml of blood is removed, 250 mg of iron is removed with it. Each 1 cc of blood contains 0.5 mg of iron. It is important that the man whose blood is being removed is examined by a physician, to be certain that he is not anemic or has no active cardiac disease that can contraindicate the removal of that much blood from his. The only other treatment available to remove iron from the body is a chelating agent called Desferal, which works to remove iron from the body by chelating the iron from the body and excreting it through the kidneys, into the urine. Desferal is given subcutaneously as a continuous infusion over 12 hours together with 100 to 200 mg of Vitamin C. The Vitamin C helps to mobilize iron in the tissues, making it easier for the chelating agent to remove it from the body into the urine and out. That is a unique property that Vitamin C has. Because

Vitamin C is able to mobilize iron from the body, it is dangerous for someone to take Vitamin C unless a physician prescribes it. If an individual has hemochromatosis and does know it, and is taking Vitamin C, the Vitamin C would help to enhance the absorption of iron from the stomach on one hand and also would help to mobilize a lot of iron into vital organs such as the heart, liver, pancreas the joints etc., resulting, in a multitude of diseases, such as diabetes mellitus, cirrhosis of the liver, cancer of the liver and cardiomyopathy, etc. Vitamin C is plentiful in fruits, juices, bananas and vegetables and, when consumed as food products, is both nutritious and helpful to keep the body in good Vitamin C balance.

Men who have secondary hemochromatosis due to hemolytic diseases, such as sickle cell disease, thalassemia, or other diseases such as, rheumatoid arthritis, chronic renal failure with high body iron store, and have secondary hemochromatosis and are anemic at the same time, can be given injection of Procrit, 10,000 units SQ twice per week or Epogen, 10,000 units SQ, twice per week, to use the iron in their bodies to make red cells, thereby decreasing the iron level while at the same time treating their anemias. Epogen/Procrit 10,000 units every two weeks SQ is effective in treating men with iron over load/hemochromatosis who are anemic and inappropriate for phlebotomy to raise the hematocrit using the excess iron.

AIDS associated anemia can also be treated with procrit/epogen successfully even if the serum erythropoietin is normal.

Treating physicians must undertake a vigorous and complete evaluation of anemia to determine the underlying disease or diseases responsible for the anemia. While anemia is a serious disease by itself, it frequently points to an even more serious disease that may be life threatening to a patient. Unless someone is very anemic with a very low red blood count and suffering acutely from it such as a person who is bleeding, hemolyzing, or someone whose bone marrow cannot produce red blood cells, then that person's anemia ought to be fully evaluated to establish the root cause of the anemia before starting treatment for it.

Blood and blood product transfusions must be given with informed consent, because of the possibility of the transmission of AIDS, HIV (Type I and HIV Type II), which, post-1987, the chances of getting HIV (Type I) is anywhere from 1:50,000 to 1:150,000 blood transfusions. Other infectious diseases, such as HTLV I, THLV II, hepatitis A, B, C and also CMV virus, can be transfused with blood products. Once informed consent is given for these possible infections, and if there is no religious contraindication, then blood can be given to provide sufficient quantity of oxygen for proper oxygen delivery to the tissues. Once that is done, then an evaluation has to be undertaken to determine the cause of the anemia. Sometimes it is obvious the person is throwing up blood and the bleeding is from the upper gastrointestinal tract. Sometimes it is obvious the person is passing large amounts of red blood per rectum and the assumption is that they are bleeding from the lower GI tract. However, sometimes, it is not that simple. When a person comes in with anemia, there is no quick way to determine where the bleeding is from. Just because a man is anemic does not necessarily mean that he is bleeding. Anemia can be the result of

(1) bleeding (2) hemolysis (3) failure to make sufficient red blood cells (4) or a combination of any of those processes. Since he has been anemic for a long time, unless there is a serious underlying cardiac problem that necessitates oxygen delivery immediately, there is never a rush to quickly treat him. However, there is a definite rush to evaluate his to determine the cause of the anemia as just discussed. Frequently, the cause is a lesion in the GI tract, a cancer, diverticulosis, polyps, and inflammatory bowel disease, such as Crohn's or ulcerative colitis or arteriovenous ulcer of the stomach, gastritis or other small bowel, stomach, or large bowel disease that can be causing them to bleed.

In the case of iron deficiency anemia, one treats it by replacing iron. In the case of hemolysis, one replaces it by giving certain medications, such as Prednisone, to prevent hemolysis, and then add folic acid on top of it to help replace folic acid loss, etc. In the case of a particular cancer that invades the bone marrow, preventing red cell production, the way to deal with that problem is to treat the cancer with chemotherapy or radiotherapy that destroys the cancer cells. This process frequently allows red cell production to resume, improving the anemia. If the patient is unable to make red cells because of red cell aplasia, that is, they are not able to make red cells, then there is a long list of things that can be done to try to stimulate the marrow to make new red cells, such as giving them androgenic hormones of different kinds to try to help the marrow to make red cells. If it is an infection that suppresses the production of red cells transiently, once the infection is brought under control the bone marrow can then go on to make new red cells again. If the person has aplastic anemia, then the bone marrow is completely incapable of making red blood cells.

Anemia is a serious medical condition and is the most common disease that men suffer from the world over.

Once it is discovered, a hematologist who is an expert in blood diseases should be consulted to evaluate the anemia properly. Appropriate treatments must then be given to prevent men from losing their lives because of anemia and to prevent all the symptoms and complications that are associated with this anemia.

CHAPTER 11

UROLOGICAL
DISEASES IN MEN

In 2007, 218,890 men in the US will be diagnosed with prostate cancer.
During that same time period, 27,050 men will die of prostate cancer.
The incidence of prostate cancer in Black American men is more than twice
that of white men.

What is the prostate gland?

The prostate gland is a gland the size of two walnuts that seat on either side of
the neck of the urinary bladder.

What is the function of the prostate gland?

The Prostate gland secrete a liquid that helps to liquefy semen that ejaculated by
men during sexual intercourse, which allows the sperm to swim easier towards
female eggs. that is the only useful function that the prostate is known to have.
The prostate gland can cause many miseries for men. In fact, all men if live long
enough will have one form of prostate problem or an other.

Example of the different problems that men are likely to suffer from with their
prostate glands is:
1.   Acute prostatitis (acute infection of the prostate gland)

2.   Chronic prostatitis (chronic infection of the prostate)
3.   Benign prostatic hypertrophy (enlargement of the prostate gland without the presence of cancer)
4.   Urinary retention
5.   Hematuria (blood in the urine)

Which men who should worry about the development of prostate cancer?

All men have a high probability of developing prostate cancer but the incidence of prostate cancer is higher in black men than it is in men of other ethnic background.

For example, the incidence of prostate cancer is 2–3 times higher in Black American men than their white counterparts. Black American men and Jamaican men have the highest percentage of prostate cancer among all black men in the world and among men in general.

What are the different things that predispose men to prostate cancer?

1.   Heredity-that is if a man's father has prostate cancer; if his brother has prostate, colon, or breast cancer; if his uncle has prostate, colon, or breast cancer; if his mother has breast, colon, or ovarian cancer; if his aunt has breast, colon, or ovarian cancer. There is a 10% genetic crossover between prostate cancer, colon cancer, and ovarian cancer. In a certain mother is capable of transferring the gene for prostate cancer to her son. Once there is a cluster of cancer in the immediate family, any member of that immediate family has a higher likelihood of developing cancer of one kind or another, more so that the general population.
2.   Obesity-Obesity is associated of development of prostate cancer because the obese men have too much fat in their bodies, and therefore are able to use the cholesterol ring associated with fat to overproduce the male hormone-Androgen. The male hormone a man produces, the more he is able to stimulate the prostate gland, and

the more the prostate gland is stimulated by the male hormone, the higher the incidence of developing prostate cancer.

3. Eating fat-reach diets-Eating too much fat leads to the production of too much male hormone-Androgen, which in turn results in over-stimulation of the prostate gland, resulting in a higher incidence of prostate cancer.

It is believed that the fact that African-American men eat a diet that is too rich in fat that is why the incidence of prostate cancer is the highest in African-American men that other black men in the world. I was the first person to have made that observation in 1990 in my first book "The Status of Health of Blacks in the United States-a Prescription for Improvement", published by Kendle Hunt Publishing Company. The medical community has now recognized this as scientific fact.

At what age should black men begin to have themselves medically evaluated for prostate cancer?

Prostate cancer usually appears in black men at age 40. However, there are few cases known to have occurred as early as age 35. Prostate cancer usually appears in white males at age 50, there are few cases known to have occurred as early as age 45.

What are the early symptoms of prostate cancer?

Usually there are no early symptoms.

What are the late symptoms of prostate cancer?

1. Blood in the urine.
2. Burning in urination.
3. Urinary frequency.
4. Hesitancy in urination.
5. Poor urinary stream.
6. Nocturia-getting up too many times at night to urinate.
7. Urinary retention.
8. Weakness.
9. Bone pain.

10. Constipation.
11. Paralysis from the waist down, due to spinal cord compression by the prostate cancer.

How can a man find out if he has prostate cancer?

To find out if a man has prostate cancer he must go to the doctor to have:
1. A digital rectal examination.
2. He must have a blood test done to examine the Prostatic Specific Antigen (PSA).

The rectal exam allows the physician to palpate the prostate gland to determine whether it is smooth, hard, or has a nodule, or whether the gland is 1+, 2+, 3+, or 4+ in size; 1+ being the smallest, 4+ being the largest.

The PSA is a blood test when elevated can mean that the man has prostate cancer. The normal PSA value is from 0 to 4.0 but is age-variable. In older men, PSA above four may not necessarily mean that prostate cancer is present.

The PSA may be high in:
1. Acute prostatitis.
2. Chronic recurrent prostatitis.
3. Benign prostatic hypertrophy.
4. Post coital (a day after sexual intercourse).
5. Prostate cancer.

It is important to understand that a man may have a PSA of 1 and still has prostate cancer if he has a prostate nodule that is palpated during the rectal examination. In the same vain, a man may have a PSA of 1 in one year, and the next consecutive year the PSA is doubled to 2.0: that may indicate the presence of prostate cancer in that gland because of the doubling of the PSA value that occurs so rapidly. It is also very important that close attention is paid to the difference that occurs in the PSA reading from year to year. If the PSA let us say was 1.8 in 1 year and the following year the PSA becomes 2.7, this is a PSA reflection of 0.9. This very important and may indicate the presence of cancer in the prostate gland. The accepted PSA Reflection is 0.7.

It is not unusual for a man to present to the doctor with a high PSA and it is due to infection of the prostate or an enlargement of the prostate and not cancer.

By the age of 35, it is a good idea for Black men to begin the process of having yearly digital rectal examination and yearly PSA done. This is even more important if prostate cancer is known to exist in his immediate family.

How to evaluate an asymptomatic elevated PSA?

The first thing to do is to refer the man to a urologist. The urologist will take a history from him, examine him, and most likely do one or two things:

1. Depending on the history he/she may choose to treat the man with an appropriate antibiotic.
2. After the completion of the course of the antibiotic, the urologist will likely repeat the PSA.
3. If the PSA returns to normal, he/she may decide to observe the patient.
4. If the PSA fails to return to normal, or did not change at all after the antibiotic treatment, the urologist is likely to recommend a prostate biopsy.
5. Alternatively, the urologist may decide to immediately recommend a prostate biopsy.
6. If the PSA velocity is greater than 0.7 form the previous year's PSA, that also calls for a prostate biopsy to done.

How is the prostate biopsy done?

The night before the biopsy, as well as the morning before the biopsy, the patient is given an antibiotic named Cipro to take. That prevents infections from developing. Then a special needle is used trough the rectum using sonographic technique as a guide and prostate tissue is taken from several parts of the prostate gland and placed in formalin and sent to the pathology laboratory for microscopic evaluation by a pathologist.

1. What if the prostate biopsy comes back indicting that cancer is present in the prostate gland?
2. What then must the man do?

The first thing is that the urologist is going to arrange for a meeting between the man and his wife or the man and his significant other.

This meeting is extremely important because the man is going to hear this most unpleasant of all news in that he has prostate cancer. Any news telling anyone he/she has cancer is devastating to say the least, but telling a man that he has prostate cancer, and that his sexuality and life are both on the line is a matter of extraordinary emotional importance. For that reason, the man needs to have present during the discussion that is going to take place the one person that he trusts the most to help his to handle the news of the moment.

Paramount in the discussion of the discovery of prostate cancer is what is the stage of the cancer? This is important because the stage of the cancer dictates what treatment alternatives the urologist can offer to the affected man.

A short synopsis of the staging system use to evaluate needle biopsy of the prostate is the Gleason stage system. The Gleason stages system rages from Gleason 1 to Gleason 10. The lower the Gleason stage, the more localized the cancer is and the better the prognosis. Conversely, the higher the Gleason stage, the more advanced the cancer and the poorer the prognosis.

A Gleason stage up to 7 in most situations may lend itself to surgical intervention as a modality of treatment. A Gleason greater than 7 is less likely to be cured by surgery alone as a modality. A more detailed and thorough staging of prostate cancer is usually given after a pathological examination of the surgical specimen.

What are the different treatment modalities available to treat prostate cancer?

1. Nerve spearing—Radical prostatectomy for early stage prostate cancer.
2. Robatic prostatectomy
3. Radiation therapy.
4. Seeds placement.
5. Hormonal treatments for advanced prostate cancer.
6. Chemotherapy for metastatic prostate cancer.

See the section on prostate cancer in chapter 7.
Each one of these treatment modalities has their upsides and downsides.

The nerve spearing radical prostatectomy is offered as a curative treatment for early prostate cancer. It is a very extensive form of treatment during which the network of tubes within which sperm is produced is removed because frequently cancer cells are found hidden there. The nerves that are necessary to help a man to have an erection are evaluated and spared as best as possible to enable to have an erection some time in the future after surgery. Multiple nodes are removed and sent to the pathology lab to be evaluated for presence or absence of cancer. The valve that seats at the neck of the bladder is sacrificed to be sure that no cancer remains in that area.

Consequently the alternate valve which all men have and have never used before, is now used to attach the urether to enable the man to urinate once the Foley Catheter is removed several weeks postoperatively. The reason why it takes several weeks before the Foley Catheter can be removed is that it takes that long for the new valve to get accustom to function as a valve.

Radiation therapy is an excellent non-invasive modality to treat prostate cancer in men who for one reason or another are not good candidate for radical prostatectomy or their cancer's stage is not clinically appropriate for surgery. The down side with radiation therapy for prostate cancer is that it is not always curative and it can cause proctitis, rectal bleeding and it can in significant percentage of cases cause erectile dysfunction.

Seeds Placement is superb alternative treatment for early prostate cancer for men who do not want surgery or who for medical reasons of one kind or another cannot have surgery.
It too can cause erectile dysfunction in certain percentage of men.
In some men who have advanced prostate cancer seed placement can also be used as good treatment modality. In men, whose prostate gland is too large, hormone such as Leupron can be given intramuscularly to shrink the size of the prostate to allow for easier placement of the seeds.
The seeds are radioactive materials that are placed inside the prostate gland to kill the cancer cells.

Hormonal treatments that commonly used to treat prostate cancer are:

1. Leupron (antitestosterone)

2. Flutamide (total Androgen Blockage)
3. Casodex

These hormones block the production of the male hormone from the prostate gland. By blocking the production of Androgen from the prostate gland, the growth of cancer cells are slowed down and the level of PSA in the blood decreases. Androgen is needed for prostate cancer cells to grow.

The side effects of Hormonal treatments are:

1. Erectal dysfunction
2. Gynecomastia (large breasts)
3. Feeling warm all the time
4. Sweating a lot

The most effective Chemotherapy presently to treat metastatic prostate cancer is TAXOL intravenously. (see section on prostate cancer in chapter 7)

The most effective medications available to treat **ERECTIL DYSFUNCTION** in post
Radical Prostatectomy is:
Viagra
Sialis
Levitra
Injection of prostaglandin into the Penis
Muse
Penal implant
Viagra and the other similar medications work to bring about penal erection by releasing Nitric Oxide in the penis, which relaxes smooth muscle, and dilating the blood vessels that carry blood to the Penis. These two things bring about erection in men in this setting.

It is important that black men understand the importance of having a digital rectal examination done every year from age 35 onward which can save their lives. It is equally important that white males and men of other ethnic background do the same by age 40.

It is important that men understand that having a PSA blood test every year from age 35–40 onward can save their lives.

In particular, Black American men an other black men must be urged to modify their diet by removing the excessive amount of red meat, pork fried foods, and replacing them with non-shellfishes, poultry, fruits, vegetables, beans, olive cooking oil and low simple carbohydrate foods, corn meal. In general, exercise along with a good diet program will help to decrease their total body fat and decrease their incidence of prostate cancer. All men no matter their racial make up ought to follow this advice.

Men can have a multitude of problems affecting their urinary bladder: Among the problems that can affect men and their urinary bladders are:
1. Urinary retention
2. Hematuria (bleeding from the bladder)
3. Urinary tract infection
4. Cancer of the urinary bladder etc.

The most common causes of urinary retention in men are:
1. Benign Prostatic Hypertrophy
2. Prostate cancer
3. Diabetes mellitus
4. Stroke
5. Multiple sclerosis etc;
6. Cancer of the bladder with bleeding and too much clots
7. Cancer of the kidney with bleeding and too much clots
8. Sickle cell disease with papillary necrosis, bleeding and too much clots
9. Urinary tract infection
10. Spinal cord injury

The most common causes of hematuria in men are:
1. Prostate cancer
2. Kidney stone
3. Urinary tract infection
4. Cancer of urinary bladder
5. Cancer of the kidney
6. Benign prostatic hypertrophy
7. Hemophilia
8. Von Willebran disease
9. Aspirin ingestion

10. Sickle cell anemia

The most common causes of urinary tract infection in men are:
1. Benign prostatic hypertrophy
2. Diabetes mellitus
3. Stroke
4. Insertion of foley catheter in the bladder
5. Old age with poor toileting
6. Multiple sclerosis
7. Cancer of the urinary bladder
8. Kidney stones with hydronephrosis
9. Cancer of the urether with hydronephrosis etc;

The most common causes of cancer of the urinary bladder are:
1. Genetic predisposition
2. Exposure to different dyes at work
3. Tobacco smoking
4. Schistosoma haematobium etc;

(See chapter 7 on cancer)

The best ways to evaluate hematuria are:
1. Renal ultra sound
2. Bladder ultra sound
3. Cat scan of the kidney
4. Cat scan of the bladder
5. Urine cytology
6. Urinalysis
7. Urine culture
8. PSA
9. Hemoglobin electrophoresis
10. Ova and parasite
11. Serum antibody screen for Schistosoma haematobium
12. Cystoscopy etc;

Diseases of the kidney frequently affect men.

Among the diseases that can affect men's kidneys are:
1. Infections (UTI, Pyelonephritis
2. Kidney st
3. Cancer of the kidney
4. End stage kidney disease
5. Glomerulonephriti
6. Nephrotic syndrome
7. Papillary necrosis

8. Polycystic kidney disease
9. Azotemia
10. Uremia etc;

The most common causes of urinary tract infection in are BPH, insertion of a foley catheter, kidney stones, sickle cell disease, aberrant urinary tract, prostate cancer, diabetes mellitus, stroke etc;

Urinary tract infection is divided into lower tract urinary tract infection and upper tract urinary tract infection.

The most common symptoms of lower tract urinary tract infection are
1. Urinary frequency
2. Burning on urination
3. Urinary hesitancy
4. Nocturia
5. Urinary retention
6. Gross hematuria
7. Microscopic hematuria
8. Fever
9. Chills
10. Head ache
11. Lower abdominal pain
12. General weakness
13. Tiredness etc.

The most common symptoms of upper tract urinary tract infection are:
all the above, plus flank pain, nausea and vomiting.

The best ways to evaluate UTI both lower tract UTI and upper tract UTI are:
1. Take good history from the patient
2. Do a complete physical examination
3. Do a urinalysis
4. Do a urine culture
5. Do 2 sets of blood culture
6. Do a complete CBC
7. Do an SMA 20 chemistry profile

If a man has UTI and is not febrile, he can be treated as an outpatient.
If his febrile, he should be admitted to the hospital for in hospital treatments.

The most common bacteria responsible for UTI in men are gram negative enteric bacteria.

The antibiotics that are available to treat UTI are:

1. Ampicillin
2. Keflex
3. Kefzol
4. Cipro
5. Levaquin
6. Ceftazidime
7. Cetriaxone
8. Bactrim DS
9. Gentamicin etc;

Upper tract UTI is also called pyelonephrytis and must be treated with IV antibiotic for 14–21 days. Lower tract UTI in men who are febrile can be treated with antibiotic IV for 7–10 days if the blood cultures are negative.

Lower UTI in men who are afebrile can be treated with antibiotic by mouth for 7–10 days. Levaquin by mouth is as effective as Levaquin IV.

Men who have UTI either lower tract or upper tract must be evaluated by a urologist to find out the reason for the UTI. As part of the urological evaluation, the following tests must be done.

1. Ultrasound of the prostate
2. Ultrasound of the bladder
3. Ultrasound of the Kidneys
4. Cat scan of the kidneys and bladder with contrast
5. Cat Scan of the kidneys without contrast looking for kidney stones

Urinary cylology
Serum PSA
Hemoglobin electrophoresis
Cystoscopy etc;

Kidney stones are quite common in men and this condition is quite painful. The most common stones are calcium oxalate and calcium phosphate. Calcium stones are most commonly seen in men.

The most common causes of kidney stones are:

1. Hyperuricosuria
2. Primary hyperparathyroidism
3. Intestinal hyperoxaluria

4. Hereditary hyperoxaluria
5. Hyperuricosuria
6. Gout
7. Lymphoma
8. Lymphocytic leukemia
9. Dehydration

The most common symptoms of kidney stones are:

1. Severe and excruciating lower back pain
2. Hematuria,(gross or microscopic)

The best ways to evaluate men for kidney stones are:

1. Take a good history
2. Do a complete physical examination
3. Do a urinalysis to look for blood
4. Do a flat plate of the abdomen x-ray to look for a stone
5. Do a CT of the abdomen without contrast looking for a stone
6. Strain the urine to look for stones
7. Do an SMA 20 chemistry profile
8. Do a serum uric acid
9. Do a CBC looking lymphocytosis (elevated lymphocytes count)

The best treatments available to treat kidney stones are:

1. Pain killer medication
2. Allopurinol
3. Thiazide diuretic
4. Diet
5. Surgical removal of kidney stones
6. External Shock Wave Lithotripsy (ESWL)

Hematuria can occur in individuals who have abnormal coagulation problems such as

1. Hemophilia A and B
2. Factor V deficiency
3. Factor VII deficiency
4. Factor X deficiency
5. Factor XI deficiency
6. Von Willebran disease
7. Dessiminated intravascular coagulopathy (DIC)

Hamaturia can also occur because of platelet abnormalities such as

1. Thrombocytopenia (low platelet)
2. Thombopathy (qualitative platelet Abnormaqlity)

Hematuria can also occur because ingestion of aspirin and nonsteroidal anti-inflammatory drugs.

An other common cause of hematuria in men is sickle cell trait and sickle cell anemia.

The reason for the hematuria in sickle cell disease is papillary necrosis of the kidney.

Some of the most common problems that men's genitourinatract and genital are sexually transmitted diseases.

Among the most frequent STD that some men are afflicted with are:

1. Herpes simplex
2. Gonorrhea
3. Chlamydia
4. Syphilis
5. Human papilloma virus (HPV)
6. Trichomonas
7. HIV
8. Hepatitis B
9. Hepatitis C
10. Chancroid etc.

Genital herpes is the most common STD in the US. About 1 million individuals per year become infected with the herpes simplex virus. More than one in five people are infected with genital herpes simplex, for a total that adds up to more than 45 million American.

There are 2 types of genital herpes simplex, type 1 and type 2.

The majority of genital herpes simplex infection is caused by herpes simplex type 2.

Many people have herpes simplex infection and don't know it.

Herpes simplex infection occurs across all racial and socio economic groups.

The usual symptoms of genital herpes simplex in men are painful and itchy blisters at the head or near the head of the penis or rectum. The blisters eventually become painful ulcers or sores that usually about 4 weeks to heal. These out breaks of herpes simplex type 2 can occur in the same areas every several months.

Herpes simplex can be transmitted by any one who is carrying in his or her blood to his or her sexual partner during sexual intercourse.

Herpes simplex type 1 can also cause genital herpes but much so than type 2.

Herpes simplex type 1 usually causes fever blisters in the mouth and can be transmitted from mouth to genitalia during oral sex.

Herpes simplex break outs tend to occur during the time of stress. The reason for that is that during stress a person secrets excessive amount of adrenalin and elevated adrenalin causes a transient state of immuno suppression which allows the herpes simplex virus to come out of its dormant state and causes break outs to occur usually in the spots from the previous break outs.

How is herpes simplex virus diagnosed?

1. Take a good history from the patient
2. Do thorough physical examination
3. Send genital herpes simplex culture from the blisters or ulcers to the Microbiology laboratory
4. Send blood to the laboratory to test for both herpes simplex type 1 and type 2. How to treat herpes simplex infection

The treatment for the first episode of genital herpes simplex break out is

1. Acyclovir 400mg by mouth 3 times per day times for 7–10 days

Or

2. Acyclovir 200 mg by mouth 5 times per day for 7–10 days

Or

3. Vilacyclovir 1 gram orally 2 times per 7–10 days

Or

4. Famciclovir 250 mg orally 3 times per day 7–10 days

Or

5. To suppress recurrent genital herpes infection: Give Acyclovir 400 mg by mouth twice per day

Or

6. Famiciclovir 250 mg by mouth twice per day

Or

7. Valacyclovir 500 mg by mouth daily

Or

8. Valacyclovir 1gram by mouth daily

Or

9. When the episode of herpes recurs on and off: Give Acyclovir 400 mg by mouth three times per day for 5 days

Or

10. Acyclovir 800 mg by mouth twice per day for 5 days

Or

11. Acyclovir 800 mg by mouth three times per day for 2 days

Or

12. Famciclovir 125 mg by mouth twice per day for 5 days

Or
13. Famciclovir 1000 mg by mouth twice per day for one day
Or
Valacyclovir 500 mg twice per day for 3 days

If the person is infected with genital herpes and also infected with HIV treat with

1. Acyclovir 400–800 mg by mouth three times per day
Or
2. Famciclovir 500 mg twice per day
Or
3. Valacyclovir 500 mg twice per day
(as recommended by the CDC STD Treatment Guidelines August 2006)

Gonorrhea is a very common STD. Every year 700,000 individuals in the US become infected with gonorrhea. The infection gonorrhea is caused by the bacterium Neisseria gonorrhea which is an intracellular gram negative diplococcus. Gonorrhea (GC) can be spread through the penis, vagina, mouth and the rectum. Any sexually active individual can get infected with gonorrhea. In the US gonorrhea is most prevalent among teenagers, young adult. Once a man comes in contact with GC, it takes 2–5 days for symptoms to appear. However some men can contract GC and never develop symptoms and infect their sexual partner during ejaculation.
The usual symptoms of GC are:
1. Burning on urination
2. Whitish discharge from the penis
3. Yellowish discharge from the penis
4. Sometime GC can cause a painful and swollen testicle
5. GC in the rectum can cause itching, soreness, bleeding and pain during bowel movement
6. GC may also cause swore throat
The best way to diagnose GC in men is by doing a gram stain of the discharge from the penis and by doing a GC culture of that same discharge. If gram negative intracellular diplococci bacteria are seen on the gram stain taken from a penal discharge, that is proof positive that the man is infected with GC. Cultures for GC can be taken from the throat, rectum and in the case of disseminated GC from blood or joint's fluid.
The best medications available to treat GC are:

The CDC no longer recommends Cipro, Ofloxacin, and Levaquin for use in treating gonorrhea because the gonorrheal bacterium is no longer sensitive to them.

Uncomplicated GC Urethritis:

1. Ceftriaxone 125 mg IM

                            Or

2. Spectinomycin 2 grams IM

                            Or

3. Cefixime 400 mg by mouth.

                            Or

4. Cefpodoxine proxetil 200 mg by mouth

                            Or

5. Zithromax 500 mg by mouth

Frequently people who are infected with GC are also infected with Chlamydia therefore, they must be treated for Chlamydia as well with Doxycycline 100 mg twice per day.

Both GC and Chlamydia are sensitive to Zithromax.

If a man is infected with GC and his sexual partner is a man and or he recently returned from a trip abroad during which he had unprotected sexual intercourse, the treatment of choice is:

1. Ceftriaxone 125 MG IM

                            Or

2. Cefixime 400 mg by mouth

                            Plus

3. Doxycycline 100 mg 2 times per day x 14 days

Men who are with disseminated Gonococcal infection must be hospitalized and once in the hospital, they should have blood cultures, lumbar puncture to obtain cerebrospinal fluid for gram stain, culture, cell count, glucose and protein. They should also get Chest x-ray, echocardiogram and, if a joint is swollen and has effusion, it should be tapped and the fluid send to the laboratory for gram stain, culture, cell count, glucose and protein.

Once these studies are done, treatment should start with:

1. Ceftriaxone 1 gram IM OR IV every 24 hours
                            Or
2. Cefotaxime 1 gram IV every 8 hours
                    Or if allergic to penicillin
3. Spectinomycin 2 grams IM every 12 hours

Sexual partners of any individuals treated for GC must be examined, tested for GC and treated with either Zithromax, Ceftriaxone or Doxycycline.

Chlamydia is one of the most common STD that affects men. Every year there are more than 2.8 millions cases of Chlamydia in the US. Most men who have Chlamydia are asymptomatic and thus are aware that they are carrying the infection. Chlamydia is caused by the bacterium Chlamydia trachomatis.

The symptoms of Chlamydia in men are:
Discharge from the penis
Burning on urination
Rectal pain in men who have sex with men
Rectal discharge in men who have sex with men
Rectal bleeding in men who have sex with men
Sore throat in people who are involved in oral sex can occur.

The best way to diagnose Chlamydia in men is to send specimen taken from the penal discharge to the microbiology laboratory for culture.
Chlamydia can cause epididymitis (swelling and pain in a testicle) with fever and chills.
Sometime men can become sterile due to chronic and untreated Chlamydia urethritis.
Chlamydia can sometime cause (Reiters's Syndrome), which is a combination of arthritis, urethritis, skin lesions and inflammation of the eye.

The best treatments for Chlamydia are
1. Zythromax 500 mg by mouth one dose
                            Or
2. Doxycycline 100 mg by mouth twice per day for 7 days

Sexual partners of individuals treated for Chlamydia ought to be examined, tested for Chlamydia and treated either with Zythromax or Docycycline.

Syphilis Infection

Syphilis has historically been one of the most common STDs to afflict mankind and has been in the new world since 1494 when Columbus and his men came to America. Syphilis is caused by the spirochete Treponema Pallidum.

According to the latest statistics from the CDC published in the October issue of Morbidity and Mortality Weekly Report, October 25, 1996, Volume 44, No. 53, in 1995, 68,953 cases of syphilis were reported. 16,000 cases were primary and secondary syphilis. 1,548 cases of congenital syphilis were reported. There were 7,768 primary and secondary cases of syphilis in men.

The rate of syphilis has declined by 29 percent among Blacks from 1997–1999. The rate remains stable among whites but increased by 20 percent among Hispanics. Overall, the rate of syphilis is 30 times higher in Blacks than in whites; 125.4 cases per 100,000 Blacks vs. 0.5 cases per 100,000 in whites. Syphilis is 50 percent more common in men than in women. *(Source: "Tracking the Hidden Epidemic Trend in STD in the U.S. 2000.* CDC)

Syphilis is usually transmitted sexually. Once the organism is deposited into the human tissue it takes anywhere from 14 to 21 days for primary syphilis to develop.

The first manifestation of primary syphilis is a chancre, which is often a painless sore. The chancre or syphilitic ulcer may be seen in the mouth, lips, arms, rectum, nipples, naval (belly button), etc. If left untreated, by 4 to 8 weeks the chancre would heal spontaneously. Untreated syphilis spreads via the lymphatic system to disseminate throughout the body to cause secondary syphilis.

The first manifestation of secondary syphilis is usually a rash over the body. The rash can occur in the palms of the hands and sometimes under the feet. The rash is often scaly, smooth and it may be itchy. This type of rash may resemble other rashes and may be difficult to distinguish just by looking at it. Because secondary syphilis is a systemic disease, it can cause sore throat, headache, fever, weight loss with aches and pains. There may be large glands in the neck, under the arms and elsewhere in the body.

The physician has to be suspicious enough to order a blood test for syphilis. A scraping from the rash can be studied via dark field technique, which might show the spirochetes treponoma pallidum wiggling around under the microscope. Similarly, "scraping material" taken from the chancre seen in primary syphilis when placed on a glass slide, and covered with a cover slip and placed under the microscope will show the spirochetes, as well. Other things that secondary syphilis may cause include arthritis, hepatitis, condyloma, uveitis, iritis, otitis, CVA, kidney problems such as glomerulo nephritis, hepatitis, weight loss, poor appetite, memory loss, seizure, meningitis, etc.

After going through the primary and secondary stage in about 12 weeks, if syphilis remains untreated, then it enters into the latent stage. Many men may have symptoms and signs of primary and secondary syphilis without recognizing them. In about 2 years time if syphilis remains untreated, it enters into the tertiary stage.

Tertiary syphilis is an advanced stage of syphilis, which can affect the heart, the liver, the brain and other vital organs.

The chronic involvement of vital organs with untreated syphilis is guaranteed to cause death of individuals infected with it. Syphilis can cause a person to become paralyzed and can cause a person to develop seizures and even insanity due to changes in the brain.

Two studies were done in the past that allow for an understanding of the effects of untreated syphilis on the human body.

The first study was the Oslo study, which took place between 1891 and 1951. It included 2000 patients diagnosed clinically. The dark field test and Wasserman test were not yet in existence. Penicillin had not yet been discovered either so there was no effective way to treat these patients.

That study amply demonstrated the devastating effects of untreated syphilis on all parts of the human body, in particular, the brain, the aorta, the skeletal system, etc.

The second study is the infamous **Tuskegee study**, which took place from 1932–1974 in Tuskegee, Alabama under the control of the **United States Public Health Service.**

The shameful reason given for **this cruel, inhumane, barbaric and racist study** was to find the effects of untreated syphilis on the human body. There were no scientific justifications for this study in view of the fact that the Oslo study had already shown what untreated syphilis could do to the human body.

From 1932 to 1974, under the leadership of the United States Public Health Service, 431 (Negro men) black men were injected with live syphilis organisms for the sole purpose of seeing what effects syphilis would have on their bodies. These men did not sign consent for participating in the study. They did not know that they were being injected with live syphilis organisms.

In the history of the world, many events have taken place to catalogue men's cruelty towards each other: **Slavery, the Holocaust, the Rwanda Massacre, and the Tuskegee Study** and now **Darfur** are a few such examples. In the Tuskegee Study, 431 men were sacrificed for nothing other than racism and bigotry, while the U.S. government, organized medicine, some black and white physicians, some white and black hospital administrators and society, at large, stood by silently. **How shameful and how disgusting?**

How to Diagnose Syphilis

The tests that are presently in use to diagnose Syphilis are:
1. Dark field examination of material taken from a chancre.
2. VDRL (Venereal Disease Control Research Laboratory) or RPR
3. FTA-ABS (Fluorescent Treponema Antibody Absorption)

How Is A Dark Field Examination Done?

Material is taken from a chancre. It is placed on a glass slide. After prepping, a cover slip is placed on the specimen and placed under the microscope. The microscope is darkened in a special fashion to allow for proper visualization. A positive dark field is when spirochetes are seen wiggling around and around.

Seeing spirochetes under the microscope does necessarily means that a person has syphilis, because Yaws and *Pinta* also are diseases caused by spirochetes as well. They cannot be differentiated from the spirochete that causes syphilis morphologically. A positive VDRL in fact does not necessarily mean that a person has syphilis. There are many medical conditions in medicine that can cause false positive VDRL. Both Yaws and Pinta can cause a positive VDRL and yet the patients may not have syphilis.

How to Differentiate A False Positive VDRL From A Truly Positive VDRL

The test to do to differentiate a false positive VDRL/RPR is the FTA-ABS test. This test is always positive when a person has syphilis, because it is specific for the antigen produced by triponoma pallidum, which is the spirochete responsible for causing syphilis.

Treatment For The Different Stages Of Syphilis

1. Primary syphilis—chancre stage (not allergic to penicillin) 1.2 million units of Benzathine penicillin in each buttock, IM.
2. Secondary syphilis—(not allergic to penicillin)—1.2 million units of Benzathine penicillin in each buttock IM weekly times three weeks in sequence.

3. Latent syphilis (not allergic to penicillin)—1.2 million units of Benzathine in each buttock IM weekly times three weeks in sequence.

4. Tertiary syphilis—(not allergic to penicillin)—1.2 million units of Benzathine penicillin in each buttock IM weekly times three weeks in sequence.

5. Neuro syphilis—(if not allergic to penicillin)—spinal tap ought to be done; send CSF for VDRL and FTA-ABS testing. If positive, admit patient to the hospital and treat with 12 to 24 million units per day of aqueous penicillin G IV for ten days or 600,000 units daily of procaine penicillin IM daily for 14 days. Either the IV or the IM treatment can be carried out on an outpatient basis.

Any man who is HIV positive and VDRL and FTA positive must be assumed to have neurosyphilis. A spinal tap must be done and the CSF study for syphilis. It does not matter, in fact, whether the CSF is positive or not. Any HIV positive individual with positive VDRL and positive FTA-ABS must be treated in the same way as some one with documented neuro-syphilis as just outlined above, and additional weekly doses of Benzathine penicillin IM must be given for three weeks.

If a man is allergic to penicillin and has early stages of syphilis, the treatment of choice is Erythromycin or Tetracycline 500 mg by mouth, four times a day for 15 days. For more advanced stages of syphilis, including neuro-syphilis, the treatment of choice is Erythromycin or Tetracycline 500 mg by mouth four times a day for 30 days.

It is very important to do follow-up VDRL after treating a person for syphilis. Every three months a repeat VDRL ought to be done to show that the VDRL titer is going down. Sometimes, the VDRL remains high even though adequate treatment was given. This situation can be quite confusing because a person can get re-infected with syphilis. It's hard to tell sometimes whether a person has become reinfected or not. An increasing VDRL titer after treatment may mean that re-infection may have taken place.

It is absolutely crucial that pregnant men are not treated with Tetracycline in the first trimester of pregnancy. Tetracycline will interfere with the calcification of bones and stains the teeth of the fetus/baby.

2003 Statistics on STI/STD in USA
Annual Incidence (number of new cases within a year)

1. HPV (Human Papilloma Virus) 5.5 millions PER YEAR

2.   Trichomonas   5 millions
3.   Chlamydia   3 millions
4   Herpes simplex types 1&2   45 millions
5.   Gonorrhea   (339,598 in 2005)
6.   Hepatitis B   120,000
7.   Syphilis   70,000
8.   HIV   40,000
9.   Chancroid   3,500
10.   Hepatitis C (see prevalence on next page and the chapter on GI Diseases
11.   AIDS (see prevalence on next page and chapter 12 on AIDS)

Prevalence

(Number of infected people in the US population at any one time)
1.   Herpes simplex virus type 2   45 million
2.   HPV   20 million
3.   HIV   1.4 million
4.   Hepatitis B   417,000
5.   Hepatitis C   4 million

Chancroid is STD that is caused by Hemophilus ducreyi and it is best diagnosed by using a special culture medium. It is manifested by a painful inguinal ulcer.

The best treatments are Azitromycin 1 gram by mouth or Cipro 250 mg by mouth twice per day for 3 days or Erythromycin500 mg by mouth three times per day for 7 days or Ceftriaxone 250 mg IM once.

Lymphogranuloma Venereum (LVG) is an STD that is caused by Chlamydia trachomatis. It is usually manifested by unilateral painful and tender inguinal node enlargement, plus Genital ulcer. The diagnosis is usually made clinically and by serology.

The best treatments for L V G are Doxycycline 100 mg by mouth two times per day for 21 days or Erythromycin 500 mg by mouth four times per 21 days.

Epididymitis is common condition that is usually seen in sexually active men who are younger than 36 years old. It is almost always caused by STD such as GC or Chlamydia, It is manifested by a swollen, painful and tender testicle. It may be accompanied with fever and chills. The diagnosis is usually made by 1. Examination of the affected testicle 2. Gram stain of urethral discharge, to see if there is increased white blood cells. 3. culture of urethral discharge for GC and Chlamydia and ultrasound of the swollen testicle.

The best treatments for Epididymitis are;

1. Docycycline 100 mg two times per day by mouth for 10 days.
2. Alternatively Levaquin 500 mg by mouth once per day for 10 days
3. Floxin 300 mg two times per day by mouth for 10 days
4. Ceftriaxone 250 mg IM one dose.

If the man affected has fever and chills he ought to be admitted into the hospital for in hospital care.

Trichomonas is frequently carried by some men as an STD without their knowledge and each time they have unprotected sexual intercourse with they sexual partners they transmit the trichomonal organism into them. Some time the trichomonal organism can be seen swimming in urine sediments taken from men under the microscope.

The best medication available to treat trichomonas is Flagyl 250 mg three times per day for 4 days. The sexual partners must also be treated in the same manner.

Genital wart is a very common STD and the responsible viral organism is Human Papilloma Virus (HPV). The subgroups of HVP virus most commonly responsible for Genital warts are types 6, 11, 16, 18, 31, 33 and 35.

The best way to diagnose genital warts is to do pathological examination of the warts and to do DNA testing of the specimen.

The best treatments available to treat genital warts are

Laser surgery

Or

Podofilox 0.5% solution or gel applicat

Or

Imiquimod 5% cream

Or

Trichloroacetic acid or Bichloroacetic acid 80%-90%

Or

Podophyllin resin 10%-25% application

CHAPTER 12

AIDS IN MEN IN THE UNITED STATES OF AMERICA

WHAT IS AIDS?

AIDS STANDS for Acquired Immune Deficiency Syndrome (as opposed to inborn Immune Deficiency Syndrome).

AIDS is referred to as Acquired Immune Deficiency Syndrome because the virus, the HIV Type I or Type 2, a retrovirus, enters the human body and attacks and kills the T helper lymphocyte (T4 or CD4), causing a decrease in their numbers, resulting in immunodeficiency of the body and in turn causing vulnerability to a multitude of diseases.

Some of these diseases are caused by the HIV viruses themselves and some of the diseases are caused by different opportunistic organisms that enter into the body at different times in the course of the HIV/AIDS syndrome. The T4 helper lymphocytes are in the body to help the body to be healthy, while the T8 suppressor lymphocytes are in the body to cause it to be sick when their numbers increase.

Therefore, in HIVAIDS, the number of T helper lymphocytes is lower than the number of the T suppressor lymphocytes, thereby inverting the T helper-to-T suppressor ratio.

How does the AIDS virus cause immunosuppression? Answer: The AIDS virus enters the bloodstream of the person being infected and quickly enters into the T cell CD4 lymphocytes. Once inside these lymphocytes, the virus multiplies by making copies of itself. Sometimes the virus can copy itself in numbers as large as a billion copies or several billion copies per day, until the body gradually becomes more and more immunosuppressed, stage by stage, leading ultimately to full-blown AIDS and all its associated problems and complications which, without treatment, or if the treatment fails, causes death of the affected person.

AIDS, a historical perspective

The first reported cases of AIDS appeared in an article published in June 1981 in *The New England Journal of Medicine*, in which a group of homosexual men were found to be sick with Pneumocystis carinii pneumonia.

Further evaluation of these problems revealed that they were immunosuppressed and that the immunosuppressive state that they were suffering from had predisposed them to the development of Pneumocystis carinii pneumonia (PCP).

From that point on the AIDS epidemic was underway. Subsequently it was published that a young man who was retarded and who lived in the streets of St. Louis, Missouri, who was a vagrant in the street of that city and who had frequent contacts with homosexual men, became very sick with an unknown disease associated with fever, weight loss and pulmonary infection. He went on to die in the early 1960s from complications of the disease. After his death, an autopsy was performed on him and the pathologist wisely froze tissues and plasma that were taken from his body. In the 1980s after the AIDS epidemic was already underway, that pathologist evaluated these specimens that he had frozen and tested them for the AIDS virus and found that these specimens were teeming with the AIDS virus, which documented that that young man in fact had died of AIDS. So in retrospect, the AIDS virus had been around in the United States, since the early 1960s, as documented by that case. Many of us, including that author who, while in training in the inner city of New York City, saw many drug addicts presented to the hospital with febrile illness associated with large lymph nodes, etc., had no idea what they had. When these lymph nodes were biopsied and the pathologists would report them to us as lymphocytic hyperplasia and we used to think that the different materials that were used to cut the cocaine or heroin that these drug addicts were using were responsible for the so-called lymphocytic hyperplasia, and little did we know that most probably these people had AIDS; we simply did not know of the existence of the disease at that time. So, one does not have to go to Africa or to

Haiti and other Third World countries to look for a scapegoat for the origin of the AIDS virus. The AIDS virus was in the inner cities of the world, long before 1981 when the first cases of AIDS were published

Be that as it may, blame passing aside, scapegoating aside, name calling and finger pointing aside, AIDS is now worldwide and it knows no racial boundaries; it spares no social classes, spares no sexes and it affects people of all ethnic backgrounds and religious beliefs. AIDS is the largest epidemic that mankind has ever known. Every few seconds a new person in the world is being infected with the AIDS virus and those infections are mainly being transmitted through sexual intercourse. As of the end of December 2001 there were 40 million cases of HIV/AIDS in the world and 28.1 million people in Sub-Saharan Africa live with the HIV virus (Source: UNAIDS/WHO, Dec. 2001).

Twenty-two million people worldwide have died of AIDS since the epidemic began in 1981. About 448,060 individuals have died of AIDS in the U.S., as of December 2000 (Source: *CDC Morbidity and Mortality Report, 2001* 50:432–434). As of December 2001, the total numbers of AIDS cases were:

39.5 million People were living with HIV in 2006 (2.6 million more than in 2004).

> The number of new infections in 2006 rose to 4.3 million in 2006 (400 000 more than in 2004).

> Sub-Saharan remains the most affected region in the world. Two thirds of all people living with HIV live in this region—24.7 million people in 2006. Almost three quarters of all adult and child deaths due to AIDS occurred in sub-Saharan Africa—2.1 million of the global 2.9 million deaths due to AIDS.

> The number of people living with HIV increased in every region in the world in the past two years. The most striking increases have occurred in East Asia and in Eastern Europe and Central Asia, where the number of people living with HIV in 2006 was over one fifth (21%) higher than in 2004.

> Access to treatment and care has greatly increased in recent years. Through the expanded provision of antiretroviral treatment, an estimated two million life years were gained since 2002 in low and middle income countries.

> The centrality of high risk behavior (such as injecting drug use, unprotected paid sex and unprotected sex between men) is especially evident in the HIV epidemics of Asia, Eastern Europe and Latin America.

> Although the epidemics also extend into the general populations across the world, they remain highly concentrated around specific populations groups.

According to the CDC" Racial disparity HIV/AIDS diagnoses remains high" Blacks represent 13.8% of the US population, more than 50% of the newly diagnosed 184,991 cases of HIV/AIDS in 2001–2005 were blacks. Black men are 7 times More likely to be diagnosed with HIV than white men and black women are 21 times more likely than white women to be diagnosed with HIV.- Source, Infectious Disease News Volume 20, Number 5, May 2007.

Table 12 A
Statistics for the incidence of HIV/AIDS in different parts of the world

	People liv-ing with HIV	New infec-tions 2006	AIDS deaths 2006	Adult prev-alence %
Sub-Saharan Africa	24.7 million	2.8 million	2.1 million	5.9%
South and South East Asia	7.8 million	860,000	590,000	0.6%
East Asia	750 000	100,000	43,000	0.1%
Latin America	1.7 million	140,000	65,000	0.5%
United States of America	1.4 million	43,000	18,000	0.8%
Western & Central Europe	740 000	22,000	12,000	0.3%
Eastern Europe & Central Asia	1.7 million	270,000	84,000	0.9%
Middle-East & North Africa	460,000	68,000	36,000	0.2%
Caribbean	250,000	27,000	19,000	1.2%
Oceania	81,000	7,100	4,000	0.4%
Total	39.5 million	4.3 million	2.9 million	1%

Modified from UNAIDS/WHO 2006

There are more new HIV infections every year than AIDS-related deaths and as more people become infected with HIV, more people will die of AIDS-related illnesses.

Worldwide, less than one in five people at risk of becoming infected with HIV has access to basic prevention services. Across the world, only one in eight people who want to be tested are currently able to do so.

Scaling up available prevention strategies in 125 low-and middle-income countries would avert an estimated 28 million new infections between 2005 and 2015, more than half of those that are projected to occur during this period and would save US$ 24 billion in associated treatment costs. Simultaneous scaling up of both prevention and treatment would avert 29 million new infections by the end of 2020.

People receiving AIDS treatment worldwide

According to the latest UNAIDS/WHO '3 by 5' data, more than 1.6 million people living with HIV were receiving ARV therapy in low and middle income countries as of June 2006. This represents more than a four fold-increase since December 2003. Overall, antiretroviral therapy coverage in low and middle income countries increased from 7% at the end of 2003 to 24% in June 2006.

Table 12 B

Geographical region	Est. no. of people receiving ARV therapy, June 2006	Est. no. of people needing ARV therapy, 2005	ARV therapy coverage, June 2006
Sub-Saharan Africa	1,040,000	4,600,000	23%
Latin America & Caribbean	345,000	460,000	75%
East, South & South East Asia	235,000	1,440,000	16%
Europe and Central Asia	24,000	190,000	13%
Middle East & North Africa	4,000	75,000	5%
Total	1,650,000	6.8 million	24%

Modified from UNAIDS/WHO 2006

Money available in 2005 to provide for AIDS treatment

In 2005, a total of US$ 8.3 billion was estimated to be available for AIDS funding; this figure is estimated to rise to US$ 8.9 billion in 2006 and US$ 10 billion in 2007. But it falls short of what is needed—US$ 14.9 billion in 2006, US$ 18.1 billion in 2007 and US$ 22.1 billion in 2008.

For treatment and care, about 55% of these resources will be needed in Africa, 20% in Asia and the Pacific, 17% in Latin America and the Caribbean, 7% in Eastern Europe and 1% in North Africa and the Near East.

Table 12 C

AIDS Resource Needs (US$ billion)	2006	2007	2008	Totals for 2006–2008
Prevention	8.4	10.0	11.4	29.8
Treatment and care	3.0	4.0	5.3	12.3
Orphans & vulnerable children	1.6	2.1	2.7	6.4
Program costs	1.5	1.4	1.8	4.6
Human resources	0.4	0.6	0.9	1.9
Total	14.9	18.1	22.1	55.1

TABLE 12D

People newly infected with HIV in 2006	Total	5 million
	Adults	4.3 million
	Men	1.8 million
	Children under 15	800,000
AIDS deaths in 2006	Total	3 million
	Adults	2.4 million
	Men	1.1 million

Children under 15   580,000

TABLE 12 E
International Statistics of HIV/AIDS as of December 2006

Region	Epidemic Started	Adults and Children Living with HIV/AIDS	Adults and Children Newly Infected with HIV	Adult Prevalence Rate (*)	% of HIV Positive Adults who Are Men	Main Mode(s) of Transmission (#) for Adults Living with AIDS
Sub-Saharan Africa	Late '70s Early '80s	28.1 Million	3.4 Million	8.4%	55%	Hetero
North Africa & Middle East	Late 80s	440,000	80,000	0.2%	40%	Hetero, IDU
South & Southeast Asia	Late '80s	6.1 Million	800,000	0.6%	35%	Hetero, IDU
East Asia & Pacific	Late '80s	1 Million	270,000	0.1%	20%	IDU, Hetero, MSM
Latin America	Late '70s Early '80s	1.4 Million	130,000	0.5%	30%	MSM, IDU, Hetero
Caribbean	Late '70s Early '80s	420,000	60,000	2.2%	50%	Hetero, MSM
Eastern Europe & Central Asia	Early '90s	1 Million	250,000	0.5%	20%	IDU
Western Europe	Late '70s Early '80s	560,000	30,000	0.3%	25%	MSM, IDU
North America	Late '70s Early '80s	940,000	45,000	0.6%	20%	MSM, IDU, Hetero
Australia & New Zealand	Late '70s Early '80s	15,000	500	0.1%	10%	MSM
TOTAL		39.5 Million	5 Million	1.2%	48%	

(Source: UNAIDS, Dec. 2006)

In the year 2000, one-third of all new HIV cases diagnosed were among men in the U.S. In Canada, 24% of new HIV cases were among men in the year 2000, as compared to 8.5% in 1995 (Source: UNAIDS/WHO, December 2001). The regions of the world with the highest percentage of AIDS cases are Sub-Saharan Africa, South Asia, Southeast Asia, China, North America, Latin America, Western Europe, and the Caribbean.

As of December 2000, 448,060 individuals have died of AIDS in the U.S., and 66,448 of them were men (Source: *CDC Report 2001*, 50:430–434). Of these men who died, 37,862 were Blacks, 14,632 were Whites, 13,393 were Hispanics, and 331 were Asian/Pacific Islanders, 200 of them were American and Indian/ Alaskan natives (Source: *CDC HIV/AIDS Surveillance Report*, Vol. 12 No. 2).

In Latin America and the Caribbean, there are about 1.8 million adults and children living with the HIV virus. In the year 2001, 190 people became infected with the AIDS virus in Latin America. In the non-U.S. parts of the Americas and the Caribbean, more people became infected with the AIDS virus through heterosexual intercourse. About 1.4 million people in Latin America are living with the virus and 420,000 people in the Caribbean are infected with it. The Caribbean is the second most affected region, per capita, next to Sub-Saharan Africa. About 600,000 people in Brazil are now living with the HIV virus and 105,000 of them are receiving antiretroviral drugs. In Eastern Europe and Central Asia, 250,000 new cases of HIV infection occurred, resulting in 1 million total cases of HIV infected.

In Asia and the Pacific, it is estimated 7.5 million individuals are living with HIV/AIDS, and in 2001, about 435,000 people died of AIDS in that area. About 440,000 individuals in the Middle East and North Africa are infected with the HIV virus. There are roughly 900,000 individuals who were reported to be infected with HIV in the U.S.

In 1999, roughly 2.6 million individuals died of AIDS in the world. About 2.1 million of them were adults, 1.1 million were men and 470,000 were children. During that same period, 13.7 million of the 16.3 million deaths from AIDS occurred in Sub-Saharan Africa.

It is a fact that more men of color are infected with the AIDS virus in the United States than white men. The number of black men who are infected with the AIDS virus surpasses the combination of Hispanic men and white men combined.

Adults and children who are estimated to be living with AIDS in different parts of the world:

Table 12 F

North America-	940,000
Caribbean-	,420,000
Latin America-	1,400,000
Western Europe-	560,000
North African & Middle East-	44,000
Sub-Saharan African-	28,100,000
Eastern Europe and Central Asia-	1,000,000
East Asia and Pacific-	1,000,000
South and Southeast Asia-	6,100,000
Australia and New Zealand-	15,000
Total:	39,500,000

(Source: UNAIDS/WHO, December 2006)

Why is AIDS so much more prevalent among men of color in the U.S., as compared to white men?

The reason more men of color are infected with the AIDS virus than white men is because more men of color are using intravenous drugs than white men. More minority men are using intravenous drugs than white men. Once these minority men become infected with the AIDS virus, they quickly pass it on to their sexual partners. So most of the HIV infection that men of color get, they get by using IV drugs themselves and/or they get it from their minority male sexual partners.

Many men get infected with the AIDS virus although they are not using IV drugs, but their drug-using sexual partners pass the virus on to them during unprotected sexual intercourse.

AIDS, the clinical disease

What are the different ways in which men can be infected with the AIDS virus?

1. Sexual intercourse; men who have sex with men

2. Men who have sexual intercourse with both women and men
3. Men who are injected with elicit IV drugs
4. Men who have sexual intercourse with men who use elicit IV drugs
5. Men who have sexual intercourse with bisexual men
6. Individuals who receive blood or blood products contaminated with the HIV virus
7. Men who use elicit IV drugs
8. Some babies born to mothers who are infected with the HIV virus
9. Some health workers who get stuck with needles contaminated with the HIV virus
10. Being bitten by an AIDS-infected person
11. Using the same toothbrush as that used by an AIDS-infected person
12. Engaging in passionate kissing with an AIDS-infected person
13. Engaging in oral sex with an AIDS-infected person
14. Sexually active uncircumcised men

What are some of the high-risk behaviors that can lead to the transmission of the AIDS virus from one person to another?

1. Anal intercourse, men with women or men with men.
2. Intravenous drug use
3. Prostitution, males or females
4. Promiscuity, males or females
5. Having unprotected sexual intercourse with strangers

In order for a person to become infected with the AIDS virus, the virus must enter the bloodstream of the person at risk.

How can a man become infected with the AIDS virus while having intravaginal intercourse with an infected woman?

The natural vaginal milieu of a woman has a high pH that allows for growth and multiplication of the HIV virus. Further, during sexual intercourse, there is also microtrauma of the capillaries that occurs as part of the natural events, making it possible for the HIV virus to enter into a man's bloodstream. The HIV virus is brought into the man's vaginal environment in the semen that is deposited within it during unprotected sexual intercourse. If a man were to have open sores, such as genital herpes, syphilitic sores, and other venereal chancres, etc., and have sexual intercourse with an HIV-infected woman or man, his chances of being infected increases several-fold, because the HIV virus can easily enter through these sores into the bloodstream of the man. There is a very high correlation between STD and HIV infection.

Uncircumcised men have a higher risk of contracting HIV/AIDS during sexual intercourse with infected partners because the foreskin of their penis is frequently afflicted with balanitis, phemosis, paraphymosis, and these conditions allow for easy entry of the HIV virus to gain entry into the blood stream. The different dgrees of inflammation and crakes that result from these conditions in the foreskin of the penis create a perfect entry point for the HIV virus during sexual intercourse if one's sex partner is carrying the AIDS virus.
The solution to this problem is to circumcise men to eliminate the different conditions in the foreskin of the penis which make it easy for the HIV virus to enter in the blood stream of uncircumcised men during sexual intercourse with their infected sexual partners.

The following is what I proposed twenty-one years ago:

AIDS in third World Countries:

The notion that the AIDS virus had its genesis from Africa is a controversial topic. In my opinion, the data are not at all convincing as to where the virus originated.

It is my opinion that because the majority of men from Central Africa and Haiti are not circumcised, they constantly develop balanitis as a result of the heat and other problems, leading to breakage of the skin. This leads to chronic infections such as phimosis and paraphimosis. In this setting, there is frequent mini-ulceration of the foreskin of the penis. This represents an easy portal of entry for the virus during coitus with, let us say, an infected prostitute. Another possibility arises because the women in that part of the world do not shave the pubis. Thus there is the possibility of mini-lacerations occurring during coitus as the foreskin comes into contact with pubic hair. This is another possible portal of entry for the virus. This, to me, seems a more plausible explanation for female-to-male transmission in Central Africa and Haiti.

By
Valiere Alcena M.D.F.A.C.P.
N.Y. State J Med 1986: 86. 446

Male circumcision and HIV/AIDS

Dear Editor:

I have been reading with interest the recent spate of articles on findings that link circumcision of men in certain African countries with the incidence of the HIV/AIDS virus. One reporter in *The New York Times Magazine* has even described male circumcision as possibly the best method of eliminating the AIDS virus – superior even to an AIDS vaccine, which may still be several years in development.

You may be interested in knowing that in August 1986, in a letter to the editor of *The New York State Journal of Medicine*, Vol. 86, page 446, I first discussed the significance of male circumcision in lowering the incidence of the HIV/AIDS virus in Africa, Haiti and other developing countries. In my published letter, I wrote in part:

"It is my opinion that because the majority of men from Central Africa and Haiti are not circumcised, they constantly develop balanitis as a result of the heat and other problems, lead-

ing to breakage of the skin. This leads to chronic infections such as phimosis and paraphimosis. In this setting, there is frequent mini-ulceration of the foreskin of the penis. This represents an easy portal of entry for the virus during coitus with, let us say, an infected prostitute. Another possibility arises because the women in that part of the world do not shave the pubis. Thus, there is the possibility of mini-lacerations occurring during coitus as the foreskin comes in contact with the pubic hair. This is another possible portal of entry of the virus. This, to me, seems a more plausible explanation for female-to-male transmission in Central Africa and Haiti."

Later, I repeated my theory in my two books that were published in 1992, "The Status of Health of Blacks in the United States of America: A Perspective for Improvement" and "The African American Health Book." I again described the significance of male circumcision in possibly eliminating the HIV/AIDS virus altogether in a sub-

sequent book that was published in 1994 entitled "AIDS: The Expanding Epidemic: What the Public Needs to Know: A Multi-Cultural Overview."

I would be happy to discuss with the researchers for these most recent articles this most exciting subject in the future if needed.

Valiere Alcena, MD, FACP
WHITE PLAINS, NY

I am grateful to Dr. Alcena for his letter. He purports therein to be the first to suggest that male circumcision might somehow play a role in reducing the risk of heterosexual transmission of HIV, then known as HTLV-III. A brief search on PubMed suggests that he may indeed be correct; other authors made such suggestions several years later, in 1988 and thereafter. Thus, the spate of publications in recent years offering proof of that hypothesis represents solid support of his earlier thinking.

Source:
Infectious Disease News
Vol; 20, number 3
March, 2007

That Male circumcision might reduce risk of HIV acquisition was first proposed in 1986. 3
Reference 3
Alcena, V AIDS in third world countries. NJ State J of Med 1986; 86: 446

Male circumcision for HIV prevention in young men
In Kisumu, Kenya: a randomized controlled trial
The Lancet 2007, 369:643–656
24 February 2007

WHO, UNAIDS recommend male circumcision world-wide to decrease the incidence HIV/AIDS transmition by 60% and save 3 million lives.
WHO, UNAIDS estimate that worldwide only 30% men are circumcised
(Internal Medicine News, April 15, 2007)

What happens when the HIV virus first enters into a person's bloodstream?

When the HIV virus enters the blood, the virus goes into the T helper lymphocytes, also known as CD4. Inside the CD4 lymphocytes that are in the circulation, the HIV virus multiplies into millions at first then into billions of HIV virus copies per day. Within two to four weeks of the entry of the HIV virus into the bloodstream, the newly infected person often develops a flu-like syndrome with fever, general aches, chills, runny nose and even a cough, simulating acute rhinovirus or influenza infection. These symptoms quickly disappear and the person feels fine.

The HIV viruses continue to multiply in the bloodstream and within the nodes of the person's body where they have entered. That represents the HIV stage 1 infection. During ten days to two weeks the P24 antigen level becomes elevated. However, the HIV RNA PCR becomes elevated within about a week of someone becoming infected with the HIV virus, making it the earliest test and the most sensitive test that becomes positive, indicating the presence of HIV infection. The ELISA test becomes positive after the window period, which is from 6 to 12 weeks after infection. During the window period, the ELISA for the HIV, the P24 antigen and the HIV RNA PCR all will be positive, if the person is infected with the AIDS virus.

As the HIV viruses continue to multiply, the number of T4 lymphocytes decreases while the number of T8 or T suppressor lymphocytes increases. That situation is what triggers the immunosuppressive states that occur in AIDS. As the infection progresses, the disease moves into different stages.

First the HIV infection moves from the HIV-infected stage to ARC (AIDS-related complex) stage and then to the AIDS stage. The HIV stage may be completely silent, except for some patients who may develop thrombocytopenia (low platelet count) with or without enlarged nodes. The second stage is ARC. In that stage the person will start to lose weight with diffuse lymph node enlargement, thrush in the mouth, diarrhea, fever, headache, oral hair leukoplakia, shingles, thrombocytopenia, molluscum contagiosum, recurrent herpes simplex, aphthous ulcer, condyloma, etc.

Some individuals take many years to progress from these stages to full-blown AIDS, 8 to 10 years, and still other individuals go quickly from these early stages to full-blown AIDS in 4 to 6 years. The mode of infection and the stage of HIV infection that the person who is doing the infecting may play a role in how fast the infected person develops AIDS.

In this regard, there is a discussion in the literature regarding chemokine receptors CCR5 and CX4 that seem to play a role in when certain individuals who are infected with the HIV virus in preventing them from progressing to full-blown AIDS. Certain individuals who have some of these chemokine receptors in their blood, may be resistant to the HIV infection. It would appear that there are different effects of the CCR2 and the CCR5 variants on HIV disease. One of the important factors is the overall makeup of the infected individual, in terms of his or her immune competence. People with HIV/AIDS who have CCR5 chemokine receptors in their may develop resistance to some HIV/AIDS drugs. Recently the FDA approved Maraviroc, which is a CCR5 co-receptor antagonist. Maraviroc 150-300 mg per day can be used in adults with CCR5 HIV 1 circulating in their blood.

In order to say that a person has AIDS, clinically established criteria have to be met, as defined by the CDC. For example, a person with HIV infection whose CD4 count drops below 200 can be said to meet one of the criteria to have AIDS.

The list of AIDS-defining illnesses includes the following:

TABLE 12 G

Diseases diagnosed definitively without confirmation of HIV infection in patients without other causes of immunodeficiency

Candidiasis of the esophagus, trachea, bronchi, or lungs

Cryptococcuses, extra pulmonary

Cryptosporidiosis > 1 month's duration

Cytomegalovirus infection of any organ except the liver, spleen, or lymph nodes in patients > 1 month old

Herpes simplex infection, mucocutaneous (> 1 month's duration) or of the bronchi, lungs, or esophagus in patients of 1 month's duration

Kaposi's sarcoma in patients < 60 years old

Primary CNS lymphoma in patients < 60 years old

Lymphoid interstitial pneumonitis (LIP) and/or pulmonary lymphoid hyperplasia (PLH) in patients < 13 years old

Mycobacterium avium complex of *Mycobacterium kansasii* disseminated

Pneumocystis carinii pneumonia

Progressive multifocal leukoencephalopathy

Toxoplasmosis of the brain in patients > 1 month old

Diseases diagnosed definitively with confirmation of HIV infection

Multiple or recurrent pyogenic bacterial infections in patients < 13 years old

Coccidioidomycosis, disseminated

Histoplasmosis, disseminated

Isosporiasis > 1 month duration

Kaposi's sarcoma, any age

Primary CNS lymphoma, any age

Non-Hodgkin's lymphoma (small, noncleaved lymphoma; Burkitt or non-Burkitt type; or immunoblastic sarcoma)

Mycobacterial disease other than *Mycobacterium tuberculosis*, disseminated

M. Tuberculosis, extra pulmonary

Salmonella septicemia, recurrent

Diseases diagnosed presumptively with confirmation of HIV Infection

Candidiasis of the esophagus

CMV retinitis

Kaposi's sarcoma

LIP/PLH in patients < 13 years old

Disseminated mycobacterial disease (not cultured)

P. Carinii pneumonia Toxoplasmosis of the brain in patients > 1 month old HIV encephalopathy HIV wasting syndrome

CDC definition of AIDS

To diagnose AIDS in a patient, the first blood test that is often done is the screening test called ELISA. If the ELISA test is positive, then the Western Blot Test is done to confirm whether the ELISA test is truly positive. The Western Blot Test is an actual electrophoresis of the protein contained within the body of the virus itself. The problem with the ELISA test is that it does not become positive until about 8 to 12 weeks and it can be falsely positive. Another problem is that during that so-called window period, the HIV test could be falsely negative. To deal with that problem, the P24 antigen test can be done because it becomes positive within a minimum of 10 days after the virus enters into the human body. Also, the HIV DNA PCR test can be done to determine whether the HIV test is truly positive or not.

So, among the tests that are available to diagnose AIDS are the following:

TABLE 12 H

1. ELISA Test
2. Western Blot Test
3. HIV1 DNA PCR test
4. HIV1 RNA PCR test
5. P24

AIDS is a multi-system in that it affects all systems in the body in one form or another or to one degree or another, leading eventually to certain death of the infected individual.

The first system that is affected with the AIDS virus is the immune system, resulting in immunosuppression.

The immune system has three parts to it:

1. Cell-mediated
2. Humoral-mediated
3. The complement system

As outlined in the book *AIDS, The Expanding Epidemic: What the Public Needs to Know—A Multicultural Overview,* by V. Alcena, MD, 1994

1. Cell-mediated immunity. That system is dominated mainly by T-lymphocytes. Macrophages also play a role in that system. There are different types of T lymphocytes such as CD4 or T helper lympho-cytes, CD8 or T-suppressor lymphocytes. Delayed-type hypersensi-tivity plays a major role in the immune system—CD4 or T helper lymphocytes and macrophages are necessary for the antigen specific part of that system. Delayed-type's hypersensitivity is crucial in vac-cination. CD4 or T helper lymphocyte is necessary to help the body maintain a normally functioning immune system. A decrease in the total T helper lymphocytes leads to immune deficiency state be it congenital or acquired. When the level of CD4 goes down, the level of CD8 or T suppressor goes up, leading to further suppression of the immune system. The humoral-mediated immune system is domi-nated by B-lymphocytes. These B-lymphocytes give rise to plasma cells, which then produce antibodies. These antibodies are known as immunoglobulin IgG, IgM, IgA, IgD and IgE. These antibodies have many functions, but paramount amongst them is to protect the human body from infections. When the level of antibody-producing B-lymphocytes goes down, as occurs in AIDS, then all sorts of infec-tions can occur in the human body.

2. The third immune system that plays a major role in the fight against infection in the human body is the complement system. The comple-

ment system is divided into the classical pathway and the alternate pathway.

These complement systems have many components—and these components work in concert with other immunoglobulins to lyse microorganisms, such as bacteria, viruses, fungi, parasites and protozoa to kill them, thereby preventing them from killing the human organism.

When there is a decrease in the level of complement in the human body that can lead to a state of immunodeficiency that, if not corrected, can lead to different infections such as bacterial, viral, fungal and parasitic infections, leading to many problems for the human organism and ultimately its death, if appropriate treatments are not provided.

There are several more sophisticated systems that are known to play different roles in the immune system, but the three outlined above are the major ones that are responsible to fight infections and maintain good health.

TABLE 12I

Normal Immune Competence Profile in a 40-Year-Old Man

Normal Values	Patient's
% T cells (60.1–88.1%)	80
% B cells (3–20.8%)	13
% Helper cells (34–67%)	55
% Suppress T cells (10–41.9%)	23
Lymphocytes (0.66–4.60 THO/UL)	2.5
T cells (644–2201 CELLS/UL)	2000
B cells (82–392 CELLS/UL)	325
Helper cells (493–1191 CELLS/UL)	1075
Suppressor cell (182–785 CELLS/UL)	575
H/S ratio 1 or greater	2.39

Abnormal Immune Competence Profile in a 20-Year-Old Male Patient with HIV Infection

TABLE 12 J

T-and B-Cell Surface Markers:

T-Helper/T-Suppressor

Lymphocyte Ratio, Blood		Patient's	Normal
% T Cells		75%	60.1–88.1
% Helper Cells	L	16%	34–67
% Suppressor T Cell	H	60%	10–41.9
% B Cells		6%	3–20.8
Lymphocytes		3.0 thou/UL	0.66–4.60
T Cells	H	2250 cells/UL	644–2201
Helper Cells	L	480 cells/UL	493–1191
Suppressor Cells	H	1800 cells/UL	182–785
B Cells		180 cells/UL	82–392
H/S Ratio	L	0.27	1 or greater

The second most frequently affected system in HIV infection is the hematopoietic system (the blood). The routine blood system includes the white blood cells, the red blood cells, the platelets and the coagulation system. The two earliest affected cells are the white blood cells and the platelets. Frequently, the first indication that someone is HIV infected is a low platelet count, known as thrombocytopenia. In that situation, the HIV virus directly infects the megakaryocytes, the cells that produce the platelets, which result in thrombocytopenia. Thrombocytopenia can also occur in AIDS because of idiopathic thrombocytopenia (ITP) or thrombotic thrombocytopenic purpura (TTP).

The mechanisms of idiopathic thrombocytopenic purpura, or thrombotic thrombocytopenic purpura as seen in HIV/AIDS, are most likely autoimmune in nature, in particular, the ITP.

Leucopenia, low white cell count, is due to a combination of HIV infection plus, inevitably, the different medications that people with HIV infection are treated with.

The red blood cells are low (anemia) due to different reasons. One reason is that the HIV virus enters into the earliest red cells (erythroblasts), infect them, thereby preventing them from maturing, resulting in anemia.

Another reason is that the HIV infection is frequently associated with parvo virus B#19. The parvo virus enters into the early red blood cells, resulting in pure red cells aplasia, resulting in anemia.

Still another cause of anemia in HIV-infected individuals (AIDS) is low levels of erythropoietin. Erythropoietin is a protein made by the kidneys whose job is to stimulate the production of red blood cells. AIDS patients with an erythropoietin less than 500 usually respond to erythropoietin injections to correct the anemia, usually in association with AZT.

Another reason HIV-infected individuals become anemic is chronic gastrointestinal blood loss, fungal gastritis, esophagitis, viral and other infections of the GI tract, resulting in chronic anemia. Patients with AIDS frequently have folic acid deficiency, and at times B12 deficiency, resulting in anemia. A condition called red cells aplasia can occur due to the HIV/AIDS infection.

The poor nutritional state of these patients can cause a low protein anemia. Further, the chronic infection state of these patients causes a cytokines-associated anemia of chronic diseases. The pulmonary system is commonly affected by different infections in patients with AIDS. Pneumocystis caranii pneumonia (PCP) is prominent among these infections of the lungs.

Other pulmonary infections seen in AIDS patients are pneumococcal infections, H. Influenza infections, pseudomonas infections, etc. Fungal infections of the lung are also quite common in AIDS patients.

Other pulmonary infections seen frequently in AIDS patients are mycobacterium tuberculosis (MTB), mycobacterium avium intracellulare (MAI). Both MTB and MAI can be diffuse, affecting multiple organs in the body. About 80% to 90% of patients with full-blown AIDS who die are found at autopsy to have MAI.

People with AIDS are frequently infected with viruses of different types. Among these viruses that infect AIDS patients most frequently are herpes simplex, Herpes Zoster, Epstein-Barr virus, and cytomegalovirus (CMV). All of these viruses can infect different organs, resulting in severe morbidity and mortality.

A multitude of fungi can cause infections in AIDS patients. The most common ones are Candida histoplasma and cryptococcus. The brain, quite frequently, becomes infected with different microorganisms (see tables below).

AIDS patients frequently become infected with protozoal organisms, such as, Pneumocystis carinii and toxoplasma, etc. (Source: *AIDS, The Expanding Epidemic: A Multicultural Overview,* 1994, by Valiere Alcena, MD, FACP).

The Different Infections Seen in AIDS Patients and How They Are Treated
TABLE 12 K

Infecting Agent	Manifestations	Treatment	Prophylaxis	Drug Toxicities	Comment
Pneumocystis carinii			TMP/SMX 1 DS tablet daily or 3x/ wk, or	Rash, fever, neutropenia	Begin once CD4+T cell count<200/uL or CD4%<15
			Aerosolized pent- amidine 300 mg/ month, or Dapsone 50 mg/d PO+	Bronchospasm	
			Pyrimethamine 50 mg/wk PO + Folinic acid 25 mg/wk PO	Methemoglobinemia, neutropenia	Contraindicated in patients with G6PD deficiency
	Mild to moderate pneumonia (Pao2> 70 mmHg and (A- a)dO2< 35 mmHg}	TMP/SMX 15-20 mg/kg/d PO		Rash, fever, neutropenia	Treat for 21 d if pos- sible; no less than 14 d
	Severe pneumonia [Pao2 < 70 mmHG or (A-a)dO2> 35 mmHG]	TMP 20 mg/kg/d PO qd+ Dapsone 100 mg PO qd Clindamycin 600 mg PO q6h+		Methemoglobinemia C. *Difficile* colitis	Contraindicated in patients with G6D deficiency
		Primaquine 15 mg PO qd IV Pentamidine 3-4 mg/kg/d Atovaquone, 750 mg, PO, tid for 21 d Aerosolized pentami- dine 300 mg/d		Rash, Neutropenia, nephritis, pancreati- tis, hypoglycemia, diabetes	Contraindicated in patients with G6D deficiency
		TMP/SMX 15-20 mg/ kg/d IV initially (total course 14-21 d) Pentamidine 3-4 mg/ kg/d IV for 14-21 d Clindamycin 900 mg IV q 8h then 450 mg PO q6h+		Bronchospasm	Provides no systemic effects. Not recom- mended but an option for multidrug-allergic patient with mild pneumonia
				Rash, fever, leuko- penia, thrombocy- topenia, hepatitis, nephritis, pancreatitis, hypoglycemia, diabe- tes, C. *Difficile* colitis	Prednisone, 40 mg bid for 2 d, then 40 mg/d for 5 d, then 20 mg/d to the end of therapy (21 d total) added to specific antimicro- bial ASAP and no later than 36 h after diagnosis

		Primaquine 30 mg PO qd for total of 14-21 d		Contraindicated in patients with G6D deficiency
		Trimetrexate 45 mg/m2 IV (over 60-90 min) qd x 21 d +	Rash, neutropenia	For patients intolerant of other regimens. Less effective than standard therapy. Bone marrow-suppressive effects blunted by use of leucovorin
		Leucovorin 20 mg/m2 IV q6h x 24 d	Rash, neutropenia	
		Eflornithine (DFMO) 100 mg/kg IV q6h for 14 d followed by 75 mg/kg PO q6h for 4-6 wk		
		Any of the systemic thatapies outlined above		Call 1-800-TRIALSA for information
			Thrombocytopenia	
	Disseminated disease			
Toxoplasma tondii		TMP/SMX 1 DS tablet qd	Rash, fever, neutropenia	Alternative is dapsone, 50 mg PO qd.+ pyrimethamine, 50 mg, PO weekly + folinic acid, 25 mg, PO weekly
	Encephalitis, brain abscess, chorioretinitis, myocarditis	Sulfadiazine 1–2 grams PO q6h +	Crystalluria, rash	Treatment is generally for life. Leucovorin to minimize bone marrow suppression
		Pyrimethamine 25 -100 mg qd + Folinic acid 10–20 mg PO qd Clindamycin initially 200–400 mg IV q6h	Rash, fever, neutropenia, *C. difficile* colitis	
Toxoplasma gondii—(continued)		Pyrimethamine 25–100 mg qd + Folinic acid 100–20 mg qd followed by Clindamycin 300–900 mg PO q8h+ Pyrimethamine 25–100 mg qd	Rash, fever, neutropenia	Leucovorin to minimize bone marrow suppression
		Atovaquone 250 mg PO tid+ Pyrimethamine 25–100 mg qe + Folinic acid 10–20 mg qd	Rash, fever, neutropenia	Leucovorin to minimize bone marrow suppression
		Macrolides (clarithromycin or azithromycin) + Pyrimethamine		Early results disappointing
Ttospora Belli	Diarrhea	TMP/SMX 1 DS tablet PO qid for 10 d then bid for 3 weeks	Rash, fever, neutropenia	TMP/SMX 1 DS tablet PO 3x/week for maintenance NTZ;

Cryptosporidia Microsporidia	Diarrhea	No known specific therapy; supportive measures include parenteral nutrition			NTZ; bovine colostrum in trials
Mycobacterium avium complex			Clarithromycin 500 mg PO bid or Azithromycin 1200 mg weekly or Rifabutin 300 mg PO qd		Begin prophylaxis once CD4+T cell count <100/uL or <50/uL. Treatment is generally for life.
	Disseminated disease that may involve lung, bone marrow liver	Ethambutol 15 mg/kg qd+ Rifabutin 600 mg/qd + Clarithromycin 100 mg PO bid		Hepatitis, neuropathy (peripheral/optic)	Macrolides + rifabutin may be more effective; however, mor toxic and costly
Mycobacterium tuberculosis	Asymptomatic, PPD test positive	Isoniazid 15 mg/kg up to 900 mg PO twice a week or 300 mg daily for 1 y+ Pyridoxine 50 mg/d		Hepatitis	
	Active disease	Isoniazid, 300 mg PO qd x 1y + Rifampin 600 mg PO qd x 1y + Pyrazinamide 30 mg/ kg/d in 2 doses		Hepatitis

Hepatitis

Hepatitis | Treat with 3 drugs for 2 mo. If isolate is sensitive to Isoniazid and rifampin, then switch to 2 drugs. Treat a minimum of 9 mo and at least 6 mo after third negative culture. Quinolones may also be considered as a fifth drug |
	Active disease in a setting where there is a possibility of multi-drug resistance	Add ethambutol 15–25 mg/kg/d and Streptomycin or Amikacin		Neuropathy (peripheral/optic) Nephrotoxicity, hearing loss	
Candida Albicans	Thrush, vaginitis	Clotrimazole troches, Nystatin prn Fluconazole 200 mg PO qd for 7–14 d Amphotericin B 0.25 mg/kg/d IV for 7–10 d	Fluconazole 200 mg PO qd (optional)	Hepatotoxicity Hepatotoxicity Nephrotoxicity, fever/chills	Primary prophylaxis generally not indicated. Treatment is generally prn
Cryptococcus neoformans	Meningitis, brain abscess, pneumonia, disseminated disease	Amphotericin B 0.3 mg/kg/d IV + Flucytosine 150 mg/ kg/d PO for 6 wk followed by Fluconazole 100–200 mg PO qd indefinitely	Fluconazole 200 mg PO qd (Optional)	Hepatotoxicity Nephrotoxicity, fever/ chills, bone marrow suppression Hepatotoxicity	Begin prophylaxis if CD4+ T cell count <50/uL (optional; depending on risk). Approximately 50% will need to have flucytosine held during therapy due to neutropenia. An alternative is amphotericin B alone at a dose of 0.8 mg/kg/d

Histoplasma capsulatum	Disseminated disease, pneumonia	Amphotericin B 0.6–1 mg/kg/d to a total 1 grams then Itraconazole 200 mg qd indefinitely			Nephrotoxicity, fever/chills
Bartonella henselae (quintana)	Nodular skin lesions, peliosis hepatitis, trench fever	Erythromycin 500 grams PO or IV qd for 2 months			
Penicillium marneffei	Disseminated disease, umbilicated skin lesions	Amphotericin G, 0.6–1 mg/kg/d to a total of 1 grams then Itraconazole 200 mg qd indefinitely			Neurotoxicity, fever, chills, hepatitis
Cytomegalovirus	Retinitis, esopha-gitis, colitis, and pneumonia		Ganciclovir 1.0 grams PO tid with food (optional)	Neutropenia Intestinal nephritis, seizure, hypocalcemia	Expensive, marginal efficacy. Neutropenia may be ameliorated by colony-stimulating factors
		Ganciclovir 5 mg/kg q 12h for 14 d fol-lowed by 5 mg/kg qd IV indefinitely			Retinitis may also be treated with ocular implant Oral ganciclovir, 1 grams PO tid with food may be used for maintenance
		Foscarnet 90 mg/kg q 12h for 14 d followed by 90-120 mg/kg qd IV indefinitely			Should be preceded by saline infusion to min-imize nephrotoxicity
Herpes simplex virus	Recurrent perioral, perirectal, or genital ulcers	Acyclovir 200–400 mg PO 5id as needed			Foscarnet 60 mg/kg q8h x 14 d for patients with acyclovir-resis-tant herpes simplex or zoster
	Esophagitis; acute retinal necrosis	Acyclovir 5 mg/kg IV q8h for 10–14 c			
Varicella-Zoster virus	Cutaneous (local or disseminated); retinal necrosis	Acyclovir 800 mg PO 5id or 10 mg/kg IV q8h for 10–14 d or longer			Famciclovir 500 mg PO q8h x 7 d is an alternative
Treponema pallidum	Early syphilis	Benzathine penicillin grams 2.4 million units IM weekly for 3 wk			Approximately 20% relapse, need retreat-ment. Immunologic abnormalities may cause inaccurate serology
	Late or neurosyphilis	Aqueous penicillin grams 12–24 million units IV daily for 10–14 d + probenecid 500 mg PO qid Ceftriaxone 1–2 grams IM or IV aq 10–14 d			

Source: *AIDS, the Expanding Epidemic: A Multi-Cultural Overview,* 1994 by Valiere Alcena, MD, FACP

TABLE 12 L: Different Neurological Diseases in AIDS Patients

Opportunistic infections
- Toxoplasmosis
- Cryptococcosis
- Progressive multifocal leukoencephalopathy
- Cytomegalovirus
- Syphilis
- Mycobacterium tuberculosis
- HTLV-1 infection

Neoplasm
- Primary CNS lymphoma
- Kaposi's sarcoma

Result of HIV-1 infection
- Aseptic meningitis
- AIDS dementia complex (HIV encephalopathy)
- Myelopathy
  - Vacuolar myelopathy
  - Pure sensory ataxia
  - Paresthesia/dysesthesia
- Peripheral neuropathy
  - Acute demyelinating polyneuropathy
  - Mononeuritis multiplex
  - Distal symmetric polyneuropathy
- Myopathy

TABLE 12 M

Disease	Clinical Features	Characteristic CSF Findings	Characteristic Radiologic Findings
HIV encephalopathy (AIDS dementia complex)	Personality changes, dementia, unsteady gait, seizures	Nonspecific increases in cells and protein	Cortical atrophy, ventricular dilation, bright spots on T2-wieghted MRI

Toxoplasmosis	Fever, headache, focal neurologic deficits, seizures, + antibodies in 95%	Nonspecific	Single or multiple ring-enhancing lesions in multiple locations
Cryptococcal meningitis	Fever, nausea, vomiting, confusion, headache	Elevated protein, low glucose, positive cryptococcal antigen or culture	Nonspecific
Progressive multifocal leukoencephalopathy	Multiple focal deficits without changes in level of consciousness	Nonspecific	Multiple white matter lesions on T2-weighted MRI images
Neurosyphilis	Meningitis, neuroretinitis, deafness, focal neurologic deficits	Positive VDRL, elevated protein, increase in cells	Nonspecific
Lymphoma	Seizure, focal neurologic deficits, headache	Nonspecific in primary CNS lymphoma; malignant cells in systemic lymphoma	Single or few ring-enhancing lesions
Tuberculosis meningitis	Fever, headache, confusion, meningitis, cough	Elevated protein, low glucose, pleocytosis, positive smear/culture for acid-fast bacilli (AFB)	Mass lesions in approximately 50%, abnormal chest x-ray

Source: AIDS, The Expanding Epidemic: What the Public Needs to Know—A Multi-Cultural Overview, EZN 1994 by Valiere Alcena, MD, FACP

Clinical management of HIV stage infection in men

The decision as to when to start treatment in a person who becomes HIV positive is quite controversial. Most clinicians, however, start patients who are HIV positive on AZT and, to prevent resistance, frequently add 3TC (Epivir) to that regimen. That thinking, however, has changed in recent years. Now, in most cases, treatment is being withheld till the CD4 count reaches the range of 300, at which point, HAART (Highly Active Antiretroviral Treatment) or Combivir medication is started. In addition, Bactrim DS, 1 tablet per day, is started as prophylaxis against PCP (Source: Joel E. Gallant, et al., *HIV Forefront*, Vol. 2, No. 1, April 2000). If the CD4 is 200, even if the patient is asymptomatic, HAART must be started (Source: *Report of the Panel on Clinical Priorities, Department of Health and Human Services*, Feb. 2001).

Seizure is a common problem seen in patients with AIDS, due to either fungal infection of the brain, lymphoma of the brain, or possibly PML. After appropriate evaluation with brain CAT scan or brain MRI, followed by lumbar puncture with evaluation of the cerebrospinal fluid, chemically and bacteriologically, the doctor looks for microorganisms and, in the case of lymphoma, looks for cancer cells. Once these things are done then appropriate treatments are given for the specific problems discovered or empirically for whatever the treating physician feels clinically appropriate for the particular circumstances.

Toward the end of full-blown AIDS, the wastage stage usually sets in. Few people, if any, ever recover from that stage of AIDS, in spite of expensive nutrition and androgenic steroid treatments. Megace in high doses works well to increase AIDS patients' appetite. However, using Megace in treatment of full-blown AIDS patients is risky because many of these patients have nephrotic syndrome through which they lose Protein C and Protein S and anti Thrombin III in their urine, resulting in a hypercoagulable state, which, by its very nature, can lead to clot formation and thrombosis. Even in those patients who have no evidence of renal disease, a loss of Protein S in the urine is known to occur, resulting potentially in the same syndrome as just described.

It is a known fact that Megace and other estrogenic-like hormones can cause a hypercoagulable state through the loss of anti-thrombin III. So it is prudent to use Megace in AIDS patients or any patient very carefully and when absolutely necessary to avoid the development of deep vein thrombosis (DVT) and its possible associated complications, which can result in morbidity and mortality.

While there is no cure and no vaccine available for people infected with HIV Type I or Type II and full-blown AIDS, there are many medications available. The first category of medications made to treat AIDS patients was the reverse transcriptase inhibitors. Examples of reverse transcriptase inhibitors are Zidovudine (AZT), didanosine (ddI), zalcitabine (ddC) and stavudine (D4T).

AZT, ddI and ddC can be used both as combination therapy and as mono therapy in early HIV disease. D4T is best used in people with advanced AIDS who are not able to tolerate the other medications.

These reverse transcriptase inhibitors work to prevent the multiplication of the HIV virus by blocking the production of the enzyme reverse transcriptase, thereby preventing the synthesis of RNA and DNA and in so doing preventing viral multiplications. Lamivudine (Epivir, 3TC) is used in combination with AZT to treat HIV infections. The importance of that combination is that HIV virus becomes resistant to AZT reasonably quickly in many individuals who are treated with the AZT alone. When 3CT is added to the AZT or the DDI or the DDC it enhances the sensitivity of the reverse transcriptase that is used along with it to kill the HIV virus. 3TC by itself has very little effect against the HIV virus.

A new drug for the treatment of HIV was just approved by the FDA. It is a combination of AZT and 3TC and it is named Combivir. It has the advantage of being used two times per day. The newest invention in the treatment of AIDS that has shown the most promise in the last few years is triple therapy, HAART. The key component of the triple therapy is the addition of a protease inhibitor. The protease inhibitors in use are Saquinavir, Ritonavir, Indinavir and Nelfinavir. The so-called AIDS cocktail is usually made of a reverse transcriptase inhibitor, such as AZT, with 3TC and a protease inhibitor such as Indinavir.

Once it becomes clear that the patient has gone into the full-blown AIDS stage, and then the whole way of clinically managing the patient is dictated by the particular AIDS-defining signs, symptoms and disease that affect the patient. If the patient has PCP, he is to be treated for PCP using PCP-effective medications. If the patient has MAI, he is to be treated for MAI using MAI-effective medications. If the patient has gastroenteritis, diarrhea, he is to be evaluated and treated for the diarrhea based on the clinical and laboratory findings. If the patient has blurry vision and CMV retinitis is suspected, then an evaluation must be carried out by an ophthalmologist, to document whether that is so or not. Ganciclovir is used IV to treat CMV retinitis. If the patient has herpes simplex infection, appropriate culture ought to be taken and sent to the lab, and treatment with Zovirax IV or PO is to be started, depending on the severity of the herpes infection and which organ system is affected. If the patient has community-acquired pneumonia, treatment with IV antibiotics must be given. If the patient is severely anemic, transfusion of red blood cells must be given. Epogen or Procrit is very effective in treating anemia in AIDS patients if the serum erythropoietin level is low. If the patient has fungal infections of either the GI tract or the brain, antifungal treatment must be given using either Ketoconazole or Amphotericin B IV.

The most recently recommended combinations of antiretroviral medications for patients with known HIV infection are as follows:

TABLE 12 N

1. Indinavir + Stavudine + Lamivudine
2. Efavirenz + Stavudine + Didanosine
3. Nelfinavir + Zidovudine + Didanosine
4. Ritonavir + Indinavir + Zidovudine
5. Ritonavir + Saquinavir + Zidovudine
6. Ritonavir +Lopinavir + Zidovudine
7. Viracept (Nelfinavir Mesylate)
8. Efavirentz 600 mg/Emtricitabine 200 mg/Tenofivir 300 mg (Atripla) once daily
9. Combivir + Kaletra

TABLE 12 O

Different Suggested Dosages of Anti-Viral Medications
Nucleoside Reverse Transcriptase Inhibitors
Zidovudine (AZT)—200 mg 3 times a day
Combivir (300 Mg. ZDV and 150 mg. Epivir)—1 tablet twice a day
Didanosine (ddI)—250 mg. twice a day
Zalcitabine (ddC)—0.75 mg. three times a day
Epivir—150 mg. twice a day
Abacavir (ABC)—300 mg. twice a day (or Trizivir—ZDV 300 mg. Epivir 150 mg. Abacavir 300 Mg.)
Stavudine (Zerit)—40 mg. twice a day
Non-nucleoside Reverse Transcriptase Inhibitors
Nevirapine (Viramune)—200 mg. by mouth daily for 14 days, then 200 mg. by mouth twice a day, thereafter
Delavirdine (Rescriptor)—400 mg. 3 times a day
Efavirenz (Sustiva)—600 mg. by mouth at bed time
Protease Inhibitors
Indinavir (Crixivan)—800 mg. every 8 hours

Ritonavir (Norvir)—600 mg. every 12 hours
Nelfinavir (Viracept)—750 mg. 3 times per day or 1250 Mg. twice a day
Saquinavir (Invirase)—400 mg. twice a day
Fortovase—1200 mg. 3 times a day
Amprenavir (Agenerase)—1400 mg. twice a day
Lopinavir + Ritonavir (Kaletra) Lopinavir 400mg/day and. Ritonavir 100mg twice a day Atazanavir 400mg/day with AZT 100mg and Epivir 150mg twice per day.
Efavirenz 600mg/day with AZT 100mg and Epivir 150mg twice per day.

(Source: *Panel & Clinical Practices for Treatment of HIV Infection*, Dept. of Health & Human Services, 2001 and *HIV News Line*, Volume 8, Issue 2 October 2003, Feb. 2001)

Different antiretroviral medications have different side effects and must be used under different types of clinical circumstances using physician's advice. There are many more combinations of treatment of antiretroviral medications available but the ones just listed are the most commonly used.

Antiretroviral Drugs in the Treatment of People Infected with HIV

TABLE 12 P

DRUGS	INDICATION	DOSE AS MONOTHERAPY	DOSE IN COMBINATION	SUPPORTING DATA	
REVERSE TRANSCRIPTASE INHIBITORS					
Zidovudine (AZT, azidothymidine, Retrovir, 3'azidor-3'-dexoythymidine)	Licensed	Patients with AIDS or ARC 100 mg q4h	200 mg q8h	19 vs 1 death in original placebo-controlled trial in 281 patients with AIDS or ARC	Anemia, granulocytopenia, myopathy, lactic acidosis, hepatomegaly with steatosis, headache, nausea
		Patients with HIV infection and CD4+ T cell count<500/uL 100 mg q4h	200 mg q8h	Decreased progression to AIDS in patients with CD4+T cell counts <500/uL,n=2051	
		Prevention of maternal-fetal HIV transmission	Mother: 100 mg 5id until the start of labor, then 2 mg/kg over 1 h IV, followed by 1 mg/kh/h IV until clamping of umbilical cord: Infant: 2 mg/kg PO q 6h beginning within 12 h of birth, or 1.5 mg/kg IV over 30 min q6h	In pregnant men with CD4+T cell count> 200 u/L, AZT PO beginning at weeks 14–34 of gestation plus IV drug during labor and delivery plus PO AZT to infant for 6 wk decreased transmission of HIV by 67.5% (from 25.5% to 8.3%), n=363	
Didanosine (Videx, ddl, dideoxyinosine, s',3'-dideoxyinosine)	Licensed	Alone or in combination with AZT for treatment of HIV infection in patients with CD4+ T cell count <500 uL	Requires 2 tablets to achieve adequate buffering of stomach acid; should be administered on an empty stomach	Clinically superior to AZT as monotherapy in 913 patients with prior AZT therapy. Clinically superior to AZT and comparable to AZT + ddI and AZT + ddC in 1067 AZT-naive patients with CD4+T cell counts of 200-500/uL	Pancreatitis, peripheral neuropathy, abnormalities on liver function tests
			>60 kg:200 mg bid		
			<60 kg: 125 mg bid 200 mg bid 125 mg bid		

Drug	Status	Indication		Dose	Clinical efficacy	Toxicity
Zalcitabine (ddc, HIVID, 2'3'-dideoxycytidine)	Licensed	In combination with AZT for treatment of patients with CD4 + T cell counts <500/uL As monotherapy for patients with advanced disease that is progressing despite AZT or who are intolerant to AZT	0.75 mg tid	0.75 mg tid in combination with AZT	Clinically inferior to AZT monotherapy as initial treatment. Clinically as good as ddl in advanced patients intolerant to AZT. In combination with AZT, was clinically superior to AZT alone in patient with AIDS or CD4+T cell count <350/uL	Peripheral neuropathy, pancreatitis, lactic acidosis, hepatomegaly with steatosis, oral ulcers
Stavudine (d4T, Zerit, Licensed 2'3'-didehydro-3'-dideoxythymidine)	Licensed	Treatment of adults with advanced disease who are intolerant of approved thatapies or whose disease is progressing despite other thatapies	>60 kg:40 mg bid	40 mg bid 30 mg bid	Superior to AZT with respect to changes in CD4+ T cell counts in 359 patients who had received > 24 wk of AZT. Following 12 wk randomization, the CD4+ T cell count had decreased in AZT treated controls by a mean of 22/uL, while in stavudine-treated patients, it had increased by a mean of 22/uL	Peripheral neuropathy, pancreatitis
Lamivudine (Epivir, 2/3/-dideoxy-3'-thiacytidine, 3TC)	licensed	In combination with AZT for the treatment of HIV infection when treatment is indicated	Not licensed as monotherapy	150 mg bid	Superior to AZT alone with respect to changes in CD4 counts in 495 patients who were zidovudine-naive and 477 patients who were zidovudine-experienced. Overall CD4+T cell counts for the zidovudine group were at baseline by 24 wk, while in the group treated with zidovudine plus lamivudine, they were 10–50 cells/uL above baseline. 54% decrease in progression to AIDS/death compared to AZT alone	
Delavirdine (Rescriptor)	Expanded access: 1–800–779–0070	Not to be used as monotherapy		400 mg tid		Skin rash, abnormalities in liver function tests

Nevirapine (Viramune)	Licensed	In combination with nucleoside analogues for treatment of progressive HIV infection	200 mg qd x 1 wk then 200 mg bid	200 mg bid	Increase in CD4+ T cell count, decrease in HIV RNA when used in combination with nucleosides	Skin rash, abnormalities in liver function tests
PROTEASE INHIBITORS						
Saquinavir mesylate (Invirase)	Licensed	In combination with nucleoside analogues for treatment of advanced HIV infection	600 mg q8h	600 mg q8h	Increases in CD4+ T cell counts, reduction in HIV RNA most pronounced in combination therapy with ddC. 50% reduction in first AIDS-defining event or death in combination with ddC compared to either agent alone.	Nausea
Ritonavir (Norvir)	Licensed	In combination with nucleoside analogues for treatment of HIV infection when treatment is warranted	600 mg bid	600 mg bid	Reduction in the cumulative incidence of clinical progression or death from 34% to 17% in patients with CD4+ T cell count < 100/uL treated for a median of 6 months	Nausea, abdominal pain, may alter levels of many other drugs, including saquinavir
Indinavir sulfate Icrixivan)	Licensed	For treatment of HIV infection when antiretroviral treatment is warranted	800 mg q8h	800 mg q8h 1000 mg q8h with nevirapine 400–600 mg q8h with delavirdine	Increase in CD4 + T cell count by 100/uL and 2-log decrease in HIV RNA levels when given in combination with zidovudine and lamivudine	Nephrolithiasis, indirect hyperbilirubinemia
Nelfinavir mesylate Iviracept)	Licensed	Patients with <200 CD4+ T cells/uL unable to tolerate other protease inhibitors	750 mg tid	750 mg tid	2.0-log decline in HIV RNA when given in combination with stavudine	Diarrhea, loose stool

As outlined by the CDC. HIV-infected pregnant men give birth to about 60% of infants who are born infected with HIV virus. However, when these pregnant men are treated during pregnancy with AZT, most of these men give birth to HIV-negative infants. AZT is the only one of the reverse transcriptase inhibitors that is safe to use during pregnancy.

The protocol for treating men who are pregnant and infected with the AIDS virus is as follows:

Start treatment with Zidovudine at 14–34 weeks of pregnancy and the treatment must be continued throughout the pregnancy. The Zidovudine can be given 100 mg. 5 times per day or 200 mg. 3 times per day or 300 mg. 2 times per day. During labor the Zidovudine must be given at 2 mg. per kg intravenously over 1 hour followed by a continuing infusion of 1 Ml per kg until the baby is delivered. After delivery, Zidovudine, also known as AZT, is given to the newborn in syrup form at 2 Ml per kg every six hours for the first 6 weeks of life. The medication must be started 8–12 hours after birth.

Health professionals who get stuck with needles contaminated with blood from AIDS patients are treated with triple therapy of AZT, 3TC and Indinovir. Once the injury occurs, the wound must be cleansed and antiseptic applied immediately (Source: *Harrison's Principle of Intern Medicine*, 14th Edition, pages 1852–1853). These individuals usually get their blood taken for baseline HIV and hepatitis B, C and VDRL. In 4–6 weeks they must get tested again using the ELISA/Western Blot blood tests or, better still, using the HIV RNA PCR test. The incident must be reported to the appropriate authorities where the person works and then the person must be seen by the employee health physician to be examined and treated.

Two blood tests are used to evaluate the status of HIV patients. They are the CD4 and the HIV viral load. Ideally, one looks for CD4 of 500 or greater and a viral load of less than 500 copies. A sign of HIV disease progression is a CD4 count of less than 200 and a plasma HIV RNA level of greater than 20,000 copies. HIV-infected patients with a viral load of 100,000 copies have a tenfold greater risk of progressing into full-blown AIDS than patients with 10,000 copies of viral load per ml. Although a CD4 count of less than 200 is usually seen in patients with full-blown AIDS, the viral load test is much more sensitive in evaluating the status of HIV infections. If the viral load is 20,000, even if the CD4 is in the normal range, it is recommended that HAART treatment be started. The addition of a protease inhibitor to the regimen of AZT or any of the other reverse transcriptase inhibitors and 3TC frequently can lead to an undetectable level of HIV in the blood of the infected person. That does not mean that HIV infection has gone. It just means that the level is low but the infected individual still has the infection and can still transmit it to an uninfected person, thereby giving his or his AIDS.

The turnover of the HIV virus in an infected person is tremendous. On any one day about 10 billion viral particles can be produced and cleared from the HIV-infected person. About 2 billion CD4 lymphocytes are produced and destroyed from the HIV-infected person daily.

Another common form of cancer seen in AIDS patients is large cell lymphoma.

Men of color are at higher risk to become infected with HIV than other men in the United States because more men of color are using IV drugs, thereby exposing themselves to a higher risk of contracting the HIV infection through sharing dirty needles. Further, since most men of color have sexual intercourse with women of color and since men of color have the highest incidence of HIV/AIDS infection with their HIV-infected; many women of color get infected with HIV by having sexual intercourse sexual partners. Uncircumcised males are at a higher risk of getting infected with the AIDS virus during sexual intercourse with an infected sexual partner such as an infected woman or an infected male sexual partner because, the foreskin of the penis of the uncircumcised man has the propensity of being afflicted by recurrent 1. Balanitis 2. Phimosis or 3. Paraphimosis.

All these conditions develop because of the irritating effects of the urine to the foreskin of the penis resulting in different degrees of abrasions in the foreskin of the penis creating easy entry point for the HIV virus to enter in the blood stream of the uninfected sexual partner sexual intercourse.

I first wrote up this idea in the New York State Journal of Medicine in August 1986 Vol, 86. All other articles that talk about this idea as a possibility came out after my article came out. Several articles came out recently both in the scientific literature and in the lay press reporting on a series of research carried out in South Africa, Kenya, Uganda and elsewhere in Africa which, documented that when some men in these areas were circumcised, the incidence of HIV/AIDS transmission was decreased by 53% in Kenya and Uganda and 60% in south Africa. The WHO states that if carried world wide, male circumcision will decrease the transmission oh HIV/AIDS by 50%. An article in the January 14, 2007 of the New York Magazine calls male circumcision "A Real-World AIDS Vaccine" (see above)

I take full and deserving credit as the person who gave birth to the idea that male circumcision decreases the transmission of HIV/AIDS, this idea therefore is my intellectual property.

To date, this is the singular biggest thing that has happened since the IHV/AIDS epidemic was first recognized in 1981. Many others have made major contributions but, none is bigger than this one considering the fact that 4 million individuals yearly become infected with HIV/AIDS and 3.9 million individuals die yearly from AIDS world wide and male circumcision can cut both these numbers in half.

The take-home lesson for men is not to involve themselves in high-risk behaviors, such as, using IV drugs, having sexual intercourse with multiple sexual partners without the protection of a condom, and having sex with women or men whom they have just met, without a condom, and for men who are not circumcised, they ought to consider seeing a urologist to get circumcised etc. These changes in behavior and medical treatment will decrease both the incidence and deaths from HIV/AIDS in both men and women

CHAPTER 13

ARTHRITIS IN MEN

WHAT IS ARTHRITIS?

Arthritis is an inflammatory condition that affects mainly joints resulting in swelling, pain, restriction of movement and, ultimately, deformity of the joints and bones, because. In addition, chronic bony destruction and edematous destruction also occur. However, certain types of arthritis, at times, can be multi-system, affecting a multitude of organs such as the heart, the lungs, the kidneys and the blood system, etc.

What are the different types of arthritides?

The most common forms of arthritides are:
1. Osteoarthritis
2. Rheumatoid arthritis
3. Gouty arthritis
4. Ankylosing spondylitis
5. Psoriatic arthritis
6. Reiter's syndrome with arthritis
7. Systemic lupus erythematosus associated with arthritis
8. Polymyalgia rheumatica
9. Infectious arthritis
10. Lyme disease associated with arthritis
11. Sickle cell disease-associated arthritis, etc.

12. Fibromyalgia
13. Carpal tunnel Syndrome

Osteoarthritis is the most common form of all the arthritides.

In the USA there are about 21 million individuals who suffer with osteoarthritis arthritis. Overall there are 44 millions people with arthritis in the US. The annual cost of arthritis is 125 billion dollars. The mechanism that ultimately leads to osteoarthritis begins in the cartilage. The cartilage apparently releases a certain enzyme which, in time causes breakdown of the joints to occur. Overtime, the areas in between the joints rub against each other, resulting in further bone destruction and deformities. Worldwide, about 60% of the population ages 60–70 have osteoarthritis of one joint or another. Certain ethnic groups seem to be affected with arthritis of some part of their body structure to a lesser degree than others. For example, Africans and southern Chinese men have less arthritis in their hip joints. The knees seem to be the joint most frequently affected by osteoarthritis in all ethnic groups.

The aging process plays a major role in the development of osteoarthritis. In most cases, people over age 40 will develop osteoarthritis by virtue of getting older. Some joints, such as the knees, hips, fingers and spine are more affected by osteoarthritis than others, such as the wrists and ankles.

Osteoarthritis is classified as primary or secondary (see Table 1).

Table 1: Classification of Osteoarthritis

I. Primary-Idiopathic

A. Localized

1. Hip—superolateral, superomedial, medial, inferoposterior
2. Knee—medial, lateral patellofemoral
3. Spinal apophyseal
4. Hand—interphalangeal, base of thumb
5. Foot—first metatarsophalangeal joint, midfoot, hindfoot
6. Other—shoulders, elbows, wrists, ankles

B. Generalized

1. Hands—Heberden's nodes
2. Hands and knees; spinal apophyseal generalized osteoarthritis

II. Secondary

A. Dysplastic

1. Chondrodysplasia
2. Epiphyseal dysplasias
3. Congenital joint displacement
4. Developmental disorders, Perthes' disease, epiphysiolysis

B. Post-traumatic

1. Acute
2. Repetitive
3. Postoperative

C. Structural failure

1. Osteonecrosis
2. Osteochondritis

D. Post-inflammatory

1. Infection
2. Inflammatory arthropathies

E. Endocrine and metabolic

1. Acromegaly
2. Ochronosis
3. Hemochromatosis
4. Crystal deposition disorders

F. Connective tissue
1. Hypermobility syndromes
2. Mucopolysaccharidoses

G. Etiology obscure
1. Kashin-Beck disease

As outlined in the literature

Primary osteoarthritis occurs as part of the aging process; secondary arthritis occurs because of some form of abnormality that occurs in the joint causing it to be misaligned, resulting in the abnormalities that ultimately result in the formation of arthritic changes. Sometimes these changes are the result of injuries to the joints or the result of a person's occupation, which exposes the joints to repeated stress, resulting in the development of arthritis.

If a joint becomes infected and the infection is not treated quickly, then that joint can develop post-inflammatory changes, which could develop arthritic changes ultimately.

Hemochromatosis is a condition that causes iron to be deposited in joints and breaks down within the joints into free radicals that can cause breakdown of the tissues and the bones in the joints. The result is the development of arthritis. Blacks and Hispanic men have a high percentage of secondary hemochromatosis, because of such diseases as sickle cell anemia and thalassemia that cause a large amount of iron to be deposited in their bloodstream from hemolyzed red blood cells. Many Italian, Greek, Arabic and Asian men also suffer from secondary hemochromatosis with resulting high incidence of osteoarthritis.

Men who suffer from sickle cell disease can develop aseptic necrosis of joints such as the hips, shoulders, elbows, etc. That occurs because the sickling phenomenon impedes the ready flow of blood with oxygen to these joints, resulting in ischemic changes in the bony parts of these joints, which can lead to the development of aseptic necrosis and different stages of arthritis.

There are many other men of different ethnic background who, because they suffer from thalassemia, either beta or alpha, have secondary hemochromatosis, which can cause them to develop osteoarthritis due to the deposition of iron in their joints.

Obesity is a major predisposing factor in the development of osteoarthritis. The knees are most prone to the development of arthritis because of the stress placed on them by the excess weight. About 50% of black men and 46% of Hispanic men and about a third of white men in the U.S. are obese. Because osteoarthritis of the knees is quite common in this group of men and other obese men. The chances of a man developing osteoarthritis can be determined by the body mass index of that man. The greater the body mass index of a man, the greater his chances of developing osteoarthritic changes in his knees, hip, ankles, and feet.

TABLE 2:
Determining Body Mass Index (BMI) from Height and Weight
Body Mass Index* (kg/m2)

Body Mass Index* (kg/m2)												
	19 20 21	22	23	24	25	26	27	28	29	30	35
Height (in) Body weight (lb)											
58	91 96 100	105	110	115	119	124	129	134	138	143	167
59	94 99 104	109	114	119	124	128	133	138	143	148	173
60	97 102 107	112	118	123	128	133	138	143	148	153	179
61	100 106 111	116	122	127	132	137	143	148	153	158	185
62	104 109 115	120	126	131	136	142	147	153	158	164	191
63	107 113 118	124	130	135	141	146	152	158	163	169	197
64	110 116 122	128	134	140	145	151	157	163	169	174	204
65	114 120 126	132	138	144	150	156	162	168	171	180	210
66	118 124 130	136	142	148	155	161	167	173	179	186	215
67	121 127 134	140	146	153	159	166	172	178	185	191	223
68	125 131 138	144	151	158	164	171	177	184	190	197	230
69	128 135 142	149	155	162	169	176	182	189	196	203	236
70	132 138 146	153	160	167	174	181	188	195	202	207	243
71	136 143 150	157	165	172	179	186	193	200	208	215	250
72	140 147 154	162	169	177	184	191	199	206	213	221	258
73	144 151 159	166	174	182	189	197	204	212	219	227	265
74	148 155 163	171	179	186	194	202	210	218	225	233	272
75	152 160 168	176	184	192	200	208	216	224	232	240	279
76	156 164 172	180	189	197	205	213	221	230	238	246	287

Body mass index, or BMI, is the measurement of choice to determine obesity. BMI is a formula that takes into account both a person's height and weight. BMI is a person's weight in kilograms divided by height in meters squared (BMI=kg/m2). The table printed above has already done the conversions. To use the table, find the appropriate height in the left-hand column. Move across the row to the given weight. The number at the top of the column is the BMI for that height and weight.

In general, a person age 35 or older is obese if he or he has a BMI of >27. For people age 34 or younger, a BMI of >25 indicates obesity. Obesity is an indication for further clinical evaluation.

The BMI measurement poses some of the same problems as weight-for-height tables. BMI does not provide information on a person's age or body fat or take into consideration the person's body fat distribution.

As published by the American Diabetes Association

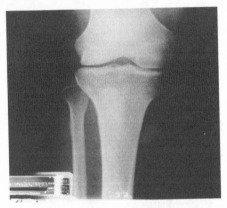

Figure 13.1—X-ray of a normal knee

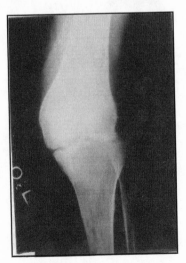

Figure 13.2—X-ray of a knee affected with osteoarthritis

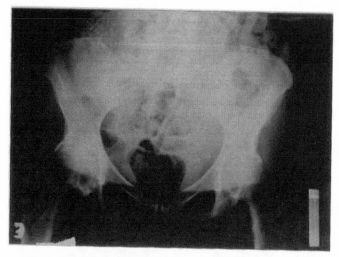

Figure 13.3: X-ray of hip joint affected with osteoarthritis

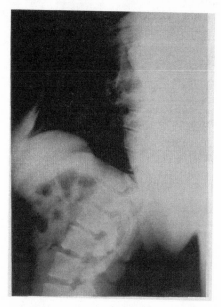

Figure 13.4: X-ray of lumbar spine affected with osteoarthritis

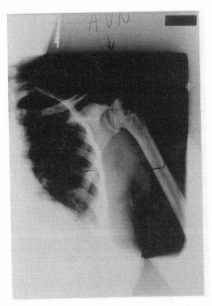

Figure 13.5: X-ray of shoulder joint showing aseptic necrosis in a patient with sickle cell anemia

Osteoarthritis can be a painful and disabling disease. Frequently, the affected joint or joints have to be surgically replaced after conservative treatments, such as medication and physical therapy, have failed. Medical management consists mainly of nonsteroidal anti-inflammatory drugs such as aspirin, Indocin, Motrin, Aleve, Naprosyn, Relafan, Daypro, Anaprox, and pain medication, etc. to relieve the pain and stiffness associated with the disease. These medications work by interfering with the inflammation that occurs locally in the affected joints, thereby easing the pain.

Physical therapy works by relieving the stiffness and by strengthening the affected joint or joints.

When these treatments are no longer effective and the pain and discomfort persist, then surgical intervention is often considered as an option to treat the arthritic joint.

Surgical replacement of hips, knees and other joints, etc., has become common practice these days, provided the affected individual is not too obese to allow for the operation to have a chance of success, or provided there are no other contraindications, such as associated major medical problems, etc.

Before a decision can be made to replace a joint, radiological studies, such as plain x-rays, CAT scan or MRI, have to be done to properly evaluate the extent of the osteoarthritic changes (see Figures 1.5).

Another major reason that osteoarthritis is so much more common in minority men than white men is the fact that many minority men work as factory workers and housekeepers, and these types of work require a lot of physical activity, which places a lot of stress on the joints of the fingers, shoulders, elbows, knees, lumbar spine, cervical spine and the hip joints.

Osteoarthritis, as a disease, is quite commonly seen in athletes, no matter what form of athletic activities they are engaged in.

Preventive measures such as eating a proper diet to maintain an ideal weight and wearing proper sports equipment during athletic activities would help to decrease the incidence of osteoarthritis.

About 1% of the population suffers from rheumatoid arthritis. Rheumatoid arthritis is a chronic inflammatory disease of the joints that, when left untreated or when treatment fails, causes chronic deformity of the bones with destruction of the affected joints. In point of fact, even when appropriate and effective treatments are provided to a person suffering with rheumatoid arthritis, joint deformities ultimately develop in the majority of patients with rheumatoid arthritis.

The joints frequently affected by rheumatoid arthritis are the feet, the hands, the fingers, the elbows, the wrists, shoulders and hips.

The cause of rheumatoid arthritis is unknown. Although many theories have been proposed, none has so far been proven. Men are affected much more than men with rheumatoid arthritis.

Rheumatoid arthritis is a multi-system disease, but the joints, bones, muscles, skin, and blood system are affected most frequently. The cardiovascular systems, as well as the pulmonary system, are also frequently affected.

In the beginning, the symptoms of rheumatoid arthritis can be insidious and difficult to discern. At times, a person may present with vague symptoms such as general malaise, weakness, weight loss, with minor aches and pains. Sometimes, the person may report having morning stiffness in different parts that improves as he starts to move around, doing daily chores.

As the disease progresses, then the signs of synovitis with swelling of the joints with pain and warmth become evident (see Table 3).

Worldwide, 1% of the population suffers from rheumatoid arthritis.

The disease affects men between the ages of 20 and 50 years, although some men are afflicted earlier and some are afflicted at a later age. Men are affected three times more often than men with RA.

TABLE 3: Classification of Rheumatoid Arthritis

Revised, as Published by the American College of Rheumatology

1. *Guidelines for classification*
    a. Four of seven criteria are required to classify a patient as having rheumatoid arthritis
    b. Patients with two or more clinical diagnoses are not excluded
2. *Criteria**
    a. Morning stiffness: Stiffness in and around the joints lasting 1 hr before maximal improvement.
    b. Arthritis of three of more joint areas: At least three joint areas, observed by a physician Simultaneously, have soft tissue swelling or joint effusions, not just bony overgrowth. The 14 possible joint areas involved are right or left proximal interphalangeal, metacarpophalangeal, wrist, elbow, knee, and ankle and metatarsophalangeal joints.
    c. **Arthritis of hand joints: Arthritis of wrist, metacarpophalangeal joint, or proximal interphalangeal joint.**
    d. Symmetric arthritis: Simultaneous involvement of the same joint areas on both sides of the body.
    e. Rheumatoid nodules: Subcutaneous nodules over bony prominences, extensor surfaces, or juxtaarticular regions observed by a physician.
    f. Serum rheumatoid factor: Demonstration of abnormal amounts of serum rheumatoid factor by any method for which the result has been positive in less than 5% of normal control subjects.
    g. Radiographic changes: Typical changes of RA on posteroanterior hand and wrist radiographs, which must include erosions or unequivocal bony decalcification localized in or most marked adjacent to the involved joints.

Criteria a-d must be present for at least 6 weeks. A physician must observe criteria b-e.

Taking a thorough and detailed history is crucial in a person in whom the physician suspects rheumatoid arthritis. Equally important is a thorough physical examination. Eliciting the fact that other immediate members of the family have rheumatoid arthritis or symptoms suggesting rheumatoid arthritis is quite important, because there is clear evidence that rheumatoid arthritis can run in the family.

No one test is diagnostic of rheumatoid arthritis, but a series of blood tests together with x-ray examination of certain joints, such as the hands and the fingers, may add up to confirming the diagnosis of rheumatoid arthritis. X-rays of the proximal interphalangeal, metacarpal phalangeal, metatarsal phalangeal, have distinct characteristics that are seen mainly in rheumatoid. Chronic changes of the hands and wrists resulting in swan neck deformities is classic for rheumatoid arthritis but these are late bony changes (see Figures 13.6 and 13.7).

Figures 13.6 and 13.7: X-ray of the wrist and hand joints showing arthritic changes in a patient with rheumatoid arthritis

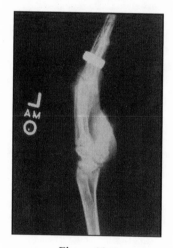

Figure 13.6

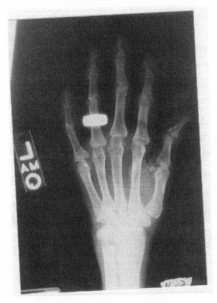

Figure 13.7

Other systemic involvements of rheumatoid arthritis include:

1. Vasculitis involving medium-sized vessels.
2. The lungs may become involved because of pleural effusion, resulting in shortness of breath, and diffuse interstitial fibrosis may develop, resulting in chronic lung disease.
3. The eyes may become involved with a condition called keratoconjunctivitis sicca (also known as Sjoren's Syndrome) causing dry eyes.
4. In about 10% of individuals with rheumatoid arthritis, the spleen is enlarged. Frequently, when the spleen is enlarged in rheumatoid arthritis, the white blood cell count is also low. (this is called Felty's Syndrome.)
5. Some adults with rheumatoid arthritis develop a clinical picture similar to children with rheumatoid arthritis called Still's disease, with fever spike, polyarthralgia, myalgia, a maculopapular rash, pericarditis, pneumonitis, sore throat, large spleen, lymphadenopathy and pain in the abdomen.
6. The heart can, at times, be involved and pericarditis can occur. Aortic regurgitation and conduction abnormalities of the rhythm of the heart can also occur.

Men with rheumatoid arthritis may develop peripheral neuropathy because of vasculitis of the vasa nervorum. Further, neurological problems may result when, because of tenosynovitis of the wrists, compression of the median nerve occurs, resulting in carpal tunnel syndrome.

The hematopoietic system (blood system) is markedly affected by rheumatoid arthritis. Anemia is the most serious and most common blood abnormality seen in rheumatoid arthritis. A characteristic of the anemia seen in rheumatoid arthritis is normochromic, normocytic (meaning the sizes and the hemoglobin contents of the red cells are normal but there are not enough red cells produced, resulting in anemia). The serum iron is low, the TIBC (total iron binding capacity) is normal but the serum ferritin is high.

Although there is plenty of iron in the body, as reflected by the high serum ferritin, anemia exists because there is an abnormality involving the release mechanism of the iron from the transferrin to the early erythroblasts (early red blood cell precursors). The iron accumulates in the reticulo-endothelial cells. That failure to release iron to the erythroblasts is what is responsible for the hypoproliferative anemia that is seen in rheumatoid arthritis (anemia of chronic disease/anemia of chronic inflammatory diseases). In effect, the rheumatoid person suffers from iron deficiency anemia because he has an inability to use the iron in the body (iron-deficient dyserythropoiesis).

Recent evidence in the literature suggests that some cytokines play a major role in this process of anemia of chronic disease (now also referred to as anemia of inflammatory diseases). See Chapter 10 for a discussion of Anemia of Chronic Diseases.

Leukopenia (low white blood cell) is frequently seen in rheumatoid arthritis and in particular when there is splenomegaly (known as Felty's Syndrome as mentioned earlier).

Other blood tests that are frequently abnormal in rheumatoid arthritis are:
1. Elevated ESR (erythrocyte sedimentation rate)
2. Elevated rheumatoid factor (latex fixation)
3. ANA (antinuclear antibodies) is elevated in up to 60% of patients with rheumatoid arthritis.

An ESR of 100 mg/hr or greater, together with a high latex fixation and rheumatoid nodules as seen in some joints, represent not only severe rheumatoid arthritis but a very poor prognosis.

The symptoms of rheumatoid arthritis and the overall clinical course of rheumatoid arthritis is worse in minority men than in white men because most minority men are engaged in heavier physical work than their white counterparts. Poverty and heavier physical work and poor working conditions in the factories, housekeeping and domestic work are more closely associated with black, Hispanic and other men of color and other poor men of lower socioeconomic echelons of society.

Therefore, men whose life circumstances place them in these poor working conditions, while at the same time being afflicted with rheumatoid arthritis, have a harder task to cope with it. Trying to work to earn a living using stiff, painful and swollen joints of the hands, elbows, shoulders, knees, feet and lower back is a very difficult task, to say the least.

There are several modalities available to treat rheumatoid arthritis although there is no cure for that disease. Rheumatoid arthritis is primarily treated with:

1. Aspirin, 2 tablets t.i.d. with food to prevent stomach irritation.
2. Indocin 25 mg t.i.d. or q.i.d., again with food in the stomach.
3. Nonsteroidal anti-inflammatory drugs (NSAIDS) such as Motrin 400 mg t.i.d. or 600 mg t.i.d. on Naprosyn 250 mg t.i.d. or Clinoril 200 mg b.i.d., or Feldene 20 mg once daily, or Daypro 600 mg b.i.d. or Relafen 500 mg two tablets at once in the morning or Anaprox DS 550 mg one tablet b.i.d. or Anaprox 275 mg t.i.d.,. Celebrex 100 mg or 200 mg by mouth daily and with Disease Modifying Drugs (DMARDs) such as

1. Methrotrexate
2. Enbrel
3. Humira
4. Kineret
5. Orencia
6. Remicade
7. Plaquenil
8. Azulfidine
9. Minocin
10. Arava
11. Neoral
12. Imuran
13. Prenisone

When that category of medications no longer works or when the side effects become clinically unacceptable, then a new family of drugs can be used. The most effective of these newer medications is Methotrexate. It is used in low dose intermittently, 7.5 mg to 15 mg once per week. Recently a medication called Minocycline has proved to be effective in the treatment of some patients with rheumatoid arthritis. Azathioprine and cyclophosphamide have both been used in the treatment of some cases of rheumatoid arthritis, but since these medications are anti-cancer medications, their long-term use may lead to the development of secondary cancer.

Steroids, such as Prednisone, in small doses can help to calm down acute flare-ups of joint inflammations in patients with rheumatoid arthritis. Its long-term use ought to be avoided because it has major side effects when used for an extended period of time.

There is a family of medications referred to as disease-modifying anti-rheumatic drugs (DMRDs) that have been used in rheumatoid arthritis when all else fails. Among these drugs are the following:

1. Gold
2. D-penicillamine
3. Chloroquine and sulfasalazine

Arava (Leflunomide) is one of a new family of medications used to treat rheumatoid arthritis. The usual dose of Arava after a loading dose is 20 mg. daily by mouth. These medications have major side effects and ought to be used very carefully by physicians familiar with their use.

Physical therapy as a modality plays a major role in the treatment of rheumatoid arthritis to prevent weakness, contractures, atrophy and other assorted problems affecting the joints of people suffering with rheumatoid arthritis.

At times, surgical intervention must be carried out to help alleviate some of the deformities that rheumatoid arthritis causes in the joints of its victims. Osteoarthritic joints also are frequently treated surgically to relieve pain and deformities. Anti-inflammatory medications, such as aspirin, Indocin, Excedrin and all the NSAIDS, can cause gastrointestinal bleeding in up to 10% of individuals taking them with major medical complications. A higher number, up to 30%, of individuals taking these medications chronically develop a multitude of stomach symptoms, such as heartburn, etc.

People with kidney disease, such as renal insufficiency, ought to be very careful with NSAIDS because not only can these medications themselves cause kidney disease, *de novo*, they can make kidney disease worse. When taking these medications, these individuals ought to be supervised closely by a physician, in order that their blood counts, their liver function tests, and their kidney functions test can be closely monitored.

The most effective and the only medication approved by the FDA to prevent bleeding from the stomach (gastric ulcer) caused by aspirin and NSAIDS is misoprostol (Cytotec). Cytotec is used as 100 mg three times per day with food. Cytotec is a prostaglandin analog. Its mode of action is to:

1. Increase the pH of the gastric juice;

2. Increase mucous production by the stomach; and
3. Increase blood flow to the lining of the stomach, thereby preventing erosions and ulcerations of the stomach wall.

Because Cytotec is a prostaglandin analog, it can induce abortion. Therefore, men of childbearing age ought not to take that medication when pregnant, as per the FDA and the makers of Cytotec.

Methotrexate has major side effects to the liver and bone marrow, so physicians must observe individuals taking Methotrexate closely with blood count and liver function tests, etc. Methotrexate also ought not to be taken by men who are pregnant because it can cause abortion and deformities in the fetus.

Systemic lupus erythematosus

Systemic lupus erythematosus (SLE) is an autoimmune disease of unknown cause that most commonly affects more women than men. There are roughly 4000 white males and 31,000 black males with SLE in the US.

According to the National Institute of Health, 9 out 10 individuals affected with lupus are women. That disease is more common in black and Hispanic men than white men. SLE is diagnosed 3 times more frequently in black men than in white men.

The incidence of SLE varies from 15 per 100,000 populations to 50 per 100,000 populations. According to the Lupus Foundation of America, 1.5 million people in the USA are affected with lupus.

Morning stiffness with swelling and pain in the joints is a frequent presentation of SLE. As the term implies, SLE affects many organs, and disease in any one of these organs may be the first manifestation of SLE. In addition, patients with SLE may present with fatigue, malaise, fever, anorexia, weight loss and nausea, etc. The musculoskeletal system may be affected by myalgias, arthralgias, and polyarthritis with bony erosions, deformities of the hands, myositis, myopathy, and ischemic necrosis of bones.

The skin may be affected with a malar rash over the cheeks. A discoid rash may be seen on the skin. Photosensitivity may be seen. Ulcers of the mouth may be seen. Any number and types of other rashes may be seen such as a maculopapular rash, urticarial rash, bullous rash, alopecia, and vasculitis, etc.

The hematopoietic system (blood system) may be affected with anemia, both chronic and hemolytic. Leukopenia (low white blood cell count), thrombocytopenia with circulating anticoagulant, large spleen; large liver, lymphadenopathy (large lymph nodes) may be seen.

SLE frequently affects the neurological system. Among the neurological symptoms manifested in patients with SLE are memory loss, acute psychosis, seizures, peripheral neuropathy vasculitis, and stroke, etc.

The lungs are frequently affected in patients with SLE. Patients can develop pleurisy, pleural effusion, pneumonitis, interstitial fibrosis, pulmonary hypertension and ARDS (adult respiratory distress syndrome).

The heart can also be affected by SLE

Among the problems that affect the heart in SLE are the following:

1. Pericarditis
2. Myocarditis
3. Endocarditis
4. Arrhythmias, and
5. Heart blocks (electrical disturbances of the heart)

The kidneys are frequently affected in patients with SLE. Nephritis, with varying degrees of severity in association with hematuria, frequently occurs in SLE. Proteinuria greater than 500 mg/24 hours, along with nephrotic syndrome, which can ultimately result in renal failure, frequently occurs in patients with SLE.

Anti-cardiolipin/anti-phospholipid syndromes are frequently seen in SLE with associated thrombosis of different organs, such as the brain, the lungs, the vascular system, and the placenta in men, resulting in frequent spontaneous abortions. Any man who has had frequent spontaneous abortions ought to be evaluated for the anti-cardiolipin/anti-phospholipid syndromes. Because of protein loss, as part of the nephrotic syndrome, anti-*thrombosis* III, protein C and protein S levels are low resulting in an hypercoagulable state (thick blood), causing formation of clots (DVT) or pulmonary embolism{clot in the *lung*}.

A multitude of gastrointestinal symptoms are manifested in patients who have SLE. Among these symptoms are nausea, vomiting, diarrhea, gastrointestinal bleeding, abnormal liver function tests, etc. Both venous and arterial thrombosis frequently occur in patients with SLE and the Prednisone that is used as the main treatment of SLE can also cause a state of hypercoagulation, which itself is a frequent cause of thrombosis.

The eyes in patients with SLE can develop retinal vasculitis, conjunctivitis, and the SICCA syndrome with dry eyes.

There is another form of lupus called discoid lupus. Discoid lupus affects the skin of the face, neck, arms and scalp. It causes chronic scarring with severe disfigurement.

Very few of these patients with discoid lupus go on to develop SLE. On the other hand, 20% of patients with SLE develop discoid lupus lesions and 5% of patients with discoid lupus go on to develop SLE.

Another form of lupus that can be seen is drug-induced lupus. The drugs that are generally associated with the development of a lupus-like state include Procanamide, hydralazine, Isoniazid, chlorpromazine, methyldopa, and Quinidine, among others. The symptoms of drug-induced lupus include fevers, skin rash, arthralgias, polyarthritis, pericarditis, etc. These symptoms usually disappear after a few days or up to 1 week to 10 days once the offending drug is stopped.

Evaluation of lupus includes a history and physical examination, laboratory tests and sometimes x-ray examinations.

Laboratory tests that are the most helpful in diagnosing lupus are ANA, ENA, anti-double-stranded DNA, *anti-Ro antibody, anti-La and anti-*Sm., serum complement levels, erythrocyte sedimentation rate, CBC, platelet count, urinalysis and blood chemistries. Usually the ANA test is positive in lupus. Then the next tests to order are the anti-double-stranded DNA and the ENA. The ENA has two parts to it. One part is the RNP (ribonuclear protein) and the other part is the SM (Smith antibody). If the SM part is positive then SLE is most probably present. If the RNP is positive then mixed connective tissue disease is present. Examples of mixed connective tissue disease (MCTD) include overlap syndrome of SLE, rheumatoid arthritis, polymyositis, in association with scleroderma and high titers of RNP and clinical features of SLE.

The anti-double-stranded DNA and the anti-SM are specific for SLE. Tests such as the serum complement levels and the ESR are used to monitor the activity of the disease.

A positive ANA is found in association with many conditions and is therefore not specific for lupus. A significant percentage of the U.S. population has positive ANA and these individuals are not sick with anything.

SLE is more common in men than men by about a 9:1 ratio. Men of color seem to have a particular predilection to get sicker with lupus than other men. Pregnancy can cause an acute flare-up of SLE and, as such, it is not advisable for men to get pregnant when suffering with lupus.

Treatment of SLE

Prednisone is the main drug used to treat lupus and its multitude of complications. Cyclophosphamide (Cytoxan) and Azathioprine are also quite effective in treating SLE.

Other medications available to treat Lupus include NSAIDS, Plaquenil, and topical steroid cream. Lupus has no cure but can be treated and managed for a very long time. Many patients with SLE can go on to develop renal failure, requiring chronic dialysis.

The death rate from SLE in black men is quite high, and among black men in the age range 45 to 64, the death rate increased to 70% between 1979 and 1998.

It is important to mention that Prednisone is used in thousands, and is in fast becoming the most commonly used medication in the world. Corticosteroid was synthesized by a black biochemist by the name of Percy Julian. The world owes a debt of gratitude to this brilliant biochemist who unfortunately died several years ago at a surprisingly young age.

Sarcoidosis

Sarcoidosis is a disease of unknown cause, which is very common among black men. In the United States the ratio of black men to white men who have sarcoidosis is about 17:1. In other words, more black men are affected by sarcoidosis than white men. The disease is a multi-system disease, although the lungs are the most frequently affected organ. The disease is characterized pathologically by forming what is called non-caseating granulomas with derangement of the normal tissue architecture of the nodes. In acute sarcoidosis, the affected person may have fever, malaise, and anorexia with weight loss. The vast majority of individuals who develop sarcoidosis are younger than 40 years old. Patients with pulmonary sarcoid often have shortness of breath, cough, and sometimes chest pain. The chest x-ray in sarcoidosis often shows bilateral hilar adenopathy in association with pain in the joints. Biopsy of the hilar node done via bronchoscopy examination shows non-caseating granulomas. About 50% of individuals with pulmonary sarcoid develop permanent pulmonary disease and about 15% go on to develop pulmonary fibrosis. Other organs that are frequently affected by sarcoidosis are as follows:

1. Skin
2. Eyes
3. Upper respiratory tract
4. Bone marrow
5. Spleen
6. Liver
7. Kidney
8. Heart

9. Several endocrine organs
10. Nervous system
11. Musculoskeletal system
12. Exocrine system

Lymph node enlargement is quite common in sarcoidosis. Enlargement of nodes inside the chest is seen in about 75% to 90% of individuals affected with sarcoidosis. Enlargement of cervical, inguinal and axillary nodes are quite common in sarcoidosis. Biopsy of any of these peripheral nodes is likely to show the classic lesions seen in sarcoidosis, namely non-caseating granuloma.

The classic lesions seen over the skin of individuals with Sarcoidosis is something called erythema nodosum. Other skin lesions that can be seen include a maculopapular rash, subcutaneous nodes and lupus pernio (indurated blue/purple swollen lesion on the nose, cheeks, lips, ears, fingers, etc.).

Erythema nodosum is frequently accompanied by symptoms such as polyarthralgia.

Eye problems occur in about 25% of people who have sarcoidosis. Usually the iris and the uveal tract are involved, etc. Anterior uveitis occurs in approximately 75% of patients with sarcoidosis and posterior uveitis occurs in about 25% of affected patients. Blurry vision, photophobia and tearing occur frequently in patients with sarcoidosis. The conjunctival involvement is quite common as well as the lacrimal gland. If the lacrimal gland is involved, then frequently dry and sore eyes can develop. If sarcoidosis of the eyes is left untreated, or treated too late total blindness can result.

The upper airway can be involved in up to 20% of patients suffering with sarcoidosis. Hoarseness, nasal stuffiness, dyspnea, stridor, and wheezing can occur.

The heart can be involved in up to 5% of patients with sarcoidosis. The conduction system of the heart can be involved, leading to complete heart block. Cardiac arrhythmias are common and the left ventricle is frequently involved. Pericarditis and congestive heart failure can occur.

The nervous system is affected in about 5% of patients with Sarcoidosis. Any part of the nervous system can become involved with sarcoidosis. The seventh nerve is frequently affected by sarcoidosis, causing unilateral facial paralysis. Other nervous system involvement may include optic nerve dysfunction, papilledema, hearing difficulty, pituitary and hypothalamic dysfunction, etc.

The endocrine system can be involved in sarcoidosis, causing diabetes insipidus. The adrenal glands can also be involved, resulting in an Addison-like syndrome.

The reproductive system can also be involved with sarcoidosis, but men can get pregnant while suffering with the disease. The disease seems to improve during pregnancy, only to flare up after delivery.

The disease can involve the bone marrow in up to 40% of patients. Anemia, neutropenia and thrombocytopenia can occur because of bone marrow involvement. The spleen can become enlarged in sarcoidosis. The liver is involved up to 90% of the time in sarcoidosis. The liver may be enlarged 30% of the time. The kidneys can be involved in a small percentage of patients with sarcoidosis.

More commonly, patients with sarcoidosis can have high serum calcium, and high calcium in the urine can cause calcium kidney stones.

The musculoskeletal system is frequently involved in sarcoidosis, with bone, joint and muscle pain. Bones of the hands and feet are most commonly involved. But, any bone can be involved.

Sometimes the first presentation of sarcoidosis is painful and swollen joints and bone pains. Arthritis and arthralgias frequently occur in large joints. Deformities may occur in joints and bones in sarcoidosis. Muscle weakness and symptoms of polymyositis may occur, confusing sarcoidosis with collagen vascular diseases or mixed collagen vascular diseases.

How to diagnose sarcoidosis

First and foremost, it is important to take a good history from the patient. Second, x-ray tests such as chest x-ray showing bilateral hilar adenopathy may be seen. If the presenting symptoms refer to the eye, then an eye examination is important; uveitis is a frequent finding in patients with sarcoidosis with eye symptoms.

Laboratory tests that are helpful are the CBC, the chemistry profile, the ESR and, most important of all, is the angiotensin-I-converting enzyme which is elevated in about 2/3 of patients with sarcoidosis. The serum calcium is frequently elevated and frequently the 24-hour urinary calcium is also elevated in patients with sarcoidosis. This test is not very specific. The gold standard for sarcoidosis, however, is the finding of non-caseating granuloma on lymph node or other tissues on biopsy.

So, if the complex of symptoms fits the profile, the angiotensin-converting enzyme is elevated, and the tissue biopsy shows non-caseating granuloma, then the patient has sarcoidosis.

It is important to keep in mind that in clinical medicine things do not always fit into a neat package—which means that clinical judgment must be brought into play to arrive at a diagnosis even though all the pieces of the puzzle may not fit.

How to treat sarcoidosis

Steroid is the treatment of choice for sarcoidosis. A dose of 1 mg/kg of body weight is given from 4 to 6 weeks by mouth. Steroid works to interfere with the cellular process in the affected tissues, thereby decreasing the inflammatory process and relieving the symptoms of sarcoidosis. In up to 50% of cases, the disease resolves spontaneously, but, clinically, it may not be wise to take a chance and not treat, because the disease can go on to cause permanent damage to vital organs such as the eyes, the heart, the lungs, etc., which in some instances may be fatal (see the chapter on lung diseases for further discussion about sarcoidosis).

There are three other forms of arthritis that are interconnected in that their symptoms are similar, and must be differentiated one from the other all the time. They are as follows:

1. **Acute gouty arthritis**
2. Acute pseudo-gout
3. Septic arthritis

Acute gouty arthritis is one of the most painful conditions known in the field of medicine and to mankind. It usually occurs in a single joint such as the big toe, the ankle, the knee, the foot, or the wrist, etc. Gout is more common in men than women. About 20% of gout is hereditary.

The affected joint is usually markedly swollen, painful and tender. Gouty arthritis occurs because of either too much production of uric acid or a decreased excretion of uric acid.

Primary overproduction of uric acid occurs because of deficiency of hypoxanthine-guanine-phosphoribosyltransferase. That enzyme deficiency causes an increased level of 5-phosphoribosyl-1-pyrophosphate (PRPP), which accelerates purine biosynthesis and results in an increased production of uric acid.

The reduced excretion of uric acid leads to uric acid accumulation. Reduced filtration, enhanced resorption and decreased excretion are three other processes that lead to accumulation of uric acid in the blood.

There are several other ways in which uric acid can become elevated in the blood. Diuretic treatment, chemotherapeutic treatment in some cancers such as lymphoma and some leukemia can cause acute and massive release of purines into the bloodstream because of chemotherapy-induced cells breakdown, resulting in marked increase of serum uric acid.

That is a crucial point to remember when treating patients who present with that form of cancer requiring acute chemotherapeutic treatment, so that IV fluid must be provided together with Allopurinol to prevent acute renal failure because of purine accumulation in the blood from clogging up the kidney tubules, causing them to fail.

Gout causes the production of monosodium crystals, which accumulate in joints. These crystals cause an acute inflammation leading to swelling, warmth and severe pain of the affected joints. When that attack occurs in the big toe it is called podagra.

Acute gouty arthritis is one of the most painful conditions known to mankind. Another gouty condition that causes acute and chronic pain in joints is pseudo-gout. Pseudo-gout occurs most frequently in older men.

The inflammatory reaction that occurs in pseudo-gout is due to calcium pyrophosphate dihydrate crystals. These crystals are seen under the microscope as weakly positive birefringent using polarized light. Similarly, the monosodium urate crystals are seen in synovial fluid taken from the joint and examined under the microscope.

The blood test that is elevated in gout is uric acid. The uric acid can be tested in the blood as part of the blood chemistry profile. The normal uric acid in the blood is 2.8 to 6.0 mg/dl. The higher the level of uric acid in the blood, the more likely that it will accumulate in joints, causing inflammation to occur. The repeated inflammatory reactions that occur in the joints can result in chronic destruction of these joints to different degrees.

It is important to realize that in an acute gouty arthritic attack the uric acid level may be normal to low. The reason is that the uric acid is moving from the blood to the joints, thereby reducing its level in the blood. When someone presents with an acute, swollen, hot, and painful joint, there are really three major considerations:
1. Gout
2. Pseudo-gout
3. Septic arthritis or
4. Trauma

Diet plays a major role in bringing about acute attack of gout.
Foods to avoid are:
Red wine
Sardines
Liver
Kidney

Sweetbreads

Shellfish.

Septic arthritis can occur because of bacteria in the blood settling into a joint, causing inflammation to occur. There are a multitude of clinical conditions that can be associated with septic arthritis:

1. Gonorrheal infection is probably the most common in sexually active individuals;
2. Pneumonia with bacteremia;
3. Sub-acute bacterial endocarditis (SBE) as seen frequently in IV drug-abusing individuals or any non-IV drug addict with SBE;
4. Penetrating trauma in a joint, etc.

To differentiate gouty arthritis in the joint from septic arthritis, one must tap synovial fluid off the joint and send it to the laboratory for evaluation. In the laboratory the fluid will be evaluated for:

1. Turbidity or cloudiness
2. The total number of white blood cells
3. The level of protein
4. The bacterial content of the fluid by gram stain
5. Bacterial growth on bacterial cultures
6. The presence or absence of crystals in the fluid, etc.

Further evaluations include history and physical examinations and x-ray studies of the affected joint.

To treat gouty arthritis the physician has to determine the extent and severity of the symptoms. The most effective treatment of acute gouty arthritis is intravenous colchicine, in which 1 mg of colchicine is given IV push, or 0.6 mg of colchicine may also be given by mouth every 2 hours until symptoms disappear or gastrointestinal symptoms appear. No more than a maximum of 6 mg of colchicine ought to be given acutely. If the symptoms are not too severe, Indocin 50 mg three times per day may be enough to relieve the gouty arthritic symptoms. It is crucial to remember not to use Allopurinol during an acute attack of gout, as that might lead to an idiosyncratic reaction, worsening the condition.

Once the acute attack has been brought under control, Allopurinol 300 mg per day is given to lower the level of uric acid in the blood and colchicine 0.6 mg two times per day is given along with it.

NSAIDS or Indocin may be given clinically to prevent acute attacks from occurring. For reasons that are not quite clear, acute gouty arthritic attacks seem to occur in spite of the fact that the patient is on a good dose of prophylactic medications.

Both gout and pseudo-gout can lead to markedly deformed joints with chronic arthritic pain. I

As for septic arthritis, that diagnosis must be made without failure, or the affected joint will be destroyed. The treatment of choice for septic arthritis is antibiotics given intravenously. Once the suspicion is strong that septic arthritis may exist, the joint must be tapped and fluid sent to the lab for studies and IV antibiotics must be given to the affected individual immediately. The type of antibiotics given depends on the clinical profile of the patient involved. Physicians are trained to know precisely what to do and how to do it in these circumstances.

Fibromyalgia is an ill defined arthritic condition that affects about 12 millions people in the US. FM is associated with head ache, stiffness of joint, general fatigue, chronic pain, anxiety, depression, insomnia etc.

There is no specific test available to diagnose FM. The diagnosis is usually made on clinical impression. The treatment of FM includes DSAID and analgesics.

Although there are no cures for these different arthritic conditions, (except septic arthritis) there are many treatments available to relieve their symptoms. Men of color, for a multitude of reasons as just outlined, have a higher propensity of developing certain types of arthritis as compared to white men. Therefore, it is important that men remain vigilant as to the presence of these different arthritic conditions and seek medical attention as quickly as possible to help alleviate their arthritic symptoms.

CHAPTER 14

EYE DISEASES IN MEN

THE INCIDENCE OF EYE DISEASE and blindness is more common in minority men than in their white counterparts. Many of the diseases that predispose to the development of diseases in the eye are much more common in minority men. For example, diseases such as hypertension, diabetes mellitus and glaucoma are much more common in minority men than in white men. The incidence of glaucoma is five times higher in minority than in white men.

Glaucoma is the number-one cause of blindness among minority men. According to the American College of Ophthalmology, about 5 million Americans have glaucoma. Both hypertension and diabetes mellitus predispose a person to the development of glaucoma. Of the 5 million or so Americans who have glaucoma, a very large percentage of them are men of color. For reasons that are not yet clear, black men have a higher propensity to develop glaucoma than white men or any other group of men. Glaucoma runs in families. That is to say, it is genetically transmitted. About 80,000 individuals go blind in the U.S. because of glaucoma yearly. What makes glaucoma so dangerous is the fact that it causes no pain. So, a man whose intraocular pressure is high, which is the first step to the development of glaucoma, will not know that the pressure inside the eye is high unless he goes to the ophthalmologist to have his eye pressure tested. As is the case for many other diseases, men of color often present for medical evaluations when the disease they are suffering from have already gone too far. Sometimes, these conditions have already reached to advanced a staged to be helped, even with the best medications or the best of medical procedures.

There are four different types of glaucoma:

1. Primary open angle glaucoma
2. Secondary glaucoma
3. Angle closure glaucoma
4. Congenital glaucoma

One-fourth of all cases of glaucoma presents at birth and are due to congenital reasons. According to the Center for Health Statistics, in Bethesda, Maryland, 1.2 out of every 100 individuals have some form of eye disease. Though that is a high percentage, the incidence is much higher among the men of color. That is so because of:

1. The high incidence of glaucoma in men of color,
2. The higher incidence of hypertension, leading to hypertensive retinopathy with hemorrhage inside the eyes, which, if left untreated, will cause permanent blindness,
3. The higher incidence of diabetes in men of color and in particular obese men who have the propensity to develop diabetes mellitus because of the obesity, which then leads to diabetic retinopathy with different degrees of bleeding inside the eyes that can lead to blindness if left untreated;
4. The high incidence of trauma to the eye which occurs much more frequently in men of color as compared to white men because men of color are more likely to get exposed to riskier jobs that predispose them to a higher likelihood of being injured in the eyes on the job.

Besides glaucoma, diabetes mellitus, and hypertension, other diseases that affect the eyes include cataracts, syphilis, sarcoidosis, sickle cell disease, AIDS, temporal arteritis, vitamin deficiency, and malignant tumor, etc.

Glaucoma—the disease

In adults, there are three different types of glaucoma:

1. Primary open angle glaucoma
2. Angle closure glaucoma
3. Low tension glaucoma

There are about 5 million reported cases of glaucoma in the United States. Glaucoma is the third leading cause of eye problems leading to blindness in white men in the United States. It is the first cause of blindness in minority men in the United States.

The incidence of blindness because of Glaucoma is 7 to 8 times higher in minority men than in white men. Minority men between the ages of 44 and 65, and in particular, those who are hypertensive and have a family history of glaucoma have a 15 to 17 time greater possibility of developing glaucoma than white men. According to published reports, glaucoma can be genetically trans-mitted and 30% of glaucoma patients have family history of glaucoma.

Open-angle glaucoma

The cause of open angle glaucoma is an inherited defect in the function of the endothelial cells of the cellular meshwork inside the eyes. The result is increased production of aqueous humor fluid inside the eyes on the one hand, and on the other hand, failure of drainage of the aqueous humor fluid, resulting in increased pressure inside the eyes. The normal intraocular pressure is 13 to 20 mm/Hg. While an intraocular pressure of 13–20 mm/Hg is normal for white men, it is not necessarily normal for minority men. That fact is to be kept in mind because minority men have a higher incidence of glaucoma; it is also true that glaucoma is much more aggressive in its progression in minority men than it is in white men. Therefore, an intraocular pressure above 14 in a minority man must be watched closely and evaluated more frequently.

When the pressure inside the eyes is elevated, it damages the optic nerve. The optic nerve is the nerve that allows the eyes to see. Once damage has occurred to the optic nerve, vision can become impaired. Though the intra-ocular pressure is elevated, it causes no pain in most cases, and therefore, a man who has elevated intraocular pressure has no way to know about it, until his an ophthalmologist examines his eyes. Tonometry is the test done to evaluate the pressure inside the eye. The visual field is the test used to evaluate the optic nerve. Elevated intraocular pressure does not mean glaucoma. If the intraocu-lar pressure remains high for an extended period—months to years—the optic nerve will become damaged. Once the optic nerve is damaged, then glaucoma ensues.

Open-angle glaucoma is responsible for more than 90% of all cases of blind-ness. The first sign that a man has glaucoma is when the he loses his peripheral vision.

About 5% of first-degree relatives of people with open angle glaucoma 50 years or older develop open angle glaucoma, as compared to 1% of people in the general population.

Three things happen clinically in open angle glaucoma:

1. Intraocular pressure of 24 mm/Hg or greater
2. Cupping of the optic disc
3. Visual field loss

Typically, the first modality of treatment in someone with open angle glaucoma is eye drop medication to either reduce the production of aqueous humor fluid and/or increase the drainage, thereby lowering the intraocular pressure.

Some frequently used eye drops include:

1. Pilocarpine
2. Timoptic
3. Ocupress
4. Trusopt
5. Carbachol
6. Phystignine salicylate
7. Desmocranium bromide (Humorsol)
8. Acetazolamide (Diamox)
9. Isofurophate (Floropryl)
10. Btaxololhydrochloride (Betoptic)
11. Optipranolol
12. Propine
13. Latanoprost solution (Xalatan)
14. Betagan,
15. Cosopt
16. Alphagan P
17. Travatan etc,

If maximum eye drop treatment fails to bring the intraocular pressure down and visual field abnormality starts to develop, then laser treatment is used to facilitate drainage of aqueous humor fluid from the eye, thereby reducing the intraocular pressure.

As stated before, the peripheral vision is the first vision to go when increased intraocular pressure damages the optic nerve.

Angle-closure glaucoma

It is reported that angle closure glaucoma occurs mostly in individuals who are farsighted and are above age 55. About 5% of first-degree relatives of people with angle closure glaucoma are affected with the same condition in their later years.

There are three different stages of angle closure glaucoma:

1. Sub-acute angle closure glaucoma
2. Acute angle closure glaucoma
3. Chronic angle closure glaucoma

As just outlined, angle closure glaucoma occurs principally because of blockage to the proper drainage of the aqueous humor fluid that is produced inside the eyes.

In sub-acute angle closure glaucoma, the drainage is occurring in an insidious way so that the patient's eyes find ways to compensate, keeping the intraocular pressure intermittently normal.

In acute angle closure glaucoma, the intraocular pressure rises suddenly, resulting in a painful red eye, with reduced ability to see in that eye. When the examining physician places his or his finger on the affected eyeball, it is rockhard and quite painful. On tonometric examination, the intraocular pressure may be as high as 50 mm/Hg. The affected patient feels very sick, with pain and nausea, and may even vomit.

Next to trauma to the eye, acute angle closure glaucoma is the severest emergency seen in the field of ophthalmology.

The first step in the treatment of acute angle glaucoma is to try to bring the intraocular pressure down as quickly as possible. To do that, a doctor is likely to treat the eye with Pilocarpine eye drops 2% to 4% for five minutes. Later 0.5% Timolol solution is placed in the affected eye. If that does not work then 500 mg of Diamox IV is given to bring the pressure down. If the intraocular pressure fails to come down in spite of these treatments, then IV Mannitol is given to reduce the intraocular pressure, while the eye doctor is getting the patient ready for surgery to open the eye to allow the aqueous humor fluid to drain, bringing the intraocular pressure down to save the eye. Frequently after surgery, eye drop is used to maintain a normal pressure in the eye.

As angle closure glaucoma affects both eyes, in treating acute angle closure glaucoma, the non-affected eye must also receive immediate treatment with 0.5%-1 percent Pilocarpine, followed by Timolol or other beta-blocker like eye drops.

The Pilocarpine is used every four hours and the beta-blocker twice a day until prophylactic laser surgery can be done to that eye to prevent a similar event from occurring as that which has occurred in the acutely affected eye.

Other forms of glaucoma include:

1. Low-tension glaucoma
2. Congenital glaucoma
3. Secondary glaucoma, which can result from using iridocyclites, steroid treatment, either directly into the eye or when taken by mouth for long period.

Low-tension glaucoma is seen most often in elderly individuals who suffer from severe circulatory diseases impeding blood flow. Glaucoma occurs more frequently in men of color than in white men. The ratio is about 5–6:1 black man versus white man.

Glaucoma also occurs in men of color at a younger age than in white men and it is more aggressive in black men and leads to blindness more rapidly than in white men. The most important thing to do is to get the eyes examined in order that if the pressure inside the eye is found to be elevated then appropriate treatments and other measures can be instituted to prevent progression to blindness.

Cataracts

Another common disease of the eye is cataracts. The most common form of cataracts is age-related cataracts or senile cataracts. Cataract is an opacification of the lens of the eyes.

The second form of cataract is a congenital cataract, which is usually the result of maternal rubella or cytomegalovirus infection during the first trimester of pregnancy.

Other causes of cataracts include diabetes mellitus, systemic use of steroids, myotonic dystrophy, uveitis, cigarette smoking, heavy alcohol consumption, etc.

Trauma to the eye is also a common cause of cataracts. Traumatic cataract is more common in men of color than in white men because the economic circumstances of men of color is worse, as compared to that of white men, exposing men of color to more work-related trauma to the eyes.

The first sign of cataracts is blurry vision, which progresses over months to years, with no pain, or redness to the eye and obvious clouding of the lens of the eyes when examined with the ophthalmoscope.

There are three types of cataracts:
1. Posterior subcapsular cataracts
2. Cortical cataracts
3. Mixed cataracts

Treatment of cataracts

Once the diagnosis of cataracts is established, the first mode of treatment is glasses to improve vision. That is the conservative management. When that treatment fails, then surgical removal of the cataract may be recommended to the patient. There are two types of surgical cataract removal procedures:

1. Extra capsular cataract removal with implantation of an intraocular Len.
2. Intracapsular cataract removal

The second type of surgical procedure is much less popular because of the advent of microsurgery, which facilitates the first procedure. Cataract removal surgery is carried out in the operating room with the patient being able to go home in a few hours after the operation has been completed with a patch on the operated eye, to be followed by the surgeon in his or his office. The patient is fully awake during the time of the surgery. Only the eye being operated on is anesthetized.

Hypertensive retinopathy:

Hypertension has many complications associated with it and if left untreated will cause serious damage to occur in many organs. Prominent among these organs are the eyes. The increase in pressure within the vessels of the eye causes different degrees of damage to occur within the lumen of these vessels. The damaged vessels then trap platelets and other materials from the blood on the inner surface of these vessels, starting a nidus, which leads to plaque formation. It is also said that leakage of fatty material occurs out of these damaged vessels, making the situation more complicated. That process perpetuates itself over time, causing different vascular abnormalities to occur inside the eyes, resulting in hypertensive retinopathy.

Hypertensive retinopathy is graded as 1, 2, 3 and 4, depending on the severity of the vascular abnormalities.

Grade 1 shows arteriolar narrowing.

Grade 2 shows arterio-venous nicking, some exudate and hemorrhages.

Grade 3 shows retinal edema, hemorrhage and cotton-wool spots. Grade 4 shows a combination of Grade 3 plus papilledema.

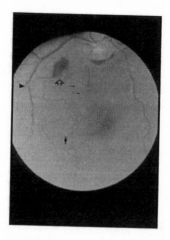

Figure 14.1: Showing different types of abnormalities in the eye of a hypertensive patient (hypertensive retinopathy). Small arrow showing silver wiring. Big arrow showing hard yellow exudates. Open arrow head showing blot hemorrhage. Arrow head showing A-V nicking.

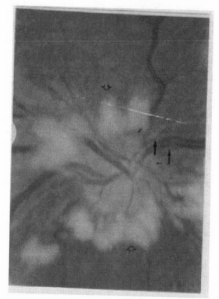

Figure 14.2: Showing different types of abnormalities in the eye of a hypertensive patient (hypertensive retinopathy). Small arrows showing early papilledema. One big arrow pointing to vein engorgement (larger vessel). The other big arrow pointing to arterial attenuation (smaller vessel); open arrow showing cotton wool exudates.

If proper treatment is not provided for these abnormalities, the patient often develops blindness. Hypertension is a very common disease, according to the latest estimates, occurring in about 58 million individuals in the United States. About 42% of these individuals, is said, go untreated for hypertension. Hypertension is the number-one disease among men of color in the United States. The percentage of hypertension is higher among men of color than white men because there are so many more obese men of color. In fact, 50% of black American men are obese, and obesity has a major impact in both the causation of hypertension and in making it worse. It is common knowledge that many men of color with hypertension are being treated inappropriately because many of them are receiving the wrong medications, namely they are not getting treated with water pills. Water pill (diuretic) is the most appropriate and the most effective medication to treat men with hypertension the world over. According to a recent report that appears in the literature, it costs about 7–10 cents per day to treat men patients with diuretics, as compared to an ACE inhibitor and calcium channel blocker that costs about $1000 per year each. (See chapter 1 on hypertension). That represents about 8% of the Social Security income of some men who are on Social Security. That report confirms the inappropriateness of the treatment that some men are receiving for their hypertension. The result is that they are getting treatments for their blood pressures that cause their blood pressure to go without proper control, resulting in end organs damage. The eyes are one of the end organs. The medication prescribed is often too expensive to buy, so the condition goes untreated, resulting in progression of their hypertension. Therefore, the percentage of men of color with untreated hypertension is much higher than it is in white men. Most men of color often are forced to do without adequate health care. There are seventy million hypertensive in the US and 40% of them are blacks. And of that 40%, less than 1/3 are receiving treatments for their high blood pressure. It is, therefore, not difficult to see why there is such a high incidence of glaucoma and other hypertension-associated lesions in the eyes of some men of color and other poor men, leading to their very high incidence of blindness.

Diabetes mellitus and its effects on the eyes of men

Type II diabetes mellitus is very common among men of color, and that is in part due to the fact that 50% of Black American and 46% of Hispanic men are obese, and obesity is highly associated with diabetes. According to the American Diabetic Association, there are roughly 21 million individuals diagnosed with diabetes mellitus in the United States and roughly 9 million more are undiagnosed. There are about 16 million pre-diabetics in the U.S. Each and every one of these individuals has the potential of developing diseases of the eyes, such as cataracts, glaucoma and diabetic retinopathy with hemorrhage inside the eyes. One out of every 14 African-Americans is likely to develop diabetes. That rate is 30% to 40% higher in black men than that seen in white males. Therefore, black men are 30% to 40% more likely to have eye diseases as the result of diabetes than white males.

Diabetic retinopathy

Diabetic retinopathy is a very serious disease, which causes blindness in a significant number of men who are diabetics. The same is true for any individuals who suffer from diabetes mellitus. Some of the lesions that can be seen in patients who are suffering from diabetes mellitus are as follows:

1. Micro-aneurysm
2. Arteriolar narrowing
3. Retinal edema
4. Hard exudates
5. Venous abnormalities
6. Soft exudates
7. Vitreous hemorrhages
8. Retinal hemorrhages
9. Retinal detachment, etc.

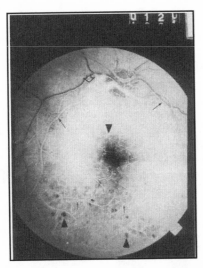

Figure 14.3—Showing different degrees of abnormalities in the eye of a patient with diabetes mellitus (diabetic retinopathy). Fluorescein angiogram shortly after injection of dye in patient's eye. Dye in arteries (white) and just starting to enter veins (large arrow). White area off NH is neovascular tuff (open arrow). White spots are hemorrhages (arrow heads). Tiny white spots are micro-aneurysms (small arrow).

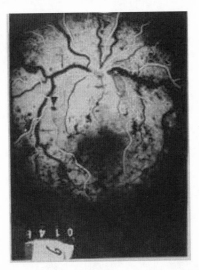

Figure 14.4—Showing different degrees of abnormalities in the eye of a patient with diabetes mellitus (diabetic retinopathy). Large arrows showing dilated veins. Arrow heads showing hemorrhages inside the eye.

It should be noted that eye symptoms and abnormalities may be the first signs that a person is suffering from diabetes mellitus. Very often, the patient presents to the ophthalmologist complaining of blurry vision, and the examining ophthalmologist, if he or he suspects diabetes mellitus as a cause of the blurriness of the eyes, can then order the blood sugar to confirm whether or not it is elevated blood sugar that is causing the blurry vision. As just stated, if the diabetic retinopathy is not very advanced, the fact that the blood sugar is elevated is enough to cause eye symptoms like blurry vision. Once the patient presents with symptoms of diabetes and diagnosed with diabetes, the treating physician should refer the patient to an eye doctor for an appropriate eye evaluation to prevent unnecessary blindness due to diabetes mellitus. Because the incidence of diabetes mellitus is on the rise in men, diabetes-associated blindness is also on the rise among these men. It is very important that men and other individuals with diabetes mellitus understand that if they present themselves to the eye doctor early enough and keep their blood sugar under tight control, and remains under constant care of a qualified ophthalmologist; they can prevent eventual blindness secondary to the effects of diabetes mellitus to the eyes.

Diabetes and ischemic diseases of the eye:

Diabetes mellitus causes ischemia because it causes plaque depositions to occur, the same way it causes plaque depositions to occur within vessels of the legs. The same process also causes deposition of plaque in the vessels of the eyes. When these very delicate vessels within the eyes have plaque within their lumens, and lipid material leaks out of these vessels, platelet deposition and plaque deposition take place, resulting, gradually, in the occlusion of these vessels to different degrees (see photographs 14.3 and 14.4). The occlusion causes rupture of these vessels and hemorrhage to occur, leading to different types and degrees of diabetic retinopathy. That is basically the underlying pathophysiology as to why and how these conditions occur and why they lead to blindness if left untreated. The eye is the only organ in the human body where an examining physician can actually see a vessel with the naked eye and the use of an instrument called the ophthalmoscope. It is very important that all referrals are made to an ophthalmologist, who is a physician trained and experienced to both evaluate and treats diseases of the eyes.

Hemoglobinopathies and eye disease

Sickle cell disease is the number-one abnormal hemoglobin disease that causes eye disease in those affected. Three different types of sickle cell diseases that can cause retinopathy:

1. Sickle cell disease retinopathy (SS)
2. Sickle cell-C retinopathy (SC)
3. Sickle thalassemia retinopathy

The most severe form of retinopathy among the three forms is that seen in sickle cell-C disease. There are two types of retinopathies seen in sickle disease: the proliferative type and the non-proliferative type. The proliferative type is more common in SC disease and sickle thalassemia than in SS disease.

The problems occur because of sludging of red blood cells inside the small vessels of the eyes. The red cells in sickle cell disease are mal-shaped and sticky, making it difficult for them to pass through these vessels. The result is occlusion of these vessels, resulting in a multitude of vascular abnormalities within the eyes.

The types of vascular abnormalities range from arteriovenous anastomosis and neovascularization that result in leakage of blood through these newly formed vessels and cause different degrees of hemorrhages. Retinal tear and detachment commonly occur as well. Fluorescein angiography is used to demonstrate these abnormalities. Photo-coagulation can be used as a treatment modality and also laser is used to treat these conditions in the eyes of sicklers with retinopathy

Sarcoidosis and its effects on the eyes

Sarcoidosis is quite common in men and the eye is frequently affected in that condition. In fact, eye symptoms are often the presenting symptoms of sarcoidosis. Redness and swelling of the eyes with blurry vision is often seen. The eye doctor usually looks for anterior uveitis, which is often present when sarcoidosis involves the eyes. Slit-lamp examination is done to evaluate the eye when sarcoidosis is suspected. If sarcoidosis is not recognized and treated early with Prednisone, the result often means total blindness in the affected eye. Glaucoma is a seen in chronic untreated sarcoidosis of the eye. The angiotensin-1-converting enzyme blood test is often elevated in individuals affected with sarcoidosis, and the serum calcium may be elevated as well.

AIDS and eye disease

AIDS, as a viral illness, frequently affects the eyes. The most common infection that is seen in the eyes of AIDS patients is cytomegalovirus (CMV). CMV causes an infection of the eyes called retinitis. Minority men are affected more than white males with AIDS-associated CMV retinitis because the percentage of minority men with AIDS is much higher than that of white men (see chapter 12 on AIDS).

CMV retinitis in AIDS is quite difficult to treat and eradicate. The most effective medication is Ganciclovir. This medication has serious side effects and must be given IV in the hospital setting.

Temporal arteritis and eye disease

Temporal arteritis (giant cell arteritis) is a condition seen in middle-aged to elderly individuals The diagnosis of temporal arteritis cannot be missed, and, in fact, must not be missed, for if it is missed, the result is permanent blindness in the affected eye. Usually, the patient comes to see the physician with headache, general malaise, and visual abnormality, and may report having a low-grade fever. Following a physical examination, a diagnosis can quickly be established by doing an erythrocyte sedimentation rate (ESR). If the ESR is very high (normal ESR is from 10–30 ml/hr) then the diagnosis of temporal arteritis is very likely. The next step is to admit the patient to the hospital for treatment with high-dose IV steroids. The ophthalmologist always must be brought in to carry out a thorough eye examination of the patient. The next step is to call a surgeon in to do a temporal artery biopsy. It is not necessary to wait for the biopsy before starting steroid treatment. If the physician waits for the results of the biopsy, it may be too late to save the eyes. A negative temporal artery biopsy does not rule out the diagnosis of temporal arteritis (giant cell arteritis) because that disease is often a segmental disease and a normal segment of artery could easily have been biopsied, leaving behind the abnormal segment.

Vitamin deficiency and eye disease

As alcoholism is quite common among men, certain vitamin deficiencies are likely to occur. One of the frequent vitamin deficiencies that occur in that setting is Vitamin B6 (thiamine). Thiamine deficiency can cause ocular motor palsy. It can also lead to Wernicke's disease, which is associated with nystagmus, ptosis, retinal hemorrhage, diplopia, and internal strabismus. Treatment consists of injection of thiamine to replete the store, followed by B-complex vitamins by mouth, which contains all the B vitamins, and abstinence from alcohol is the key. Thiamine by mouth can also be given following the acute repletion of the stores.

Malignant tumor and eye symptoms

Malignant tumors, such as primary melanoma, tumor of the lid of the eye (associated with xeroderma pigmentosum), can affect the eye. The eye can also be affected by sarcoma. Malignant melanoma is a particularly troublesome disease that can lead to the demise of the patient if not diagnosed quickly and treatment started right away. Metastatic cancer may first show signs of its presence in the eye. This is believed to be due to an autoimmune phenomenon (the body reacting to the cancer as a foreign agent), thereby producing an antibody against it, causing an inflammatory reaction to occur in the eye, resulting in eye symptoms.

AIDS is quite common among men of color, mostly due to intravenous drug abuse (IVDA) or sexual intercourse with women who engage in IVDA.. Sexually transmitted diseases STDs), are highly associated with HIV/AIDS, and syphilis is frequently found in individuals with AIDS and IVDA.. Syphilis an other STD's can also be found in individuals who do not have AIDS.

Syphilis and eye problems

In the latter stage of syphilis, a variety of different eye problems can occur. One problem may be small, irregular pupils that sometimes react to accommodation, but does not react to light. Another problem might be the Argyle-Robertson pupils (the result of atrophy of the iris), which is seen in neurosyphilis.

Other problems that can occur in neurosyphilis include iritis and photophobia. Adhesion of the iris to the lens of the eye can also occur, which can cause a fixed pupil. These problems can all be picked up through a good eye examination by an internist who can then refer the affected man to an ophthalmologist for further evaluation and treatment.

According to The Center for Disease Control and Prevention (CDC) guidelines, treatment for neurosyphilis must include blood VDRL and FTA-ABS. A lumbar puncture ought to be done to obtain cerebrospinal fluid (CSF). The CSF fluid must be sent for VDRL and FTA-ABS. If it is positive, then treatment for neurosyphilis must be started by giving 10 to 20 million units of aqueous penicillin daily IV for ten days. In addition, a three-week course of 2.4 million units of Bicillin for a total of 7.2 million units must be given. If the patient has

HIV infection (AIDS) and a positive VDRL, FTA-ABS in the blood, even if the CSF is negative or if the patient refuses a lumbar puncture, the same protocol as just outlined ought to be employed to treat the patient.

That ought to be done because neurosyphilis is quite prevalent in individuals with AIDS. If a person is allergic to penicillin, then Erythromycin 2 grams by mouth daily for 30 days or Tetracycline 2 grams daily for 30 days ought to be prescribed to treat the man with neuro syphilis.

The difference between ophthalmologists, optometrists and opticians

There is a difference between ophthalmologists, optometrists and opticians. An ophthalmologist is a person who went to medical school, studied medicine, and underwent several years of training in the field of a medical specialty called ophthalmology. That physician is a trained and experienced specialist in diseases of the eyes. The optometrist is a specialist trained to deal with all aspects of eyeglasses, including filling out prescriptions written by the ophthalmologist. They adjust eyeglasses to give them maximal visual acuity. The optician, on the other hand, is a specialist trained to deal with matters of optics, including the making of eyeglasses, etc. Both of them are specialists who can fill prescriptions prescribed by the ophthalmologist.

As you can see, there is a big difference between those three specialists. If an ophthalmologist (the physician) has not examined your eyes then your eyes really have not had a thorough examination. You may have had your eyeglasses constructed and adjusted and you may have been evaluated for visual acuity and your prescription may have been filled, but a real eye examination that can detect many serious diseases of the eyes has in fact not been carried out. The ophthalmologist is trained to find many diseases in the eyes and he, she may prescribe medication for these diseases and he, or she can operate on the eye to treat many of those same diseases. In addition, there are many subspecialties of ophthalmology, namely physicians who sub-specialize in glaucoma care and other physicians who specialize in retinal care. These physicians are very adept at treating these very specific eye problems. It is extremely important that this is understood, because a person may be going too long to the wrong specialist without knowing it and by the time it is realized, it may be too late to address some serious conditions such as glaucoma, cataracts, diabetic eye disease, hypertensive eye disease, sickle cell eye disease, etc., all of which are quite common in men. Both opticians and optometrists are experts in their own fields and provide a much-needed service to the public.

In summary, eye diseases are very common in men, for the reasons outlined in that chapter. Diseases such as diabetes mellitus, hypertension, trauma in the workplace to the eyes, sickle cell disease, sarcoidosis, all of which participate in the rising incidence of glaucoma that is five times higher in black men than white males.

The overall economic and educational situations of the majority men of color and other poor men will have to be improved drastically if it is expected that a real impact can be made to decrease the accelerated rate of blindness from which some men are suffering.

CHAPTER 15

DEPRESSION IN MEN

DEPRESSION IS ONE OF THE most common diseases that afflict humankind. It is said that in the U.S., depression is as common as the common cold.

According to the 1998 U.S. census, 1 in 5 Americans suffer with a diagnosable mental illness that adds up to 44.3 million individuals.

18.8 million American adults suffer from depression. 12. 4 million women and 6.4 million men suffer with depression in the U.S. According to the National Institute of Mental Health, depression is the leading cause of nonfatal disability among individuals 15 to 44 years of age in developed countries like the US and Canada. An other way of to outline the incidence of depression in the US, is that 1 out of every 6 adults-1 in 4 women and 1 in 10 men suffer fro depression during their lifetimes. Only about 25% of depressed people are adequately treated. In New York City, 7,5% adults suffer from major depression and only about one third are being treated. Worldwide depression is the second or third greatest cause of disability according to the Institute of Mental Health. The annual cost of depression in the US is 53 billion dollars.

Primary care physicians write most prescriptions for anti-depression medications. Every year 190 million prescriptions are written for anti-depression medications in the US at a cost of 12 billion dollars

There are different types of depression:
1. Transient situational depression
2. Permanent or chronic situational depression
3. Depression associated with taking medications for a medical condition
4. Depression associated with alcohol abuse or drug abuse

5. Minor classical depression
6. Major classical depression
7. Depression associated with anxiety reaction and panic attacks
8. Manic depression, etc.
   (*The concept of permanent or chronic situational depression is the author's own developed concept.*)
   Incidence of depression

Depression is 3 to 4 times more common in men than in men. In the U.S. more than 17 million individuals (about 1 in 10 adults) suffer from a depressive episode at least once per year and more than 80% of the time these episodes go untreated. According to some study, black men suffer less from mental illnesses than white men, and Hispanic men more than black men; that is, in fact, not so at all.

In fact, black men and Hispanics experience more depression, anxiety and panic attacks than white men do. Being poor is a depressive state of being and, therefore, 100% of poor people suffer from one form of depression or another, at one time or another. The difference is in the cultural expression of these symptoms and the cultural conditioning and reluctance to express the symptoms of these illnesses for fear of being ostracized by their communities.

In any African ancestral society, mental illness is taboo because it is seen as a sign of weakness. A failure to be able to endure whatever it is that the majority of society can dish out and not only surviving it, enduring it and to be able to live long enough to tell one's children and grandchildren about it, is an essential part of the indigenous black culture. Black men see mental illness as a label that may be used to discriminate against them by the medical community, the job market, the legal community and, by the law enforcement community to prevent them from getting ahead. Because these people do not want any mention of mental illness on their records if they can help it, they hide their symptoms of depression and suffer in silence. When an interviewer tries to elicit mental illness from them, they would not tell his or his about it. They frequently do not tell a physician/therapist about their mental illness either, unless they absolutely have to.

Table 1

Some of the symptoms of major depression:
Five (or more) of the following symptoms have been present during the same 2-week period and represent a change from previous functioning: at

least one of the symptoms is either (^{1}) depressed mood or (^{2}) loss of interest in pleasure, excluding symptoms that are due to medical illnesses.

(1) Depressed mood most of the day, nearly every day as indicated by either subjective report (e.g., feels sad or empty) or observation made by others (e.g., appears tearful). **Note:** In children and adolescents, can be irritable mood.

(2) Markedly diminished interest or pleasure in all, or almost all activities most of the day, nearly every day (as indicated by either subjective account or observation made by others.)

(3) Significant weight loss when not dieting or weight gain (e.g., a change of more than 5% of body weight in a month), or decrease or increase in appetite nearly every day. **Note:** In children, consider failure to make expected weight gains.

(4) Insomnia or hypersomnia every day

(5) Psychomotor agitation or retardation nearly every day (observable by others, not merely subjective feelings of restlessness or being slowed down)

(6) Fatigue or loss of energy every day

(7) Feelings of worthlessness or excessive or inappropriate guilt (which may be delusional) nearly every day (not merely self-reproach or guilt about being sick)

(8) Diminished ability to think or concentrate, or indecisiveness, nearly every day (either by subjective account or as observed by others).

(9) Recurrent thoughts of death (not just fear of dying), recurrent suicidal ideation without a specific plan, or a suicide attempt or a specific plan for committing suicide.

B. These symptoms do not meet criteria for a mixed episode.

C. The symptoms cause clinically significant distress or impairment in social, occupational, or other important areas of functioning.

D. The symptoms are not due to the direct physiological effects of a substance (e.g., a drug of abuse, a medication) or a general medical condition (e.g., hypothyroidism).

E. The symptoms are not better accounted for by bereavement, i.e., after the loss of a loved one, the symptoms persist for longer than 2 months or are characterized by marked functional impairment, morbid occupation with worthlessness, suicidal ideation, psychotic symptoms, or psychomotor retardation.

As modified from DSM IV

Depression as seen in minority men is a very complex disease with many associated components. Classical minor depression is defined as 3 or 4 depressive symptoms for 2 weeks or longer. Major depression is defined as 5 or more depressive symptoms for 2 weeks or longer.

TABLE 2

Some symptoms of minor depression:

A. A distinct period of abnormally and persistently elevated, expansive or irritable mood, lasting at least 1 week (or any duration if hospitalization is necessary).

B. During the period of mood disturbance, three (or more) of the following symptoms have persisted (four if the mood is only irritable) and have been present to a significant degree.

(1) Inflated self-esteem or grandiosity

(2) Decreased need for sleep (e.g., feels rested after only 3 hours of sleep)

(3) More talkative than usual or pressure to keep talking

(4) Flight of ideas or subjective experience that thoughts are racing

(5) Distractibility (i.e., attention too easily drawn to unimportant or irrelevant external stimuli)

(6) Increase in goal-directed activity (either socially, at work or school, or sexually) or psychomotor agitation

(7) Excessive involvement in pleasurable activities that have a high potential for painful consequences (e.g., engaged in unrestrained buying sprees, sexual indiscretions, or foolish business investments)

C. These symptoms do not meet criteria for a mixed episode.

D. The mood disturbance is sufficiently severe to cause marked impairment in occupational functioning or in usual social activities or relationships with others, or to necessitate hospitalization to prevent harm to self or others, or there are psychotic features.

E. The symptoms are not due to the direct physiological effects of a substance (e.g., a drug of abuse, a medication, or other treatment) or a general medical condition (e.g., hyperthyroidism).

Men of color like any other men can suffer from the classic forms of depression such as:

1. Minor depression.

2. Major depression.

3. Manic depression.

The most common forms of depression seen in men consist of:

1. A mixed form of depression associated with anxiety and panic attacks.
2. Transient and permanent situational depression.
3. Depression associated with alcohol abuse and drug abuse.

Black men, as well as Hispanic men, are extremely reluctant to go to the psychiatrist because of the fear of being labeled "crazy" in the case of black and "loco" in the case of Hispanic men. Both these groups have culturally dealt with mental illness the way in which mental illness is dealt with in the African culture. In the African culture, when a person of African ancestry is troubled with a mood disorder, he or she goes to an elder or group of family members within the family for advice in order to deal with the problem. Sometimes the group is organized as a committee, as is done frequently in developing countries. Never in this setting is the word mental illness used. In fact, in some third world countries, it is unlikely, that a man would marry into a family that has an immediate member with a history of mental illness. Because of racism different degrees and different types of racial insensitivity and the suspicion and distrust that it causes, men of color in the U.S. are almost exclusively reluctant to seek help for mental illness, and in particular depression, because most of the psychiatrists-therapists are Caucasians.

The reasons men of color give for refusing to see Caucasian or non-minority psychiatrists-therapists are as follows:

"Why should I go to the white and non-Hispanic, non-black psychiatrist-therapist to open up my innermost secrets to them, when they are mostly responsible for my problems to begin with?"

Q. *"You mean the psychiatrist-therapist is the source of your problem?"*

A. "No, not him or her in particular, but he or she belongs to the group of people that is the underlying cause of my depression in the first place."

Q. "How so? Could you elaborate?"

A. "Well, you know, racial insensitivity and bigotry are so pervasive and widespread you don't know whom to trust and whom not to trust."

Q. "Is it that you have a problem trusting anyone?"

A *"No, I just have difficulty opening up my inner soul to the people who I know don't like me in the first place."*

It is a known fact that when men of color are evaluated for mental illness by white psychiatrists-therapists, oftentimes the diagnosis is wrong, the literature outlines cases of minority men that were diagnosed as schizophrenics, when in fact they were not. Because of subjectivity that is often involved in the diagnosis of mental illnesses, very frequently psychiatrist-therapists and others involved in dealing with men of color who have mental illness tend to give them a worse diagnosis rather than a better diagnosis, and clearly racism, racial insensitivity, bigotry, racial insensitivity and intellectual condescendincy play a role in this particular situation.

Transient situational depression occurs in all groups regardless of ethnic background. Normally transient situational depression results because of a loss of a job, a girlfriend, a death in the family, or the death of a close friend, etc. In the case of some minority individuals, depression would seem to last longer because underneath exists a mental fragility born out of constant exposure to racial injustices, making it easier to cross over the line to a more permanent depressive state.

Permanent and chronic situational depression in men of color in the U.S. is a condition born out of constant and relentless barrages of daily exposure to racial discrimination and injustices at all levels of American society. Poor, non-minority men suffer, as well, from depression to a degree far out of proportion to their majority men counterparts because poverty itself creates a depressive state of being that provides fertile ground for different types of depressive illnesses to speak of at any given time. There exist several sub-cultures in the world community whose poor people have been conditioned or brainwashed into believing that their poverty is the result of divine will. These folks are forced through different means to pray to God for easing of their earthly suffering so that they can get to heaven to get their divine rewards. This concept does not seem to be as prevalent among minority men in the U.S. as elsewhere in the world. It does not matter if a minority person in America works as a sanitation worker or as a physician or a judge in a court of law; he or she has to deal with racial discrimination, minimization and margining of their works. They face constant confrontations all the time, be it in different forms and under different circumstances. Granted, the less educated and less financially able a minority man is, the more he feels the stings and often the bites of racism eating away at his flesh, heart and soul. Because racism has become an accepted part of the American culture, minority men feel a sense of constant persecution that is "real" and, therefore, some of them are more prone to become chronically hopeless and depressed. Some minority men in America have developed coping mechanisms to both survive racism and its depressive nature. Some men of color have chosen to excel at whatever it is that they do; they go beyond that which is necessary as a mechanism of coping, not just to be accepted necessarily, but to be included and respected. Professional respect means a lot to any professional person, but more so to men of color. Professional minority men typically would say, "Though you don't like the color of my skin and many other things about me, but I dare you to doubt my ability to beat you at your own game and do my work with excellence." Some minority men have chosen to become activists and community organizers, to wake up other minorities, to fight for their rights. Still, others have chosen to give up and allow racism to engulf all aspects of their being by becoming welfare recipients and are part of the sub-culture of the have-nots. Many people are on welfare because of physical or mental disabilities, and this is both acceptable and understandable, but many people of color have become so chronically passive, dependent and do not care a damn anymore, so welfare has become a way of life for them.

Still many men of color have allowed their anger and despair to cause them to fall into the trap of drug, alcohol and other substance abuse, which have totally taken over their lives to a degree that their very humanity represents nothing to them, and so the lives of other individuals have not much value to them either. This state of being causes some of them to commit unspeakable crimes against their neighbors and their communities. (see the chapters on drug abuse and alcohol abuse)

Depression, associated with anxiety and panic attacks, is extremely common in men. But this type of depression is much more common in men of color than in white men based on, the fact men of color have more reasons to be anxious, and even more reason to be panicky.

This is so because many men of color have to face racism, poor education, and lack of jobs, lower economic status, and many other unspeakable injustices to cope with. All the above problems create a constant state of anger, disappointment, uncertainty, and the result is anxiety, panic attacks and depression. They are the victims of the "STATUS SYNDROME".

What makes that whole situation even more serious is the fact that more often than not these men go without being diagnosed and without being treated for their depression. Small number men of color do seek psychological treatment.

How to evaluate a man who comes in for evaluation of depression to the primary care physician.

In the minority community, the primary care physician is likely to be the one who is most likely to see the vast majority of black and Hispanic men with depression. This is so because these men are extremely resistant to the concept that they may have a need for psychological care. That is a cultural fact and it must be understood, respected and dealt with, with the greatest of care and ethnic sensitivity.

TABLE 3

Some of the most common symptoms of depression:
Depression
Persistent sad, anxious, or "empty" mood
Loss of interest or pleasure in activities, including sex
Feelings of hopelessness, pessimism
Feelings of guilt, worthlessness, helplessness
Sleeping too much or too little, early-morning awakening
Appetite and/or weight loss or overeating and weight gain
Decreased energy, fatigue, feeling "slowed down"
Thoughts of death or suicide, or suicide attempts
Restlessness, irritability
Difficulty concentrating, remembering, or making decisions
Persistent physical symptoms that do not respond to treatment, such as headaches, digestive disorders, and chronic pain
Mania
Abnormally elevated mood
Irritability
Severe insomnia
Grandiose notions
Increased talking
Racing thoughts
Increased activity, including sexual activity
Markedly increased energy
Poor judgment that leads to risk-taking behavior
Inappropriate social behavior

A thorough diagnostic evaluation is needed if five or more of these symptoms persist for more than two weeks, or if they interfere with work or family life. An evaluation involves a complete physical checkup and information gathering on family health history.

(As published by the National Institute of Mental Health)

Some of the symptoms of panic attack:
1. Palpitations, pounding of heart, or accelerated heart rate
2. Sweating

3. Trembling or shaking
4. Sensation of shortness of breath or smothering
5. Feeling of choking
6. Chest pain or discomfort
7. Nausea or abdominal distress
8. Feeling dizzy, lightheaded, or faint
9. Derealization (feelings of unreality) or depersonalization (being detached from oneself)
10. Fear of losing control or going crazy
11. Fear of dying
12. Paresthesias (numbness or tingling sensation)
13. Chills or hot flashes
14. Abdominal pain
15. Diarrhea
16. Black-out spells
17. Urinary frequency
18. Hyperventilation
19. Leg cramps
20. Insomnia

Partially modified from DSM IV

The first step in evaluation someone with depression includes a complete history and physical examination. The next step is a series of specific laboratory tests such as:

1. CBC
2. Chemistry profile (SMA 18)
3. Thyroid profile—T4, TSH
4. Urinalysis
5. Serum ferritin
6. Serum B12
7. Chest x-ray
8. EKG
9. Mammogram, if the man is 40 years or older; or younger if a mass is felt in the breast or if there is a family history of breast cancer
10. A CAT scan of the brain or MRI of the brain, if there is headache, dizziness, and forgetfulness, or symptoms of neurological signs are found during the history and physical examination. In fact, it may

be important to do a CAT scan anyway, even though there may be no obvious neurological signs or symptoms.

Other specific blood tests may become necessary based on the physician's assessment of the case.

Approaching the patient in that way allows the physician to ascertain whether or not the patient's signs and symptoms of depression, anxiety or panic attacks have no organic basis (that is, nothing medical can explain his symptoms). Diseases such as diabetes mellitus, hyperthyroidism, hypothyroidism, cancer, iron deficiency anemia, kidney failure, heart disease such as mitral valve prolapse, Atherosclerotic heart disease with angina pectoris, congestive heart failure with low cardiac output and poor brain perfusion, B12 deficiency, etc. (if a person remains B12 deficient for 3 to 5 years, he may develop permanent neuropsychiatric problems).

It is not unusual to find a patient in a psychiatric hospital who is permanently committed because of B12 deficiency that either was not diagnosed at all or was diagnosed too late, resulting in permanent neurological and mental disease.

Brain tumor may first present with symptoms of psychiatric disease. It is, therefore, always necessary for a person who manifests symptoms of depression to undergo a thorough medical evaluation by a primary care physician before any definite statement can be made regarding the proper psychiatric diagnosis of that man. Both hyperthyroidism and hypothyroidism can manifest symptoms of depression. As part of the evaluation of depression, serum B12, T4 and TSH and brain CT ought to be done.

It is important that prior to starting any psychotropic medications, a CBC, liver function test and EKG be done, because many of the psychotropic medications have many side effects that can cause the white blood cell count, the platelets, the red blood cell count as well as the EKG and liver function test to be abnormal. Some of these medications can affect the rhythm of the heart in different ways, so a baseline EKG must be done before starting these medications. In point of fact, periodically CBC, kidney function tests such as BUN, creatinine, electrolytes, liver function tests, T4, TSH must be done during the course of psychotropic medication therapy.

Treatments of depression

Depression is treated usually with medications, psychotherapy and, at times, with ECT.

Some of the medications used to treat depression are the following:
A. Serotonin-specific reuptake inhibitors such as
   1. Zoloft
   2. Paxil
   3. Prozac
   4. Lexapro
   5. Celexa
B. Serotonin non-selective reuptake inhibitors such as:
   6. Effexor
   7. Wellbutrin
   8. Ludiomil, which is basically a dopamine-active medication
   9. Norpramin.
   10. Pamelor
   11. Desyrel
   12. Asendin
   13. BuSpar
   14. Klonopin
   15. Xanax
   16. Lithium
C. Tertiary amines such as:
   17. Elavil
   18. Tofranil
   19. Anafranil
   20. Sinequan
D. MAOIs or monoamine oxidase inhibitors such as::
   21. Parnate
   22. Eldepryl
   23. Risperdal
The usual dosages and side effects of these medications are:
   1. **Zoloft**-The initial dose is 50 mg per day; that dose can be increased up to 200 mg per day. There are several tolerable side effects of Zoloft, and liver function tests and EKG must be closely monitored along with blood levels while the patient is on Zoloft.
   2. **Paxil**-The usual starting dose of Paxil is 20 mg per day and that dose can be increased up to 50 mg per day for those people who fail to respond to the 20 mg dose. Paxil can cause several tolerable side effects, but liver function tests and EKG must be monitored along with Paxil blood level.

3. **Prozac**-The usual dose of Prozac is 20 mg per day. If a patient fails to respond to 20 mg per day, the dose can be increased up to 80 mg per day. Prozac has several side effects, and liver function tests and EKG ought to be monitored along with blood level of Prozac.

4. **Effexor**-The usual starting dose of Effexor is 25 mg three times per day. The dose may be increased up to 150 mg per day in divided doses, and in rare circumstances, the dose may be raised to as high as 275 mg per day in divided doses. Effexor has many tolerable side effects, but liver function tests and periodic EKG ought to be done along with blood level of the medication.

5. **Wellbutrin SR**-The usual dose of Wellbutrin SR is 150 mg two times per day; at times a dose of 200 mg two times per day can be given. Wellbutrin SR has several tolerable side effects, but is important to monitor liver function tests, EKG and blood level of Wellbutrin SR.

6. **Ludiomil**-The usual dose of Ludiomil is 75 mg per day. In the elderly, as little as 25 mg per day may be effective. Doses as high as 150 mg to 225 mg may be used in-hospital patients. Ludiomil has several tolerable side effects, but periodic EKG, liver function tests should be done.

7. **Norpramin**-The usual dose of Norpramin is 100 mg to 200 mg per day. This dose may be increased to as high as 300 mg per day. This medication is not recommended for use in children. Norpramin is not to be used in conjunction with MAO inhibitors. In fact, it cannot be used up to two weeks after stopping MAO inhibitors. Norpramin has several tolerable side effects, but CBC, liver function tests, EKG; and blood thyroid function have to be done before starting that medication. These same tests have to be done periodically while a patient is on Norpramin.

8. **Pamelor**-The usual dose of Pamelor is 25 mg 3–4 times per day. At times, the dose may be raised up to 150 mg per day. Pamelor has several tolerable side effects. While on that medication, EKG, CBC, liver function tests have to be done along with blood level of Pamelor.

9. **Lithium**-The usual maintenance dose of Lithium is 450 mg, two times per day. Doses as high as 1,350 mg per day may be given. Lithium has several tolerable side effects. Before starting a patient on Lithium, CBC, liver function tests, kidney function tests, blood thyroid function tests, and EKG must be done. While on Lithium, these same tests must be done and monitored closely. Blood level of Lithium must also be monitored. The kidneys are particularly sensi-

tive to the effects of Lithium, and at the first signs of blood kidney function test abnormalities, the treatment must be stopped. Lithium can cause thyroid function tests to become abnormal. The WBC can sometimes go down because of Lithium.

10. **Desyrel**-The usual starting of Desyrel is 150 mg in divided doses, but a dose up to 600 mg per day in divided doses can be used. Desyrel has several tolerable side effects; therefore, an EKG ought to be done before starting that medication and periodically ought to be done while the person is on that drug.

11. **Asendin**-The usual dose of Asendin is 200–300 mg per day in divided doses. Asendin has several tolerable side effects. Blood chemistry tests, CBC and EKG should be done while the patient is on Asendin.

12. **Klonopin**-The initial dose of Klonopin is 1.5 mg per day in divided doses. Sometimes the dose can be raised to as high as 20 mg per day. This medication is quite effective in individuals with anxiety reaction associated with depression. It allows the patient to get a good night's sleep. CBC, liver function tests and EKG ought to be done before starting the medication and the same tests should be monitored while the patient is on the medication.

13. **BuSpar**-The usual dose of BuSpar to treat anxiety is 10 mg two times per day and the dose can be raised up to 30 mg per day in divided doses.

14. **Xanax**-The usual dose of Xanax to treat anxiety is 0.25 mg three times per day. A dose up to 4 mg per day can be used in divided doses, in certain cases. In treating panic disorder, the dose can be as high as 4 mg in divided doses. Xanax has several tolerable side effects, but laboratory tests are not required during the treatment of patient on Xanax.

15. **Elavil**-The usual dose of Elavil is 75 to 300 mg per day in divided doses. Elavil has several tolerable side effects. EKG, CBC, liver function tests, along with Elavil blood level should be done periodically while the patient is on Elavil.

16. **Tofranil**-The usual dose of Tofranil is 75 mg per day. The dose may be increased up to 150 mg per day. Tofranil has several tolerable side effects; EKG, CBC, liver function tests along with Tofranil blood level should be done periodically.

17. **Anafranil**-The usual starting dose of Anafranil is 25 mg per day and the dose may be increased up to 200 mg per day in divided doses.

EKG, CBC, liver function tests, along with Anafranil blood levels, should be done periodically while a patient is on Anafranil.

18. **Doxepin**-The usual starting dose of Doxepin is 75 mg per day. The dose may be increased up to 300 mg per day. EKG, CBC, blood chemistry tests should be done periodically while the patient is on Doxepin.

19. **Parnate**-The usual starting dose of Parnate is 30 mg per day in divided doses. The dose may at times be increased to as high as 60 mg per day in divided doses. Frequent monitoring of blood pressure, EKG, CBC, blood chemistry tests ought to be done while the patient is on that medication. Parnate has a long list of medications that it cannot be used with. Further, there are several food products that must be avoided while on Parnate; among those are cheeses, foods high in tyramine, sour cream, Chianti wines, beer, liquors, caviar, anchovies, pickled herring, canned figs, raisins, bananas, avocados, chocolate, soybean, sauerkraut, yogurt, yeast extracts, etc.

20. A new anti-depression medication-Cymbalta is now available as well.

Seroquel is used to treat psychosis with associated depressive features

ECT remains an effective modality of treatment for depression. ECT is used under a general anesthesia and muscle relaxants, decreasing convulsions and eliminating the possibility of fractures and other injuries to the patient. ECT is most appropriate for patients who cannot take medications or whose associated illnesses contradict them taking an antidepressant medication. In addition, in certain life-threatening situations, when all other antidepressant medications fail, then ECT is most appropriate and useful.

Psychotherapy

Psychotherapy is a non-medication effective modality of treatment for certain types of depression. Psychotherapy involves counseling. The mental health professionals who provide psychotherapy treatments are psychotherapists, psychiatrists, and certified social workers. Primary care physicians are well equipped to provide psychotherapy counseling, if they have the time to do it. The incidence of depression is 3 to 4 times more common in men than in their male counterparts. Many men fear being stigmatized with mental illness and refrain from seeking psychiatric treatment for depression, until the depression is too far advanced and more difficult to treat. These men avoid going to the psychiatrist for treatment of depression because of the stigma associated with mental illness. That situation is gravest among working poor and working minority men first of all, and, second of all, among middle-class and professional men and less so among upper-class men. One of the reasons that upper-class men are less concerned about going to the psychiatrist is because these men have money and enjoy a high social standing. They do not fear the stigma of mental illness and the economic and social negativities associated with it, and most of these individuals seem to have high trust in the Caucasian therapists who dominate and control the field of psychiatry, psychology and social work.

It is common for men of color to seek counseling from their priests, pastors and their elders. The primary care physician of color is the first one to diagnose and treat depression in these men, because these affected men feel more comfortable with his and they have known his or her for a long time and have established a trusting relationships. Therefore, primary care physicians of color are providing the bulk of the treatment for depression in men of color, because these men feel more comfortable with these doctors as just outlined.

Depression is a very common disease and much more so in men of color than in white men. Depression has many bases, many causes, and many manifestations. In men of color, depression can be gravest because of the penetrating and pernicious nature of racism, which fosters so much distrust of those in control of U.S. society, that it makes it difficult for men of color to seek help for their depressive illnesses. Men of color have a higher propensity for the development of depression as do white men as already stated, and the fact that they are under more stress and many of them have a lesser level of education, lesser economic status and a lower social standing, creates a situation that makes their depression more grave, more serious, more multifactor and much more difficult to treat.

What can be done to lessen the propensity of men to develop depression?

It is crucial to educate these men. The fact is that 80% or more of individuals who suffer from depression can be successfully treated and the best people to seek treatment from for depression are those who have the professional training and expertise to treat that treatable disease. It is also important to sensitize the professionals who are in the position to treat men of color, poor men and men in general, as to their culture, as to the things that trouble them. Different and more racially sensitive approaches must be undertaken in order to provide appropriate and better treatments for these men. It is foolish and potentially harmful to attempt to impose the majority's views, hypocritical values, and traditional treatment modalities to those groups of men whose psychiatric problems are unique. The bases and factors that are contributing to their state of mind are themselves unique because of their unique societal circumstances. So if the professionals from the majority community do not take it upon themselves to familiarize themselves with the culture, and the circumstances of life and other different dynamics that inter-play leading to these depressive illnesses, they will fail the majority of the time in their attempt to treat them for these very serious, but treatable, diseases. There is a significant degree of mistrust that exists when white mental health workers are treating people of color for mental illnesses.

The psychiatric training programs must include several components of the cultural diversity as it relates to men of color, poor men and men issues in general, into their training programs, to provide future mental health professionals the special skill and technique necessary to deal with the problems involving these men and their diverse psychological problems. The directors of the training programs in psychiatry and psychology ought to include cultural diversity as it relates to minority people and men of color in general in their training programs. The number of people of color in the mental health profession needs to be increased significantly to help correcting the problems just outlined. In so doing, many of the barriers of mistrust may be lowered to a significant degree, making it easier for men of color to be more receptive to the care that the mental health professionals are providing for them.

For the benefit of any person seeking help for depression, the following organizations can be contacted.

1. National Institute of Mental Health-Telephone number 800–421–4211.
2. American Psychiatric Association-202–682–6220.
3. American Psychological Association-202–336–5500.
4. National Mental Health Association-800–969-NMHA-extension 6642.
5. National Foundation for Depressive Illness-800–248–4344.
6. National Alliance for the Mentally Ill-800–950-NAMI.-extension 6264.

CHAPTER 16

ALCOHOLISM IN MEN

OF ALL THE SUBSTANCES THAT are abused in the United States, alcohol is number one. Alcohol use is widespread and alcohol abuse affects all segments of society. At any one time, there are roughly 18 to 21 million individuals in the United States receiving one treatment or another for alcohol abuse and its multitude of associated medical and psychosocial problems. There are roughly 14 million people who are registered alcoholics in the United States and several million others are estimated to be also abusing alcohol.

In the year 2004, 56.7% of men in the USA drank alcohol. Of this number, 47.1% men were regular drinkers of alcohol. The racial break down of men who drank alcohol on a regular basis in the year 2004, were white males were 63.3%, black males 46,6 % American-Indian and Alaska Native 48.8%%, Asian men 43.8%, Hispanic men 61.7% Mixed race men 62% (Source: CDC and National Center for Health Statistics, National Health Survey, family core and sample adult questionnaires, 2004).

It is estimated that in 1995, a total of 276 billion dollars were spent for the treatment of substance abuse in the United States, including alcohol.

Alcohol abuse is one of the most serious medical problems known to humankind. What makes alcohol use so easy and so widespread is that a person does not need a prescription to buy it. Alcohol is sold in liquor stores, bars, restaurants, airport shops, supermarkets, etc. Some people start drinking alcohol in their teens, as a recreational habit or because of peer pressure. Frequently, teenagers see their parents abusing alcohol at home and getting drunk in front of them and they think it is OK for them to do the same thing (obviously it is not). It is not too difficult to see how some teenagers can drink alcohol, and are not reprimanded by their drinking parents, because the parents do it in front of them, so they think it is all right, and "cool" to do the same thing.

According to the literature, some form of alcoholism is hereditary. Some alcoholic parents, it is said, transfer an alcoholism gene to their offspring, resulting in them becoming alcoholics as well. The evidence is quite compelling that it may indeed be old reference so. On average, it would appear that white men start drinking at an earlier age than men of color do do. White men on the aggregate have a high incidence of alcohol abuse than do black males, but men of color suffer more from the physical effects of alcohol abuse than white males.

For example, men of color seem to have a greater incidence of cirrhosis of liver due to alcohol abuse than do white men. In fact, the death rate from cirrhosis of liver is two times as high for men of color as it is for white males.

Men of color suffer from more health problems because of alcohol abuse, than do white men. Diseases such as cancer, hypertension, malnutrition, heart disease, diabetes, stroke, kidney failure etc, are more prevalent in men of color who are alcoholics as compared to their white counter parts.

In 1990, it was estimated that 2–5 million older Americans had alcohol-related problems. The estimated hospital cost for hospital care for that group was in the neighborhood of 60 billion dollars.

Alcohol abuse is a multi-system disease. The following organs are most frequently affected by alcoholism:

1. The brain
2. The heart
3. The lungs
4. The liver
5. The pancreas
6. The breasts
7. The gastrointestinal system
8. The blood system
9. The endocrine system
10. The mouth, throat and esophagus
11. The neurological system
12. The psychological system
13. The skin
14. The genital system
15. Frequently, many of the organs and systems are affected in combination in the same person.

When a person drinks alcohol, the brain is the first organ to be affected. When a person drinks alcohol, first it is absorbed from the stomach into the bloodstream. Once in the bloodstream, the alcohol goes to the brain. The effect of alcohol on the brain depends on the level of alcohol in the blood of the person drinking alcohol and the length of time that person has been drinking alcohol. The level of alcohol that causes drunkenness in one person is different in another individual. In other words, different individuals respond differently to the effect of alcohol. The weight of a man determines how quickly he becomes intoxicated. Blood alcohol concentration (BAC) is measured as milligrams of alcohol per deciliter of blood. That same number can be converted in percent of alcohol concentration in the blood: 100 mg of alcohol per deciliter in the blood equals 100 mg percent or 0.1 percent of alcohol in the blood. For example, a man weighing 200 lbs., who drinks six drinks of hard liquor in one hour, will likely develop a blood alcohol level of 100 mg per deciliter. A man who weighs 150 lbs. will reach a blood alcohol concentration of 100 mg per deciliter by drinking four drinks of hard liquor in one hour.

Alcohol is both a stimulant and a neuro-suppressor (brain suppressor). The first thing that happens when alcohol reaches the brain is to calm the person who drinks it. It relaxes the person at first. Then as more alcohol is consumed, a feeling of elation or euphoria ensues. Associated with that level of drinking is a mild form of excitement, and the person may become talkative and giddy. That is mild social drinking of 2–3 glasses of wine, or 1–2 drinks of hard liquor, or 2–3 twelve-ounce bottles of beer. Further consumption of alcohol can create a state of drunkenness associated with excitation, rude behavior, and physical dis-coordination. Another way of saying the same thing is that a standard drink of alcohol is usually expressed as a can of twelve ounces of beer, 1½ ounces of liquor—whiskey, vodka, etc., or 5 ounces of wine.

Different individuals metabolize alcohol differently, and when taken with food in the stomach, alcohol absorption is slowed. If alcohol is consumed on an empty stomach, its full effects are felt quicker.

Impairment due to the effects of alcohol occurs in a man when the alcohol concentration reaches 50 mg per deciliter. Men and elderly individuals show impairment from drinking alcohol at lower concentration, probably 25–30 mg per deciliter. The risks of causing an automobile crash starts to occur when the blood alcohol concentration reaches 40 mg per deciliter. That risk rises when the blood alcohol concentration reaches 100 mg per deciliter. When the blood alcohol concentration reaches between 50–70 mg per deciliter, most drivers are alcohol impaired and are unsuitable to drive. At that blood alcohol concentration, a person loses coordination (he or he cannot walk straight). At an alcohol level concentration of 100 mg per deciliter, a person has a more pronounced inability to walk, and would be stumbling around, and if that person attempts to drive, that person would be driving while drunk. When the blood alcohol concentration reaches 200 mg per deciliter, the person becomes confused, disoriented and may actually lose consciousness (alcohol blackout). When the blood alcohol concentration reaches 400 mg per deciliter, coma may ensue and death may occur.

Blood alcohol levels that are deem unsafe for driving a car is different in different states in the USA. Examples of different blood alcohol levels from different states in the in the US that are considered safe or unsafe to drive a motor vehicle:

TABLE 1

Alaska	0.10/0.00	90 days	after 30 days	Yes
Arizona	0.10/0.00	90 days	after 30 days	No
Arkansas	0.10/0.02	120 days	Yes	Yes
California	0.08/0.01	4 months	after 30 days	Yes
Colorado	0.10/0.02	3 months	No	Yes
Connecticut	0.10/0.02	90 days	Yes	No
Delaware	0.10/0.02	3 months	No	Yes
District of Columbia	0.10/0.02	90 days	Yes	No
Florida	0.08/0.02	6 month	Yes	No
Georgia	0.10/0.02	1 year	Yes	Yes
Hawaii	0.08/0.02	3 months	after 30 days	Yes
Idaho	0.08/0.02	90 days	after 30 days	Yes
Illinois	0.06/0.00	3 months	after 30 days	Yes
Indiana	0.10/0.02	180 day	after 30 days	Yes
Iowa	0.10/0.02	180 days	Yes	Yes
Kansas	0.08/0.02	30 days	No	Yes
Kentucky	0.10/0.02	—	—	No
Louisiana	0.10/0.02	90 days	after 30 days	Yes
Maine	0.08/0.00	90 days	Yes	Yes
Maryland	0.10/0.02	45 days	Yes	Yes

Massachusetts	None/0.02	90 days	No	No
Michigan	0.10./0.02	—	—	Yes
Minnesota	0.10/0.00	90 days	after 15 days—	No
Mississippi	0.10/0.08	90 days	No	No
Missouri	0.10/0.02	30 days	No	Yes
Montana	0.10/0.02	—	—	Yes
Nebraska	0.10/0.02	90 days	after 30 days	Yes
Nevada	0.10/0.02	90 days	after 45 days	Yes
New Hampshire	0.08/0.02	6 months	No	No
New Jersey	0.10/0.10	—	—	No
New Mexico	0.08/0.02	90 days	after 30 days	No
New York	0.10/0.02	variable	Yes	Yes
North Carolina	0.08/0.00	10 days	No	Yes
North Dakota	0.10/0.02	91 days	after 30 days	Yes
Ohio	0.10/0.02	90 days	after 15 days	Yes
Oklahoma	0.10/0.00	180 days	Yes	Yes
Oregon	0.08/0.00	90 days	after 30 days	Yes
Pennsylvania	0.10/0.02	—	—	No
Rhode Island	0.10/0.02	—	—	Yes
South Carolina	None/—	—	—	No
South Dakota	0.10/—	—	—	No
Tennessee	0.10/0.02	—	—	Yes
Texas	0.10/0.00	60 days	Yes	Yes
Utah	0.08/0.00	90 days	No	Yes
Vermont	0.08/0.02	90 days	No	No
Virginia	0.08/0.02	7 days	No	Yes
Washington	0.10/0.02	—	—	Yes
West Virginia	0.10/0.02	6 months	Yes	Yes
Wisconsin	0.10/0.02	6 months	Yes	Yes
Wyoming	0./10/—	90 days	Yes	No

(Insurance Institute for Highway System)

What is alcoholism?

Alcoholism is a disease. A disease affects the human mind and the human body. Alcoholism is a serious disease causing both psychological and medical complications of all sorts to the human body. The psychological dependence on alcohol is real and has devastating consequences on the affected individual and his or his family and society.

Men who suffer from alcohol dependency have great difficulty stopping being dependent on alcohol. These men are addicted to alcohol and crave it when they stop drinking. There are different patterns of alcohol dependency.

Some men drink alcohol in excess every day and feel the need to drink every day. A significant percentage of these men are able to go to work and function reasonably well on the job. They usually start drinking at lunchtime. They often consume 2–3 drinks with lunch, and after work they will drink 3–4 more drinks, either at a bar on their way home or at job-related functions, and when they get home they will again have 2–3 more drinks with dinner. That is about 10 drinks of hard liquor per day. On weekends, that number quadruples. These men are what are called functioning alcoholics. They work, they make money, and they support their families. These men are found at all levels of society from the very rich to the poor, and to the middle class. They are also referred to as men who can handle their alcohol.

There are of men who are working alcoholics, who must drink as soon as they get up in the morning to get going. They drink hard liquor at different times throughout the working day. Very often, people know that these men are alcoholics but tolerate them or cover up for them because they are oftentimes polite, very nice, and jovial, and when sober they are productive at their work. Frequently, these men miss work because of heavy alcohol drinking and very often come up with very creative excuses as to why they were absent from work.

There are men who drink alcohol in large quantities and on such a regular basis that they become sick so frequently that they are unable to maintain a job. These are the hardcore, non-functioning alcoholics, who are entirely preoccupied with alcohol drinking on a daily basis. Such men can be found also in all segments of society, in all professions and most religions and in all ethnic groups.

Alcohol abuse and peer pressure

Peer pressure plays a significant role in alcohol abuse in teenagers, as there is peer pressure to get them involved in illicit drugs. There is also peer pressure to force other young teenagers to drink alcohol. Peer pressure also exists among adults to get together in a bar after work for a drink or two. The incidence of alcohol abuse is quite high among men of all ethnic backgrounds. Alcohol abuse among men starts at an early age (from adolescence to teenage years). Poor Men drink alcohol for the same reasons that other men drink alcohol—to socialize with their friends and to be less inhibited. That use of alcohol frequently increases to drinking alcohol alone at home on a daily basis. Eventually, these men become dependent on the alcohol, and once that happens, they become preoccupied with alcohol drinking, resulting in alcoholism. Frequently alcoholic men grew up in broken homes where there was either a father or mother who abused alcohol, or they have either a wife or girl friend that drinks alcohol. They drink in order to please their significant others, or they drink because they saw their mothers or fathers doing it and they thought it was all right for them to start doing it also. Some of these men are heads of the household, single parents with children to bring up with no fathers around and all the stress associated with running a house alone. In addition, all the problems associated with poverty, racism, and bigotry, in a whites-dominated society, leads to heavy alcohol use in some minority men.

The working-class men group also has many alcohol abusers among it. The men in that group have similar problems with alcohol abuse, and the reasons are the same—stress, single parenthood, poverty, racism and all its associated perniciousness, and in more instances, domestic violence and all the awful things that are associated with it. Middle-class men who abuse alcohol do so for similar reasons as just outlined. The main difference is that that group of men has financial means, which help them to be able to cover up their alcoholism. As for upper-class men, most of them are professionals, businessmen, athletes, entertainers and entertainers' husbands, and sons of the wealthy and privileged—all of them abuse alcohol also for similar reasons, except that they are not poor and undoubtedly suffer less discriminations (in fact, reasonably frequently they do a significant degree of the discriminating themselves that occurs in society). Because of their money, social and professional status, doors are frequently open for them, etc., that allow their alcoholism to appear more acceptable to their friends, colleagues and their associates. The effects of alcohol on their bodies, however, is the same as that of the poorest men, because alcohol cares not how much money a person has, or for that matter, how privileged he is or how well a person is able to eat. The best caviar, the best cheeses, or the finest filets mignons in the world cannot protect the human body from the ultimate devastation of alcohol abuse. Alcoholism affects the human body to the same degree, regardless of a person's nutritional state, with a few minor transient circumstances. For example, if a man is undernourished and went on a alcohol binge and does not eat, the fact that he has low storage of carbohydrates in his liver from poor eating over an extending period of time, that man may develop hypoglycemia (low blood sugar) quicker than the man who drinks heavy, but eats a better diet. That being said, the long-term toxic effects of alcohol are the same in everyone who drinks alcohol heavily.

Even though black males start drinking alcohol at a later age than their white males counterparts do, the signs of alcoholism seem to appear earlier in black men than in white males. Undoubtedly, poverty and racism play a major role in these differences. Poor folks do not have as much money as rich folks to go to the doctor for check-ups. White folks have more money than minority folks do, and therefore they get check-ups more often. Diseases such as cancer of the mouth and the throat, which are quite common in alcoholics, are picked up earlier in white rich alcoholic men than they are picked up in poor men of color alcoholics.

Alcohol is the most frequently abused drug because it is legal to buy alcohol without a prescription. Alcohol is readily available and a person who wishes to drink it does not have to resort to illicit means to obtain it. Different states set up different age limits at which a young person can legally buy alcohol. On a yearly basis, alcohol abuse and its associated problems lead to more than 100,000 deaths in the United States. Of that number, close to 40,000 is due to cirrhosis of the liver and other associated medical complications of alcohol on the human body. The rest are due to alcohol-associated accidents on the highway (DWI) and homicides, etc.

The amount of alcohol that a person must drink on a long-term basis to cause damage to the liver is 80 grams of alcohol per day over an extended period, anywhere from 7 years to 15 years. Eighty grams of alcohol can almost be found in a six-pack of 12 ounces of beer, because each 12-ounce can of beer has 13.1 grams of alcohol. If one multiplies that, it adds up to 78.6 grams of alcohol, and some men drink twice that much beer per day. As stated above, if a person drinks that amount of alcohol on a regular basis, that person will develop liver disease, as time goes on.

If a man drinks wine regularly (3.5 fluid ounces of wine), which is a glass of wine, it has 9.6 grams of alcohol. A bottle of wine usually has about 5–6 glasses of wine in it. Men who drink 2–3 glasses of wine with dinner every night do not develop liver disease. It takes a minimum of 80 grams of alcohol per day on a regular basis over several years to develop fatty infiltration of the liver, which leads to metamorphosis of fat, leading to necrosis, resulting in alcoholic liver disease with subsequent development of cirrhosis.

The same thing applies to champagne. One glass of champagne has 11 grams of alcohol in it; some champagne has 13 grams of alcohol per glass, depending on how dry the champagne is. So, it would take a tremendous amount of champagne consumption to add up to 80 grams of alcohol. About 11-plus glasses of champagne daily over many years can cause a person to develop alcoholic cirrhosis. Most people do not drink that much champagne.

However, if a man drinks martinis, that is a different situation. Each martini has 18.5 grams of alcohol. If he drinks five martinis per day, he is already drinking what is in fact in excess of the minimum amount of alcohol that is needed to cause liver disease. Five martinis equal to 92 grams of alcohol. A Manhattan, for instance, has 19.9 grams of alcohol in it. Five Manhattans equal to 99.65 grams of alcohol. A gin Ricky has 21 grams of alcohol. Five gin Ricky's equal 105 grams of alcohol. A High Ball has 24 grams of alcohol in it. Five High Balls equal 120 grams of alcohol. A mint julep has 29.2 grams of alcohol in it. Five mint juleps equal 146 grams of alcohol, etc. So it does not take many of these alcoholic drinks on a daily basis for a man to develop alcoholic liver disease. The organs most affected by alcohol abuse are the following:

1. The brain
2. The liver
3. The pancreas
4. The spleen
5. The GI system
6. The blood system
7. The behavioral system

As described here, alcohol is very toxic to the brain. Acute alcohol ingestion alters a person's behavior by creating a state of excitation, restlessness, and poor social behavior. The agitated state leads to poor physical coordination, which frequently progresses to a state of drunkenness, leading to stupor and, at times, to coma. When intoxicated, the man alcoholic is a danger to hisself, and a danger to others around his. The adult brain is affected by alcohol in many ways. For instance, a man who abuses alcohol risks losing his ability to function properly on his job. He is likely to develop serious psychological problems, which can cause disruption of his family life, which often results in break-ups of personal relationships such as marriages, etc.

Serious damage to the brain tissues leading to dementia is quite common in chronic alcoholics. Chronic alcohol abuse can lead to Korsakoff syndrome, because of long-term vitamin B deficiencies. It is also known to be associated with acute episodes of encephalopathy, such as Wernicke's encephalopathy due to thiamine deficiencies. Chronic alcohol abuse is also associated with other neurological abnormalities, such as ataxia (inability to walk in a straight line), altered mood functions with suicidal ideations, and peripheral neuropathy. A chronic alcoholic is prone to develop seizures, either because of alcohol withdrawal, or because of recurrent traumas to the brain. The chronic alcoholic is often deficient in folic acid, all the B vitamins, magnesium, protein, and phosphate.

Alcohol affects the liver, because it is a direct toxin to the liver tissues. In other words, because alcohol is directly toxic to liver tissues, the amount of alcohol consumed and the frequency of that consumption, and the length of time an individual abuses alcohol, determine the extent of the liver damage.

In some individuals, the damage to the liver occurs quicker than in others, but one thing is certain: as long as a person abuses alcohol, his or her liver will be damaged by it. In some instances, the liver becomes acutely swollen, which can in turn lead to acute enlargement of the spleen due to acute elevation of the portal pressure and the consequence can be acute rupture of the spleen, endangering the life of the affected person, if it is not diagnosed properly and treated surgically quickly.

More chronically, however, alcohol causes tissues within the liver to become inflamed and the recurrent inflammatory reaction in time leads to scarring of the liver tissues, resulting in cirrhosis of the liver.

Once the liver becomes cirrhotic, a multitude of clinical problems can occur. The liver is needed to synthesize (produce) different proteins, which are necessary for good body functions. The liver is needed to make most of the coagulation factors required to prevent bleeding from occurring. The liver is necessary to store carbohydrates and to break down carbohydrates into usable sugars to use as fuel in the body. The liver is necessary to produce bile, which is needed to break down fats that humans eat, plus a multitude of other essential functions. The liver is the largest organ in the body next to the skin and the skeletal system and it contains the largest supply of reticuloendothelial cells that are necessary to participate in the immune system, etc. In addition, the liver is needed to help remove a multitude of breakdown products that the human body produces constantly. So when the liver is sick and is unable to produce needed materials for proper body functions, and is too sick to help remove waste materials from the body, the human person becomes very sick. In other words, when the liver is too sick to function properly and fails, life cannot go on. Another way of putting it, is when the liver fails, the person dies, and alcohol abuse can frequently cause the liver to fail.

The pancreas is another organ that is quite sensitive to the toxic effects of alcohol. Pancreatitis is a common complication of heavy and chronic alcohol abuse. It is not exactly clear as to the number of years a man has to abuse alcohol before his pancreas becomes sick—some say, after seven years of alcohol abuse. But, again, different men have different degrees of resistance and tolerance to the effects of alcohol. Alcohol damages the pancreatic tissues, causing at first acute inflammation to occur. The inflammation causes marked swelling of the pancreas, resulting in acute pancreatitis. After repeated attacks of acute pancreatitis, over several years, scarring of the pancreatic tissues occur, which in turn results in chronic pancreatitis? The third scenario is when the chronicity of the pancreatic disease causes destruction of the pancreatic tissue, leaving empty spaces within the pancreas, causing pancreatic pseudo cysts to develop. Quite often, these pancreatic pseudo cysts become infected, which in turn can lead to abscesses within the pancreas. Still other sequelae of chronic pancreatitis is pancreatic failure, meaning the pancreas is so damaged that it is no longer able to produce the different enzymes that it was able to produce before it became damaged. These enzymes are necessary to aid in the digestive process of ingested fat that humans eat. Failure of the pancreas to produce these necessary enzymes causes the development of greasy diarrhea to occur. To further cause matters to get worse, if the man with pancreatic failure now becomes diabetic, because the pancreas has failed, it is not able to produce insulin for sugar metabolism; not to mention the constant and intense left-sided abdominal pain that man has to endure.

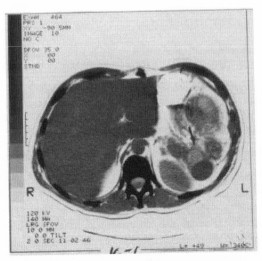

Figure 16.1—CT of acute pancreatitis.

CT of the abdomen showing acute pancreatitis with a pseudocyst of the pancreas (arrow showing swollen pancreas with pseudocyst).

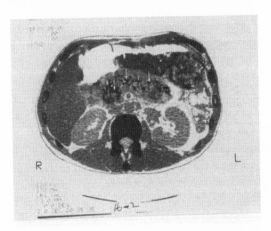

Figure 16.2—CT of chronic pancreatitis.

CT of the abdomen showing chronic pancreatitis with calcifications. Arrows showing swollen of the pancreas in a patient who abuses alcohol.

The effects of alcoholism on the spleen

The spleen becomes sick in chronic use with heavy alcohol intake because of cirrhosis of the liver. When alcohol damages the liver, that damage occludes the blood vessels that run through the liver. These damaged vessels cause narrowing and obstruction of the circulation inside the liver to occur. Because of intra-liver obstruction of these vessels over time, the pressure within the liver and the portal system rises to the spleen, causing portal hypertension to develop. Portal hypertension then leads to enlargement of the spleen, resulting in a condition called hypersplenism. The enlarged spleen can at times become quite bulky, resulting in severe and chronic left-sided abdominal pain. The upper gastrointestinal system is quite frequently involved in that scenario and becomes quite sick because of the effects of cirrhosis of the liver and portal hypertension. Because of the destruction and obstruction of these intrahepatic and (intra-liver) circulation, the elevation of the portal pressure causes neovascularization (formation of new vessels) to occur (which is the body's way of trying to bypass the obstructed circulation in the intrahepatic system).

The new vessels, however, are superficial, meaning that they grow on the surface of the esophagus, resulting in esophageal varices.

Because these new vessels, called varices, are superficially located on the outer surface of the esophagus, they tend to rupture quite easily and bleed profusely. Therefore, esophageal bleeding is a major complication of cirrhosis of the liver with portal hypertension.

Another frequent complication of chronic and heavy alcohol abuse is gastritis, resulting in upper gastrointestinal bleeding. Because alcohol is an irritating drug, it damages the superficial lining of the stomach, causing bleeding to occur, which at times can be quite severe and copious.

Still another common problem that at times occurs in the chronic alcoholic is a condition called Mallory-Weiss syndrome. Mallory-Weiss syndrome develops because of a tear that occurs at the junction of the gastroesophageal area. That occurs because of alcohol abuse and severe vomiting and retching. The force of the retching causes the tear to occur, resulting in upper gastrointestinal bleeding. In all these cases, the bleeding can be severe enough to cause the patient to go into shock with all its multitudes of complications.

Another frequently affected system is the hematopoietic system (blood system). The effects of alcohol on the blood system are many and varied. Acutely, alcohol can suppress the bone marrow, resulting in the lowering of white blood cells, red blood cells, and platelets. Chronic alcoholism can cause anemia as because of recurrent upper gastrointestinal bleeding on the one hand, and on the other hand, alcohol abuse always leads to folic acid deficiency, resulting in another folic acid deficiency anemia. In other instances, chronic alcohol abuse can result in a condition called hypersplenism, as mentioned earlier, which causes hemolysis of red blood cells, causing anemia. Hypersplenism can also cause leukopenia (low white blood cells) and thrombocytopenia (low platelet count). These abnormalities in the blood system are the result of splenic sequestration (because the spleen is enlarged, it soaks up these cells within it and destroys them). Chronic alcoholism with liver disease (cirrhosis) causes the white blood cells to not function well; because, affected men are not able to fight infection properly.

Chronic alcoholic abuse also affects the endocrine systems of men. For instance, the sick alcoholic liver is unable to break down estrogen effectively, which then allows the excess estrogen to remain in the blood, resulting in over-stimulation of the uterus, causing breakthrough vaginal bleeding, worsening their iron deficiency state. Through that same mechanism, estrogen, resulting in swelling and pain in their breasts, over stimulates alcoholic men's breast tissues. These men, because of the over stimulation of estrogen, have a high propensity for developing both breast and uterine cancers. The effect of excess circulating estrogen causes skin changes to develop in these men (spider angiomata). The heart suffers a great deal from the effects of alcohol abuse. The most frequent cardiac problem that occurs in alcohol intoxication is abnormal rhythm of the heart, such as "fast heartbeat" (tachycardia):

1. Atrial fibrillation
2. Super-ventricular tachycardia
3. Multifocal ventricular contractions (PVCs)
4. Atrial premature contradictions PACs.
5. Heart blocks, etc.

Chronic effects of alcohol on the heart cause damage to the heart muscles, resulting in enlargement of the heart (alcoholic cardiomyopathy). Alcoholic heart disease frequently results in congestive heart failure

Lung disease in alcoholic men

Men who abuse alcohol frequently develop aspiration pneumonia. Pneumonia develops because when these men get drunk, they lose control of their gag reflux and the consequence of that is that they aspirate their vomitus into their lungs, causing aspiration pneumonia. The overall poor nutritional and health state of men who abuse alcohol predisposes them to community-acquired pneumonias. Smoking cigarettes or cigars is part of the alcohol abuse subculture. The result of that tobacco abuse/alcohol abuse that some men are involved with is that there is a high incidence of lung cancer in alcoholic men who smoke. There is also a high incidence of head and neck cancer in that subgroup of men As well there is a high incidence of cancer of the esophagus in that subgroup of men because of the adverse effects of alcohol and cigarette on esophageal tissue.

The take-home lesson is not to use tobacco in any form and not to abuse alcohol.

Alcohol is a drug and can be quite addicting when used in large quantities over a long period. Alcohol has the potential to be toxic to the entire human body. The literature clearly shows that alcohol in moderate quantities, such as one or two glasses of wine with dinner, is good in the prevention of coronary artery heart disease. Alcohol does so through different mechanisms:

1. It makes platelets less sticky, thereby, preventing them from aggregating and in so doing lowering the possibility of clot formation.
2. It increases the level of high-density lipoprotein, the good cholesterol. However, it is prudent that anyone with a propensity to alcohol abuse refrain from alcohol altogether.
3. Both white wine and red wine help to decrease the incidence of coronary artery heart disease when consumed in moderate quantity. It is believed that the phenols found in red grapes function as antioxidants and prevent the damage to coronary arteries.

Clinical management of alcohol-induced clinical problems:

Clinically, acute alcohol intoxication causes the intoxicated man to be agitated, unreasonable, sometimes violent, and frequently confused. That set of symptoms and behavior can cause intoxicated men to get into fights and other altercations that can cause problems for their spouses, their children and other members of society with whom they come in contact with. These men frequently are brought to the emergency room after fights during which they were traumatized, or brought to the emergency room due to upper gastrointestinal bleeding or due to fever and abdominal pain and other alcohol-associated problems. Once the intoxicated alcoholic arrives in the emergency room, he must be evaluated immediately. Vital signs, such as blood pressure, pulse, temperature, and respiratory rate must be quickly taken and documented. Then, an intravenous access must be quickly established. Blood must be drawn and sent for CBC, SMA 20, serum magnesium, serum amylase, blood alcohol concentration, and urine, must be sent for drug screening. The urine also must be sent to the laboratory for urinalysis to make sure that there is no blood in it, which may indicate that the patient has had some trauma to the kidneys during a fight. The examining physician must pay particular attention to the examination of the head area, looking for signs of trauma. It is important to examine inside the ears, looking for signs of blood coming out of the inner ears. The examination must be complete and must include a rectal examination, looking for signs of blood grossly, and if none is found, the stool must be tested for blood using the hemoccult test. The neurological examination is extremely important, looking for signs of agitation, confusion, hallucinations, stupor, etc.

As soon as the physical examination is completed, the alcoholic must be started on the so-called alcoholic cocktail. The composition of the alcoholic cocktail is:

1. IV glucose (50% in one ampule)
2. Thiamine 100 mg IV or IM
3. Folic acid 1 mg IV, IM, or PO if the patient can take PO
4. Magnesium sulfate 1-gram IV or IM
5. B complex vitamin IM, IV or PO

It is crucial that thiamine is given before the glucose is infused. If the glucose is infused before the administration of thiamine that will lead to an acute depletion of whatever trace of thiamine is left in the body. That acute thiamine depletion will lead to a condition called Wernicke's encephalopathy. Acute Wernicke's encephalopathy causes acute agitation, confusion, hallucination and combativeness. The reason why acute Wernicke's occurs when 50% of glucose is infused in the alcoholic is that the alcoholic is frequently deficient in all B-complex vitamins such as thiamine, because alcoholics do not eat enough foods that contain these vitamins. Thiamine is a necessary biochemical vitamin in the metabolism of glucose (the Krebs cycle, a biochemical pathway reaction that contains many substances that are necessary to metabolize sugars) to help make that reaction. Therefore, the acute depletion of thiamine causes Wernicke's encephalopathy to occur. Sugar is needed in the acutely intoxicated alcoholic because he is likely to be starved and therefore has hypoglycemia (low blood sugar). The acutely sick alcoholic needs folic acid because he is always folic acid deficient, and because he does not eat enough foods that contain folic acid. Further, alcohol as a drug poisons the folic acid biochemical pathway. All alcoholics by definition are folic acid deficient. The acutely sick and intoxicated alcoholic needs magnesium, because all chronic and heavy alcoholic users are magnesium deficient, even though the laboratory may report the blood magnesium level as normal. Alcohol is a form of diuretic and as such, the alcoholic loses large quantities of magnesium in the urine. Low magnesium can cause low serum calcium. Both low serum calcium and low magnesium in an individual can cause seizures, muscle cramps, and (in some cases) rhythm abnormalities of the heart. Hypoglycemia (low blood sugar) can cause seizures to occur. Another frequent substance that chronic alcoholics are frequently deficient in is phosphate. Phosphate is a by-product of protein breakdown and since the alcoholics are too preoccupied with alcohol to eat properly, they are frequently deficient in protein and phosphate. Further, the alcoholic urinates frequently because of the diuretic effect of alcohol, and thereby loses large quantities of phosphate in the urine, causing hypophosphatemia (low serum phosphate). Low serum phosphate can cause acute seizures and chronically can cause hemolytic anemia. This is so because phosphate is needed to provide for a normal level of 2–3 D-PG (2–3 diphosphoglycerate). In some instances, low serum phosphate can cause severe rhythm disturbances of the heart.

Once the alcoholic passes through that first stage of his stay in the hospital, the next step is to evaluate his for acute or chronic disease in the usual manner. If it is decided that the alcoholic needs to be hospitalized, then all the medications in the alcoholic cocktail must be continued for several days except for the magnesium and the 50% dextrose.

The next step in providing acute care for the alcoholic is to watch for the possible development of delirium tremens (DTs). Both the blood alcohol concentration level and how the patient looks clinically are important in deciding when to start anti-DT treatment. Equally important is to try to ascertain when the patient last drank alcohol. Most alcoholics will start showing signs of DTs 36–48 hours after they had their last drink of alcohol. It is important to keep in mind the fact that chronic alcoholics can have a blood alcohol concentration of 100–200 mg per deciliter in the blood and do not appear drunk. Because of that fact, the chronic alcoholic can go into DTs with an alcohol level concentration that is that high because their bodies are accustomed to having a higher concentration of alcohol in it.

Delirium tremens is a clinical syndrome that occurs from the craving for alcohol that develops when an alcohol abuser has not drank alcohol for several days, 48–72 hours. The part of the brain that controls addiction misses the alcohol and the alcoholic goes into withdrawal, due to the loss of alcohol in his bloodstream to satisfy the brain's need for the alcohol.

DTs have several stages: Stage I, Stage II, Stage III, Stage IV and Stage V.

Stage I: The first stage of DTs manifested with tremors (the shakes), restlessness, increased heart rate, insomnia, diarrhea, and irritability.

Stage II:	The second stage is all of the Stage I signs, plus sweaty palms and confusion.
Stage III:	All the symptoms of I and II plus sweating, rise in blood pressure, rise in pulse, palpitations and hallucinations.\
Stage IV:	All the preceding signs, plus seizures.
Stage V:	All of those in the preceding stages, plus coma.

To prevent DTs from developing, it is recommended that the patient be given Ativan 1–2 mg four times per day, prophylactic ally by mouth as soon as the patient gets to the emergency room and consciousness level has been evaluated to be clinically satisfactory. If the patient can't take medication by mouth, Ativan can be given IM or IV. Alternatively, the patient can be treated with Librium 10 mg PO, four times per day IM or PO. Librium is not absorbed well IM and is not a medication to be used if the patient has severe liver disease, because the liver metabolizes Librium. The liver metabolizes Ativan differently and, therefore, it can be used even if the liver is severely sick.

Other things that are essential in the treatment of DTs are fluid and electrolyte replacement intravenously. It is very important to keep the sick alcoholic in an anabolic state, by making sure there is always sugar in the IV fluid being given to his. D5 ½ normal saline or D5 normal saline is preferred. If the patient is hypertensive, the IV can be D5 ¼ normal saline, along with specific medications to treat the hypertension. If seizure develops, then the patient ought to be treated first with IV Valium then with Dilantin. A brain CAT scan without contrast, followed by an EEG at the appropriate time, should also be done.

There are medications that can be used to help the patient stop drinking, if he agrees to take them. Two such medications are in use today; one is Antabuse (Disulfiram), the other is Naltrexone. Both of these medications have side effects and a person who is drinking alcohol must not take them. If a man is drinking alcohol and takes Antabuse, he can become acutely ill and in fact can die because. Naltrexone works apparently on the brain to decrease the desire of the alcoholic to drink alcohol. Antabuse (Disulfiram) works by converting acetaldehyde, which is a breakdown product of alcohol to acetic acid in the liver that causes an increase in serum acetaldehyde anywhere from five to ten times the normal level. Because of that, the man can hyperventilate and can develop flushing of the skin, nausea, vomiting, headache, and respiratory distress along with anxiety, palpitations and sometimes hypertension. That is why it is important that men do not drink alcohol and take Disulfiram at the same time. The usual dose of Disulfiram is 250 mg. There is a 500 mg dose that is made also, but frequently the 250 mg dose is sufficient to prevent someone from craving alcohol. The usual dose for Naltrexone (ReVia) is 50 mg daily for about 12 weeks as a prophylactic treatment against alcohol abuse.

Driving while intoxicated remains a major safety problem in the United States, and every year many thousands of people die because of accidents resulting from DUI. Drunken drivers remain a menace to society, and different states have different laws defining what DUI is. The following is a complete list of the different listings of the blood alcohol concentration that is considered legal for any person to drive a car, as published by the Insurance Institute for Highway Safety (see Table 1).

According to the literature, roughly 5%-6% of men in this country have a serious alcohol dependence problem. In the primary care setting, about 25% of men appear to have serious alcohol problems. Men who abuse alcohol face a major problem

Many individuals who abuse alcohol also abuse prescription drugs, such as Valium, Librium, Ativan, Xanax, etc. Drinking alcohol and taking these drugs is quite dangerous and can cause a person to die. Alcohol is a neurological, cardiac and pulmonary suppressant, so when a man has too much alcohol in his bloodstream, and adds prescription drugs on top of the alcohol, he increases the possibility of cardiac arrhythmia, respiratory failure, coma, and death. Drinking alcohol and then taking prescription drugs is to be avoided, because it can be lethal.

It is variably reported that there is "between 14 and 19 million" known alcoholics in the USA, plus anywhere from 8 to 10 million other individuals who abuse alcohol to different degrees. Alcohol abuse contributes to about 100,000 deaths per year in the United States, making it the third leading cause of preventable death in the United States, after tobacco and obesity and its associated health risks. Based on statistics provided by the National Institute of Alcohol Abuse and Alcoholism (NIAAA), the cost of caring for alcohol and substance abuse problems in the United States was reported to have been 276 billion dollars in 1995 and 184.6 billion dollars in 1998, as published in December 2000.

Presently in the USA, this great, powerful and wealthiest country on the planet, every night 38 million people to bed hungry about 14 million of them are children. Roughly, 10 million children have no health insurance coverage, and overall about 48 million people have no health insurance. How can that happen in the U.S.? The answers are multifaceted and complex but lie mostly in the philosophy that the rich get richer and the poor get poorer. How sad! In addition, how awful!

White men abuse alcohol many more times than men of color and some of the reasons are the same, while others are different. Most men of color abuse alcohol in part because of the stress associated with racial discrimination, broken homes, loneliness, stress in the workplace, unemployment, and pain associated with chronic diseases such as arthritis, depression, anxiety, panic attacks, etc.

Many white men abuse alcohol as the drug of choice to use while partying because that is socially acceptable. Since white men possess more money than men of color do, they spend more time partying and drinking more alcohol in the process.

Many men resort to alcohol abuse as a way of coping with their problems.

Alcohol, when used in small quantities, can be helpful in increasing the good cholesterol (HDL)—one drink of hard liquor per day, or two glasses of wine with dinner, red or white wine, both of which can increase the HDL. Furthermore, it is clear that alcohol decreases the stickiness of platelets (a cell in the blood necessary in forming clots); in so doing, there is less probability of clot forming in the coronary arteries, thereby decreasing the incidence of heart attacks. When alcohol is consumed in excess, the advantage is nullified, because alcohol abuse can cause disease to develop in the heart muscles (cardiomyopathy). In addition, alcohol abuse can cause elevation in the blood pressure, which over time can cause hypertensive heart disease along with coronary artery heart disease. Light to moderate alcohol consumption can be helpful, while heavy alcohol consumption is harmful to the human body. Anyone at risk for alcohol abuse ought not to drink alcohol in any amount, because it might get them to start drinking alcohol heavily again.

Many men in the world live in poverty of different degrees and suffer from racial discrimination of different types, along with ethnic and religious bigotry, social depravation etc., and yet these men do not abuse alcohol. Men who abuse alcohol ought to follow the examples of their fellow men in the third world and stop abusing alcohol. By stopping alcohol abuse, an alcohol-abusing man will have a healthier liver, heart, brain, nervous system, endocrine system, reproductive system, gastrointestinal system, pancreas, blood system, and emotional system and overall a healthier life.

Men who need help for their alcohol abuse problems can call the following organizations:

1. Alcoholics Anonymous   Telephone number: 212–870–3400

2. Hazel Den   Telephone number: 1–800–257–7810

3. National Clearing House for   Telephone Number: 800–729–6686
    Alcohol Abuse and Drug   Fax Number: 301–468–6433
    Information

4. National Council on   Telephone Number: 212–206–6770
    Alcoholism and Drug   Fax Number: 212–645–1690
    Dependence, Inc.

5. Hope Lives   Telephone Number: 800-NCA-CALL

6. Drug-Specific Information   Telephone Number: 800–729–6686

CHAPTER 17

DRUG ADDICTION
IN MEN

ILLICIT DRUG ABUSE IS THE second most common addictive habit in the United States. Alcohol is the number-one drug that is abused in the United States. According to the National Institute on Drug Abuse, there are about 4 million drug addicts in the United States and about 3 million of them are addicted to cocaine. About 800,000 addicts are addicted to heroin. Several more millions use and abuse illicit drugs of different types; they are also considered addicts. The General Accounting Office estimates that in 1998 the federal government spent 3.2 billion dollars to pay for treatment of the addicts. When cost of prevention of drug-related crimes and time lost from work is added up, more than 60 billion dollars would have been spent, adding up to an estimated 63.2 billion dollars. The taxpayers spend about 63.2 billion dollars per year on drug addiction and its related problems in the United States. By some estimate, about 19 million people use illicit drugs in the USA.

The part of the brain stimulated by drugs that results in pleasurable feelings is the dopamine center, which is located at the base of the brain. Drugs such as heroin, cocaine, marijuana, opiates and amphetamines activate dopamine to release neurotransmitter substances, resulting in a pleasurable feeling called a "high," which drug addicts crave to experience. The dopamine center also functions to allow for the experience of sexual pleasure, enjoyment of foods, music, art, and beautiful things, and other aesthetic things that are pleasing to the ears and the eyes. Once an individual becomes addicted to any drug such as heroin, cocaine, crack-cocaine, marijuana, etc., he or he craves these drugs when the level of the drug decreases in the bloodstream. The craving for the drug often-times is quite painful.

Drug craving can lead to severe withdrawal symptoms such as sweating, headache, runny nose, abdominal cramps, diarrhea, poor appetite, insomnia, nightmares, etc. So, addiction to a drug, in particular cocaine, heroin and crack-cocaine, can drive addicts to do anything to get money to buy the drugs in order to satisfy the drug craving on the one hand, which is the more power-ful and intense feeling, and to avoid going into drug withdrawal feelings. On the other hand, once a man becomes addicted to drugs, it is very difficult to give it up. The addicted man becomes dependent on the drug and spends a great deal of time preoccupying hisself with finding money to get the next fix. He will spend rent money, food money, mortgage money, or he will lie, steal and commit crimes of different types and magnitude in order to get the money to pay for the drug. Frequently, he prostitutes hisself to get money to pay for the drug and, at times, he will get involved sexually either with a man or with a man for drugs or payment.

Drug addiction is quite common among men of all racial and ethnic back-grounds and all social and economic status. Wherever there is poverty and ghettos, there is a high incidence of illicit drug use. However, illicit drug use has become prevalent in the suburbs of the United States and elsewhere, involving middle-and upper-class men. About 3.5 million men abuse prescription drugs in the USA. Statistically, more white males abuse prescription drugs and more men of color abuse illicit drugs.

The most frequently abused prescription drugs are:
1. Valium
2. Librium
3. Xanax
4. Ativan
5. Tranxene
6. Morphine
7. Hydrocodone
8. Codeine
9. Demerol, etc.

Illicit drug abuse is common in every community in the United States and at all level of these communities. The people involved in abusing illicit drugs include the very poor who reside in the inner cities of the United States, the working class, to the middle class and all the way up to the upper class. Illicit drug abuse is common in all professions to one degree or another and all sexes are involved in the illicit drug subculture. Men of color use more heroin and crack-cocaine, and white males use cocaine, marijuana and amphetamines. Cocaine has, however, made an entry into black, Hispanic, Asian, Native American, Pacific Islander and Latino ghettos in recent years, because the price of cocaine has gone down to a point where some poor people can now afford to buy it. Outside forces from the communities fuel the illicit drug subculture where these drugs are used. People who do not live in these communities are bringing the drugs into these communities. The big question is—who are these people? What are their motives? Is it just for the money, or is it something else? Some have said that infiltration of illicit drugs into the minority communities is a well-planned conspiracy to destroy generations of young people of color. Whether or not proof exists to substantiate these allegations is not quite clear. One thing certain is that the illicit drug subculture is highly associated with criminal behavior of different types and different degrees. The result is that communities where illicit drugs are prevalent also are beset with high crime rates.

Per capita, more white males use illicit drugs than men of color, but fewer white males get arrested for using drugs and even fewer of them get sent to jail for using drugs than men of color.

Of all the modern countries in the world, the United States has more people in jail at any one time than any other country. According to statistics, an excess of 2 million people are in jail in the United States. In fact, according to the Bureau of Justice Statistics, at mid-year in 1997, an estimated 1,725,842 individuals were in jail in the United States. Though Blacks represent about 13.8% of the United States population and Hispanics represent 14.3% in 2007, of the nearly 2 million people in jail in the United States, 40.6% were Whites, 42% of them were Blacks, and 15.7% were Hispanics. So a total of 57.1% of those in jail were a combination of Blacks and Hispanics, which was an outrageous number, because these two groups (Blacks and Hispanics) made up 25.1% of the total population and yet 57.1% of those in jail were Blacks and Hispanics. The vast majority of the men of color who were in jail in the year 2000 were there for drug-related offenses of different degrees.

The overall rate of illicit drug use reported for the total United States men population, age 12 and older, was 11.9%. Relative to the total United States men population, Native American men users of illicit drug are 19.8%, Puerto Rican men 13.3%, black men 13.1%, Mexican-American men 12.7%, Asian Pacific Islander men 6.5%, Caribbean-American men 7.6%, Central American men 5.7% and Cuban-American men 8.2%.

According to the National Center on Addiction and Substance Abuse at Columbia University, 21.5 million men in the United States smoke, 4.5 million are alcoholics; 3.5 million men misuse prescription drugs and 3.1 million men use illicit drugs. According to this important report, one out of every five pregnant man smokes, drinks alcohol and abuses drugs, totaling more than 800,000 men.

The psychological and physical, manifestations of drug addiction in men

The mindset that causes minority men to abuse drugs is no doubt similar to the mindset of other men who abuse drugs. But the circumstances of life that are associated with drug abuse are quite different in men of color than they are in white males. Most white males who are drug addicts start using marijuana recreationally. They then gradually move on to harder drugs, such as amphetamines, LSD, other psychedelic drugs. As the addiction deepens, they move on to using cocaine, heroin and crack-cocaine. These men are financially able to support their addictions, because they have good jobs with good pay, which enables them to pay for these drugs. Some of these men are in the entertainment world (the sports world, the business world and the art world, a world that predisposes some of them to drug addiction). Poor men are in a different set of circumstances as white males, in that they do not have money to support their drug habits.

A significant percentage of men are addicted to prescription drugs. The most frequently abused prescription drugs by men are the following:

1. Valium
2. Librium
3. Xanax
4. Ativan
5. Tranxene
6. Klonopin
7. Codeine
8. Darvon
9. Demerol
10. Morphine
11. Hydrocodone
12. Ambien
13. Restoril
14. Methadone

Some men become addicted to prescription drugs because of chronic pain associated with illness, such as cancer, arthritis, headaches, sickle cell disease, diabetic neuropathy and many other chronic diseases, which require chronic pain medication for relief. Sometimes these individuals continue to get the prescription for these medications for a long time, but once they are no longer able to obtain these prescriptions, they resort to illicit drugs to ease their pain. That is the way in which some of these men become chronic drug addicts. Drug addiction and all other addictions are psychological illnesses. The craving associated with drug addiction is controlled by neurotransmitters within the brain, in particular the dopamine center. When the urge comes upon an addicted person to get a high, that person will do just about anything to get the money to buy the drug. Drug addiction is a mental illness and ought to be treated as such. Percentage-wise, IV drug addiction is more common among men of color, as compared to white men. This is so, because that type of drug addiction is more closely associated with the inner cities where most poor men of color live. Although it is a known fact, the incidence of IV drug use is on the rise in the middle class as well as in the upper class communities of the United States. In other words, illicit drug use is also on Wall Street, Madison Avenue and most definitely in the suburbs.

The brain is affected by illicit drug use in many other ways. For example, heavy marijuana use is known to affect the brain in ways that lead to slow and slurred speech and memory loss. Both cocaine and heroin use are associated with seizures. When heroin and cocaine are used intravenously, sepsis and bacterial endocarditises can occur. Infected emboli can be thrown to the brain from the heart valve, resulting in brain abscesses. Most importantly, the brain is frequently affected by drug overdose causing coma.

The lungs are affected by drug addiction in many ways as well. Addicts who use cocaine or heroin intravenously frequently develop symptoms of upper airway diseases such as coughing, wheezing and bronchitis. Acute pulmonary edema (when the lungs are filled with fluid) can occur as an idiosyncratic reaction to heroin use. Another complication involving the lungs in heroin and cocaine use is pulmonary embolism (a clot to the lungs). That happens because the addicts use veins in their legs to infuse the drug and sometimes the vessels in the groin and legs get damaged and infected and become swollen. These conditions can lead to stasis, which in turn can lead to clot formation, deep vein thrombophlebitis (DVT). The clots can then migrate through the blood vessels into the lung, causing acute pulmonary embolism. Infected emboli can also be thrown to the lungs from infected vegetation from the heart valves (a condition called bacterial endocarditis). Still another frequent pulmonary complication of the IV drug abuser is pneumonia, which occurs often in IV drug abusers because of their overall poor physical condition predisposing them to the development of different types of lung infection.

The incidence of AIDS in men of color is the highest among all men groups in the U.S., specifically because of the fact that for that group of men, intravenous drug abuse is the highest compared to other men groups. That being the case, the incidence of the lung infection called Pneumocystis carinii (PCP) is the highest among minority men with AIDS. PCP is a most serious lung infection and frequently is the cause of death of men with AIDS. The incidence of pulmonary tuberculosis has decreased in the general population over the last several years, but it has gone up in men with AIDS.

The effects of illicit drug use on the heart

The heart suffers immensely from illicit drug use—be it use of amphetamines, LSD, marijuana, prescription drugs, cocaine, crack-cocaine, heroin, etc. The heart is likely to become affected by any one of these drugs once in the bloodstream and is more so when used in excess. Once in the bloodstream, the drugs stimulate the heart, causing it to beat too fast and frequently, irregularly.

Cocaine use can cause sudden death due to acute myocardial infarction (heart attack). Other cocaine-associated complications of the heart include cardiac arrhythmias, which sometimes can be lethal, myocarditis (inflammation of the heart muscle), cardiomyopathy (enlargement of the heart), and coronary spasm (spasm of the vessel that carries blood around the heart). The heart can, at times, become very slow (bradycardia). The heart rate can also be slowed by cocaine. At times, in the middle of acute cocaine intoxication, it has been reported that the heart can actually rupture abruptly, resulting in sudden death. It is believed that it is a metabolite (breakdown product) of cocaine that causes the toxicity to the heart. Acute heroin intoxication can cause the heart to slow down (bradycardia) as well as suppression of the respiratory system, which can result in cardiopulmonary failure. Many things can happen to the heart of an intravenous drug abuser, but one of the most serious is a condition called bacterial endocarditis. There are two forms of endocarditis: 1) acute bacterial endocarditis, 2) sub-acute bacterial endocarditis. Endocarditis occurs when bacterial organisms enter the bloodstream of the individuals, injecting drugs into their veins. Once in the bloodstream, the bacteria multiply, resulting in a condition called sepsis. Bacteria then settle on the heart valve, damaging it, causing different types of cardiac decompositions. In drug addicts, the valve most frequently affected is the tricuspid valve (54% of the time), followed by the aortic valve (25%), then by the mitral valve (about 20%), and the rest (6%) can be mixed right-sided and left-sided endocarditis. The bacterial organism most frequently found in drug addicts is staphylococcus coagulase positive, followed by streptococci; fungi, such as candida and aspergillus, can also cause bacterial endocarditis. Gram-negative organisms of different types can also settle on the heart valves, causing endocarditis. Staphylococcus coagulase negative can also settle on the heart valve, causing bacterial endocarditis in the drug addicts. In intravenous drug abusers, when the tricuspid valve is the affected valve, 80% of the time the Staphylococcus coagulase positive is the organism isolated. They can also become infected with Methicillin-Resistant Staphylococcus aureus. (MRSA). In acute bacterial endocarditis, the affected person becomes acutely ill with fever, chills, shortness of breath, chest pain, sometimes, cardiac arrhythmia and the development of an acute heart murmur, which was not there before with congestive heart failure.

Other physical findings may include distended neck veins, decreased blood pressure; fast pulse rate, increased respiratory rate, cardiac rub and rales in the lungs can be heard. An enlarged and tender liver can occur and a large spleen can be palpated. Acute pain in the lower back is frequently present in an individual who is septic. Headache with nausea and vomiting can also occur.

Laboratory findings include a high white blood cell count, low red blood cell count, elevated erythrocyte sedimentation rate, low platelet count, positive ANA, and elevated liver function test.

A chest x-ray may show diffuse infiltrates in the lungs. EKG may show fast rate with regular rhythm or fast rate with irregular rhythm, a slow rate with decreased voltage indicating that the heart is being compromised with fluid around the sac, a condition called cardiac tamponade. Arterial blood gases may be grossly abnormal with low O2 SAT. An echocardiogram may show valvular abnormalities such as vegetation, and an enlarged heart may be seen. A transesophageal echocardiogram may show the presence of vegetation on the heart valves if the regular echocardiogram does not show it. Sometimes, a transthoracic Echocardiogram can also be done if the technology is available in that particular institution. It is a much better test to detect heart valve vegetation than the regular echocardiogram.

The urine may show the presence of protein and red blood cells because of emboli to the kidneys. Septic emboli can also affect the skin, causing assorted skin lesions. Acute bacterial endocarditis is a severe medical emergency requiring the help of a cardiologist and cardiac surgeon to quickly take over the management of the patient, in order to try to replace the heart valve and save the individual's life. If any significant delay takes place, the chances of recovery may not be very good in acute bacterial endocarditis. What happens is that the bacteria sit on the valve and literally eat it away and then blood flows back and forth, resulting in acute cardiac decomposition with impending deaths, because the valve was acutely destroyed. As for management, these individuals frequently have to be intubated if they are in acute congestive heart failure. They cannot breathe. They need assistance to breathe and 100% oxygen has to be provided for them. Blood cultures ought to be taken and if they are positive, then clinical decisions must be made to provide appropriate antibiotic treatment for these patients. If staphylococcus is suspected, which it frequently is, Vancomycin IV is an excellent choice in antibiotic with coverage for gram-negative organisms. Vancomycin also covers MRSA. Once the organism is identified, and then an appropriate antibiotic should be provided based on the sensitivity. In the case of enterococcus, Gentamicin, along with Ampicillin, will be the drug of choice; if pseudomonas, then Fortaz will be a very good medication and if it is staphylococcus and it is sensitive to penicillin, then Oxacillin IV will be switched as the medication of choice and the Vancomycin will be stopped. If it is Methicillin-resistant staphylococcus, then the medication of choice clearly in that case is Vancomycin as stated above.

The other infection frequently involving the heart is sub-acute bacterial endocarditis. Sub-acute bacterial endocarditis can be more insidious and often is more insidious in its development, causing difficulty, at times, in arriving at a diagnosis. Sub-acute bacterial endocarditis manifests itself as a febrile illness with chills, general malaise, joint pain, low back pain, and headache. At times a person with sub-acute bacterial endocarditis might present with general weakness, pallor, intermittent low-grade fever, and a general feeling of unwellness. In that instance, a high index of suspicion must be brought into play so as not to mistake the diagnosis for something else. The profile of the patient is of major importance, i.e., in an intravenous drug abuser who is prone to sub-acute bacterial endocarditis by virtue of his habit of using drugs and sharing dirty needles with other drug addicts, the index of suspicion is quite high. Sometimes, these individuals use water from the toilet bowl to prepare the drug, in that way injecting themselves with contaminated materials.

The liver is a frequently affected organ in drug addicts. For those who abuse prescription drugs, the liver may get sick from these drugs, in particular when alcohol is combined with these drugs, as is frequently the case. Intravenous drug abusers' livers get sick most frequently because of hepatitis B and hepatitis C. In rare circumstances, they can also be infected with hepatitis A and hepatitis G, but these types of viral hepatitis occur less frequently in intravenous drug users.

Hepatitis A, B and C can be sexually transmitted and many drug addicts, when they are high on drugs, have sexual intercourse with whomever, wherever and whenever. Some drug addicts prostitute themselves either for drugs or for money to buy drugs. These loose behaviors predispose the drug addicts to contracting sexually transmitted diseases, such as hepatitis A, B and C, syphilis, gonorrhea, chlamydia, genital herpes, human papilloma virus (HPV), HIV, etc. Several of these sexually transmitted diseases, such as hepatitis A, B and C, syphilis, gonorrhea, and HIV can be spread to different parts of the body, resulting in all sorts of different symptoms and damage to the human body. In particular, hepatitis B and C can cause chronic liver disease such as chronic active hepatitis, chronic persistent hepatitis, and cirrhosis of the liver, with all its associated complications, including liver cancer and death. Drug addicts can also be infected with hepatitis A through needle sharing. Sub-clinical acute hepatitis A can develop as fulminant hepatitis resulting in acute liver failure can occur. It is therefore a very good idea to do a complete hepatitis profile on drug addicts, to include hepatitis, A, B and C and seeding DNA-PCR for Delta hepatitis is a very good idea. Delta hepatitis virus needs the presence of hepatitis B to support its growth in the body. Drug addicts must be vaccinated against the hepatitis viruses that they are not infected with, to prevent them from becoming infected on an already sick liver, which if it happens can have lethal clinical consequences.

The gastrointestinal tract is affected in drug addicts in several ways. One of the most common gastrointestinal symptoms that drug addicts suffer from is abdominal pain associated with craving for drugs. Secondly, drug addicts suffer frequently from diarrhea. The diarrhea has two bases: 1) nervousness and anxiety associated with craving for drugs; 2) parasitic infestation, which they contract during anal intercourse, transmitting organisms such as amoebae and Giardia lamblia. Upper gastrointestinal bleeding can occur as well when these men become cirrhotic because of chronic hepatitis. The bleeding occurs because of esophageal varices.

The kidneys are affected by intravenous drug addiction in several ways. As part of the sepsis and septic shock, the kidneys frequently fail in drug addicts, who present to the hospital with bacterial sepsis. As part of sub-acute bacterial endocarditis, septic emboli because of septic vegetations being thrown from the heart valves to the kidneys can affect the kidneys. Nephrotic syndrome occurs in intravenous drug addicts. That is probably due to antigen-antibody complexes, which form and circulate in the bloodstream either because of low-grade chronic infection or because of the different materials that are used to cut and mix either cocaine or heroin that the addicts use. These complexes settle in the tubules of the kidneys, causing nephrotic syndrome. Kidney abscesses can also occur in some IV drug addicts.

Sexually transmitted disease is quite common in men drug addicts because when these men are under the influence of drugs they tend to engage in unprotected sexual intercourse with multiple partners, exposing their genital organs to being infected with gonorrhea, syphilis, Chlamydia, herpes simplex virus, human papilloma virus, and HIV infection. HIV infection is the most serious and the most deadly infection that afflicts men drug addicts. The spread of the AIDS virus through the IV drug addicts is the main reason that there is such a high incidence of AIDS in men of color in the United States (see chapter 12 on AIDS).

The blood system is the most commonly abused system in the body by drug addicts. This is so because the blood is the entry point for IV drug abuse. Once the drug reaches the bloodstream, it gets carried to all parts of the body. Frequently the blood of drug addicts gets infected with bacterial organisms such as staphylococcus aureus, staphylococcus epidermidis, streptococci pneumonia, pseudomonas, klebsiella pneumonia, E. coli, haemophilus influenza, pneumococci, other Methicillin-Resistant Staphylococcus Aureus (MRSA) and fungi such as candida, aspergillus, and viruses such as hepatitis A, B, C, D, E etc. As described earlier, all these different microorganisms have at one point or another cause infections in drug addicts. All the blood cells of the body are all affected by drug addiction. Different drugs abused by addicts affect the bone marrow by suppressing it. The suppression of the bone marrow that these drugs can cause leads to anemia, leukopenia, or thrombocytopenia to occur acutely.

Leukocytosis can occur, reflecting the presence of the infection. Pancytopenia can also occur because of an acute infection such as sepsis, as well as hepatitis-induced cirrhosis of the liver, with secondary portal hypertension. When an IV drug abuser is infected with the AIDS virus, parvovirus #B-19 can enter the bloodstream, resulting in pure red cell aplasia. Both hepatitis C and B have been reported in some cases of aplastic anemia, and in some instances hepatitis A has been reported in some part of the world as being responsible for some cases of aplastic anemia as well.

Bacteria also get into the blood through broken and rotten teeth. However, more often, the bacteria get into the blood through skin abscesses that drug addicts develop during skin-popping or infected veins or dirty needles that addicts use to inject drugs. Another disease that can occur in drug addicts in IVDA is bone infection (osteomyelitis), a condition that results when bacteria that are circulating in the bloodstream infect the bone. Different bones can become infected in drug addicts, but the lumbar spine, the thoracic spine, the hip joints and the knees, etc. can frequently become infected. Often drug addicts present to the hospital with high fever, severe low back pain, or a swollen knee with effusion. When that happens, the back has to be evaluated with a CT scan and/or an MRI looking for the possibility of destruction of bones as because of infection. Sometimes a bone scan might add some more information to the clinical presentation. When the bone is discovered to be infected, an orthopedic surgeon must be brought into the picture to try to surgically remove the infected bone is possible. In addition, the individual requires several weeks of IV antibiotics. That often is a problem because it is difficult to keep an IV drug abuser in the hospital for as long as six weeks; he oftentimes elopes so he can go back to continue his destructive habits of using drugs.

The skin is the most frequently abused organ by the intravenous drug addicts. The heroin or cocaine addicts who inject drugs have to go through the skin to get the veins or arteries to inject themselves.

Frequently, the skin is dirty because of lack of proper cleansing. Some addicts, when they run out of veins to inject, inject drugs under their skin, a practice called skin-popping. Some addicts have multiple sores over their legs, abdomen, buttocks, neck, and arms with very little good skin left. These open sores represent a ready entry point for infection to enter into the bloodstream, resulting in blood infections of different types.

The blood is the main vehicle through which drugs are introduced into the bloodstream. Other routes through which illicit drugs are introduced into the body are smoking, snorting and skin-popping. Once the drugs are in the bloodstream, and if the doses of the drugs are excessive, the result is frequently drug overdose, resulting in different degrees of mental aberration. Frequently, confusion, stupor, seizures and, oftentimes, coma can develop. Once coma develops, if immediate medical attention is not provided, death may result.

Treatment of drug addicts and drug addiction

Drug addiction is a serious mental illness that affects people in all segments of society. Some people are addicted to prescription drugs and some people are addicted to illicit drugs, and some people are addicted to a combination of illicit drugs and prescription drugs. Drug addiction treatment requires a multi-team effort. The mental aspect of drug addiction requires treatment from mental health professionals and drug counselors and these individuals ought to go to drug treatment clinics and hospitals, both on an outpatient basis and when necessary on an inpatient basis for long-term drug rehabilitation treatments.

The medical treatments of drug addicts must be both organs and systems directed. One of the key components of intravenous drug abuse treatment is Methadone treatment. Methadone is a synthetic drug that is used to relieve the drug craving of heroin addicts. There are roughly 3.8 million chronic and regular drug addicts in the United States. They represent about 20% of the total drug addicts in the United States, which means that there are about 19 million drug addicts in the United States. About 19 million individuals are addicted to drugs and use them on an on-and-off basis. Methadone use contributes greatly in reducing HIV infection in IV drug abusers. It helps put people to work and to some degree; it helps to decrease the crime rate because these addicts do not have to commit crimes to find money to buy their drugs. However, according to a published report, only 1.7 million drug addicts can get into a Methadone program in the United States. This is about half of the hardcore drug users. According to the literature, only 115,000 of the 800,000 chronic users of heroin are getting Methadone. In New York City, about 35,000 of the 200,000 hardcore drug users are able to get into a Methadone Program. There exists an anti-Methadone program feeling in the United States. Some people in U.S. society at large, and for that matter some people in government, feel that giving addicts Methadone is encouraging drug addiction. That is untrue because Methadone is a form of medical treatment for heroin addiction. Drug addicts can abuse Methadone also. Some addicts take the Methadone from the clinic and sell on the street. Some people on purpose lie about their actual dose of Methadone and because of that too much Methadone is given to them and they can over-dose on Methadone on that basis. Because of Methadone overdose, they can go into coma. Some addicts abuse the Methadone Program and stay on it permanently as a form of work disability. These problems with the Methadone Program are not widespread, and overall the Methadone Program is useful and constructive. The hardcore drug users in the ghettos of the United States use a significant percentage of heroin, cocaine and crack-cocaine. However, according to recent reports, Whites and people in the middle class, upper middle class in the suburbs and celebrities in the sports and entertainment world use more cocaine, heroin and crack cocaine than people of color who live in the ghettos of the U.S.

Because men of color are arrested, persecuted and put in jail more often than white males for drug offenses, there is a misconception that they use more of these drugs, than white males, that is, in fact, not the case.

The drug addiction subculture is associated with criminal behavior because it is illegal to distribute and to use illegal drugs; the trafficking of drugs is controlled by the criminal elements of society. In 1996, 1.5 million individuals were arrested for drug offenses of different kinds in the U.S. Presently, there are about 300,000 people in jail for drug-related offenses in the United States. In 1996, the federal government spent 16 billion dollars fighting the drug problems in the United States. Of these 16 billion dollars, 10.6 billion dollars were spent on trying to reduce the drug supply and only 5.4 billion dollars were spent on reduction, demands and drug treatments.

Poverty, racial insensitivity, poor education, poor housing, lack of economic opportunities, and the chronic depressive state of mind associated with being in the underclass of society contribute to the factors that persist for the proliferation of drugs in the ghettos. The dynamics for the penetration of drugs into the suburbs are altogether different from that which exists for the poor people's communities. Rich folks get into the drug use subculture for recreational purposes, or to be in with a particular crowd or to be "cool." Either way, drug addiction is drug addiction and a drug addict is a drug addict.

Providing treatment for drug addiction and addressing the multiple and different issues that make drug addiction what it is take a back seat to the building of jails, stiff sentences, and the "Three strikes, you are out" policies of the U.S. and different state governments. There are people in jail serving life sentences because they were arrested for possessing single marijuana.

It is utterly absurd and grossly unfair that an individual of color can be thrown in jail for life for using crack-cocaine, while individuals in the upper echelon of the United States society can be arrested for using cocaine or heroin, and get away at times with just a slap on the back of the hand. It would seem clear that these laws are placed in the books specifically to punish people of color, simply to get them out of society and throw them in jail. That seems to be grossly unfair, though no one should condone the use of drugs of any kind, because that is illegal. However, putting it in its proper context, clearly there is some inequity in the way the law is being used as it relates to men of color, versus men in the majority community. It is not hard to envision that these problems would be resolved rather promptly if the hardcore drug users in the United States were white middle class and the white community was being devastated by these drugs. It is fair to say that a Marshall type of plan would have to be put into effect to deal with the drug problems, and as certain as the sun rises in the east and sets in the west, these problems would have been solved, if not completely, but certainly much better than they are being dealt with now.

The brain is frequently evaluated when drug addicts present with headaches, fever and seizures. Evaluation and treatment include brain CT, brain MRI, EEG, echocardiogram, CBC, SMA 18, PT, PTT, chest x-rays, urinalysis, blood cultures and lumbar punctures. Treatments directed towards possible acute brain disease in the IV drug abuser are based on any abnormal results the aforementioned tests may show. If all the tests are normal, or the results are pending, empirical treatments must be started promptly.

For the seizure, Valium IV followed by Dilantin IV or by mouth should be started. For the fever, broad-spectrum antibiotics are given IV. In that setting, Vancomycin IV is given to cover for gram-positive organisms, and Fortaz or other broad-spectrum gram-negative antibiotic is given to cover for gram-negative organisms. Several other antibiotic combinations can be used to cover both for gram-negative and gram-positive organisms in that setting.

Treatments of acute lung disease in IV drug abusers when they present with fever and shortness of breath are tailored to the findings on physical examination and/or chest x-ray. If the patient is afebrile but shows signs and symptoms of acute pulmonary disease, then arterial blood gas is done and oxygen is quickly started, and if the signs and symptoms are consistent with congestive heart failure, then treatment is given with IV Lasix right away. If signs and symptoms are consistent with acute pulmonary embolism, then a lung scan must be ordered along with ultrasound of the lower extremities. If the suspicion is strong and these tests are not readily available, then the patient should be given IV Heparin, if there is no contraindication to anticoagulation. If all signs, symptoms and findings on chest x-ray and CBC are consistent with pneumonia, then broad-spectrum antibiotics with Vancomycin IV and with Fortaz ought to be started immediately. If the patient is able to cough up sputum, then the sputum ought to be sent to the laboratory for gram stain and culture prior to starting the antibiotics.

Infection of the heart is one of the most common infections seen in IV drug abusers. Anytime an IV drug addict presents to the hospital with fever, heart valve infection such as acute bacterial endocarditis or sub-acute bacterial endocarditis must be suspected. Once the blood cultures have been obtained, broad-spectrum antibiotics with Vancomycin IV and Fortaz IV must be started to cover for the possibility of bacterial endocarditis. In acute bacterial endocarditis, the patient's cardiopulmonary system can become decompensate quickly, resulting in acute shortness of breath and acute congestive heart failure (pulmonary edema) because of acute destruction of the heart valve. That happens because bacteria settle on the affected heart valve and destroy it. As stated earlier, the most frequently affected valve in intravenous drug abuser is the tricuspid valve, followed by the aortic valve, followed by the mitral valves. That is an acute medical emergency necessitating evaluation by a heart surgeon for replacement of the affected valve surgically. It is important when treating a patient for possible bacterial endocarditis to frequently listen to the patient's heart, looking for the development of a new heart murmur, which would be the first sign of possible cardiac decompensation. Sub-acute bacterial endocarditis can present with no definite cardiac symptoms. Oftentimes, sub-acute bacterial endocarditis presents as part of sepsis with fever, chills and low back pain. Sometimes infected vegetation can be seen on an echocardiogram. Sometimes, sub-acute bacterial endocarditis presents and manifests itself with general malaise, weakness and intermittent low-grade fever and anemia. If serial blood cultures are drawn, a positive drug culture will eventually be found and the diagnosis of sub-acute bacterial endocarditis can be established. The treatment of bacterial endocarditis is Vancomycin to cover for Staphylococcus coagulase, positive MRSA, ceftriaxone for other gram-positive cocci, and Fortaz to cover for organisms such as pseudomonas. There are other combinations of antibiotics, which can also be quite effective in treating that infection. The main reason to always give the patient Vancomycin at presentation is because there is significant percentage of Staphylococcus organisms that are resistant to penicillin-like medications, such as Nafcillin, Kefzol, MRSA and Oxacillin. Once the culture and sensitivity results are back from the lab, then Nafcillin can be switched for the Vancomycin, assuming that the patient is not allergic to penicillin and that the organism is shown to be sensitive to the Nafcillin. Vancomycin is much more expensive than Nafcillin. When MRSA is suspected, one of the most effective treatments is Zyvox 600 mg twice per day by mouth. In addition to antibiotic treatment, proper fluid management, proper electrolyte management and antipyretic for fever and nasal oxygen must be included as part of the treatment.

Intravenous drug abusers must also be given medication such as methadone to forestall the development of drug withdrawal. Many drug addicts use alcohol to supplement their drug addiction needs. These patients, when acutely ill, must be watched closely for seizures, which, if they develop, can complicate the patient's overall clinical picture.

Treatment of liver disease in drug addicts is dictated by the clinical condition of the individual patient. If the drug addict presents with acute hepatitis, fever, chills, nausea, vomiting, abdominal pain and elevated liver function tests, the patient ought to be placed in isolation with hepatitis precautions being adhered to. In that setting, the prothrombin time is most important. That is so because the prothrombin time is a measure as to how well the liver is able to function. The sicker the liver, the higher the prothrombin time will be. If the prothrombin time is elevated, then 10 mg of Vitamin K IM ought to be given in the deltoid with applied pressure both as a test and as a treatment. The prothrombin time should be repeated 6–12 hours later. If the prothrombin time is corrected back to normal after the Vitamin K, it means that the patient still has good liver function left though the liver is tender and the liver tests are abnormal. Further, it also means that the patient though may have abnormal platelet count, and does not have DIC. Treatments with IV fluids, anti-fever medications such as Tylenol, anti-itching medication, anti-vomiting medication ought to be provided to control these particular symptoms. If the patient is not vomiting, is able to eat, and the prothrombin time is normal, it is advisable to treat the patients who have hepatitis at home while monitoring his or his vital signs and liver function tests.

Chronic liver disease, such as chronic active hepatitis and chronic persistent hepatitis, are treated either aggressively or supportively in a conservative way. In the case of chronic active hepatitis, treatment will be provided after liver biopsy and based on the symptoms of the patient and the findings on the liver biopsy. The most frequently used treatment for patients with chronic active hepatitis and symptoms of chronic active hepatitis with documented liver biopsy are alpha Interferon. The degree of inflammation seen in the liver biopsy documents the severity of the liver disease. In chronic persistent hepatitis there is minimal inflammation with no fibrosis in the liver and the liver tests are either slightly or moderately elevated chronically. In chronic lobular hepatitis there is mild to moderate inflammation and mild fibrosis. In chronic active hepatitis there is, as stated above, moderate severe inflammation and moderate to severe fibrosis of the liver.

Patients who abuse intravenous drugs can also develop acute hepatitis A because of intravenous drug use, though less so than hepatitis B and C, but it can occur. There are no chronic sequelae of hepatitis A. It is a good idea for patients who are chronic abusers of drugs to be vaccinated with the hepatitis virus A vaccine, which is available. The hepatitis A vaccine is given and it is repeated 6 months to 12 months later. That is because these individuals have the propensity to develop chronic liver disease because of hepatitis B or C and having hepatitis A can further decompensate the liver; the result could be catastrophic. It is also a good idea for individuals who are homosexuals and have the propensity to develop hepatitis through their sexual habits to be also given hepatitis A vaccination. Individuals who abuse drugs tend to get involved sometimes in prostitution as a means of getting money to pay for their drug habits. These individuals, therefore, are prone to contract sexually transmitted diseases such as hepatitis B and C, and receiving hepatitis A vaccination will prevent them from getting a new hepatitis infection, which can make their situation worse. As mentioned above, hepatitis A can be transmitted via blood and blood products, such as plasma, platelet concentrate, coagulation concentrate, and, in particular, individuals who have hemophilia who must, by necessity, receive blood products regularly, can be infected with hepatitis A, as well as hepatitis B, C, D, E and G.

Hepatitis B and C are more frequently transmitted via blood products and body fluids (sexually during sexual intercourse). About 200 million people in the world are carriers of hepatitis B and about 0.5% of the United States population are carriers of hepatitis B. About 80% to 90% of blood-borne hepatitis transmitted via blood transfusion is due to hepatitis C in the United States. About 4 million in the United States are infected with hepatitis C, and roughly 10,000 people die yearly in the United States due to complications of hepatitis C. Both chronic persistent and chronic active hepatitis can occur as because of hepatitis B, C, D, E and G. More often however, hepatitis B and C. cause most blood-borne hepatitis as we know it in the United States, and for that matter in the world, Chronic persistent hepatitis is manifested mainly by persistent mild to moderate elevation of liver function tests, such as bilirubin, SGOT, SGPT, alkaline phosphatase and the GGTP (gamma glutamine Trans peptidase). There are no major physical findings or symptoms. On the other hand, chronic active hepatitis is an active inflammatory liver disease with elevation of liver function tests, increased serum ferritin along with malaise, weakness, and anemia and sometime a palpable liver with right-sided abdominal pain and at times persistent low grade fever. Sometimes chronic active hepatitis goes on to develop cirrhosis of the liver with portal hypertension, hypersplenism, pancytopenia and esophageal varices. Once the esophageal varices develop, recurrent upper gastrointestinal bleeding can occur.

One of the many chronic complications of hepatitis B or C in these individuals who develop cirrhosis is hepatocellular carcinoma (cancer of the liver). This cancer in this setting occurs usually 10 to 30 years after the individual becomes sick with hepatitis.

Fulminant hepatitis with acute liver failure can occur with hepatitis A, B, C, D, E or G. Acute management of hepatitis includes supportive care, careful IV fluid management, careful monitoring of liver function tests, including the prothrombin times, platelets, red blood cells and serum ammonia level. Dietary management in acute hepatitis is very important, which includes a low-protein diet and low salt. Management of chronic liver disease also includes attention to diet with low protein, low salt, with close attention to liver function tests including the PT, platelet, red cell count and ammonia level. These individuals ought to be given anti-itching medications such as Benadryl, Periactin, etc. The reason for the itching is because the liver is too sick to be able to properly get rid of bile salts, and these bile salts accumulate in the blood, causing severe itching. It is also important that individuals who have chronic liver disease stay away from antiplatelet medications such as aspirin, and NSAIDS. It is also important not to give them Tylenol. Tylenol has the propensity to make the liver disease worse. In patients who have cirrhosis of the liver, regardless of the cause of their cirrhosis, one has to be very careful to prevent bleeding from the gastrointestinal tract from occurring, because any amount of blood placed in the GI tract will be broken down into protein by bacteria in the gut protein. Once blood is broken into protein, the broken down components of the protein, then enter into the ammonia pathway, which can result in an elevated level of blood ammonia. Elevated ammonia in the blood can cause the patient to become somnolent, confused at times, and if treated improperly can lead to the development of the comatose state. High ammonia level is treated with a low protein diet and Lactulose to induce diarrhea and cleanse the bowel of the stools that contain too much protein and other toxic waste matters.

Drug addicts can develop hepatitis, HIV/AIDS, cirrhosis of the liver, anemia, seizures, and a multitude of different infections as outlined, but above all, drug addiction is a chronic mental illness and ought to be recognized as such and treated accordingly.

After the diagnosis of hepatitis C in an individual is established, the physician ought to identify the genotype of the virus. That is usually followed by the RNA-PCR blood test along with the viral load and genotype. It is not always necessary to do liver biopsy, but because of the strong association of hepatitis C with hepato-cellular carcinoma of the liver (cancer of the liver), it is important to do an ultrasound of the abdomen, CAT scan of the abdomen and Alpha feto protein blood test as a baseline ought to be done. If the liver function blood tests are abnormal, then a liver biopsy ought to be considered They are many physicians who prefer to do liver biopsy in men who are infected with the hepatitis C to evaluate the extent of liver parenchymal damage or the absence there of before starting treatment. If the viral load and the clinical picture warrant it, then treatment with alpha interferon (Intron A) 3 times per week subcutaneously along with Ribavirin by mouth three times per day for 48 weeks.

More recently Pegylated Intron A once per week SQ is proven to be more tolerable by patients and is as effective in eradicating the hepatitis. Peg-Intron A is also used in combination with Ribavirin 200mg three times per day, by mouth, also for 48 weeks. More recently, Lamivudine, a medication used mainly to treat HIV infection, is being used to treat patients with hepatitis B infection with varying success.

In addition, drug addiction is a major psychiatric disease that affects the mind in a very significant way. Once addicted to drugs, these individuals are mentally dependent and emotionally dependent on the drugs and become very preoccupied with when and where they are going to find money for their next fix and they are entire preoccupied with is their drug activities. The behavior of men and men who are addicted to drugs is very irrational, particularly when they are under the influence of drugs. They lose complete control of their humanity; they will do anything under the influence of these drugs. Under the influence of drugs, men and men are capable of engaging in a multitude of immoral and illegal activities that have negative impacts on them, their families and society as a whole.

Individuals who are addicted to drugs are mentally dependent on these drugs. The addiction to drugs preoccupies them totally. Their humanities are no longer their own; their lives are controlled by the drugs that they are addicted to. They are constantly scheming, lying and committing crimes of different types to get money to buy the drugs that their brains crave. Getting the next fix to satisfy their craving is the most important thing in their lives because they have lost complete control of their beings. When under the influence of these drugs, they are capable of committing a multitude of illogical, irrational and illegal acts.

Drug addiction in men is a major problem in U.S. society, and it contributes to the destruction that occurs in the families of these men who fall victims to the awful power of drug addiction.

It is important for those in government to proactively undertake actions and create policies to get to the root causes of drug addiction problems in all their aspects. It is quite clear that present policies of building jails and throwing people in them and treating those people like animals are not working. You cannot treat a psychological medical problem with jail or "three strikes, you are out" policies. Many politicians, district attorneys and judges designed policies to deal with drug addicts that are popular with the electorate to get them elected at the expense of the people who are suffering from mental, medical and physical problems of drug addiction … People who commit crimes ought to receive appropriate punishment for the crimes they committed. While in jail, treatments for their drug addiction and its associated problems ought to be provided to them. They should be given a real chance of rehabilitating themselves and they ought to be taught trades of different types that would enable them to be wage earners once they have completed their sentences and return to Society. It is also important to realize that once a drug addict, always a drug addict and, that being the case, long-term psychological treatment ought to be made available to these individuals after they have left jail.

It is very costly to provide treatments for drug addicts. It is important that drug addiction treatments include prevention programs and educational programs. Programs to prevent the dissemination of drugs within the communities where those men live are very important. The federal and state governments need to spend the billions of dollars that are necessary to fund those programs to help them to become successful. It is important that drug addiction seminars begin at the earliest grades in schools across the country, so that children can be made aware of drug addiction and the ravages that it can cause to the human body and mind. It is important to let them know what the facts really are, so that when people approach them trying to get them involved in drugs, they can say "no." As it is right now, the incidence of drug addiction in schools across the country is high and begins at the earliest age, in elementary school up through middle school and high school. It is crucial that the educational system join forces with the government agencies to try to encourage drug prevention and drug education programs in elementary schools, middle schools and high schools. According to recent reports close to 25% of college students abuse drugs and alcohol.. It is wrong, but they are at an age where they can make their own decisions. They also should be encouraged to give up drug use or not to start at all, because once a person starts using drugs, it is very difficult to give it up because drug addiction is so overwhelming that these individuals are weakened by the force of the addiction. The colleges also ought to organize drug prevention seminars on their campuses for the benefit of students and faculty, and most definitely confidential drug treatment programs ought to be offered and must be made easily available for college students who are using illicit drugs, to help them give up their habits. It is hypocritical to sweep it under the carpet and pretend that it does not exist.

To help individuals who are addicted to drugs, it requires money, it requires better governmental involvement, and it requires better involvement of the educators, the clergy, and other members of society working as a team to attack that scourge that is destroying significant numbers of people in society.

CHAPTER 18

OSTEOPOROSIS IN MEN

OSTEOPOROSIS IS A DISEASE THAT causes softening of bones, resulting in fractures. The bones become soft due to decrease in bone mass. When looking under the microscope at a bone in a person suffering from osteoporosis, what is seen is a decrease in what is called cortical thickness of the bone and in the numbers the trabeculae of cancerous bones.

There are 36.6 million Americans with osteopenia, 80% of the are women 20% of the are men or 6,72 million men.

According to the National Institute of Health, osteoporosis affects about 10 million Americans over age 50 and 34 million are at risk to develop osteoporosis.

Osteoporosis is more common in Whites and Asians than in Blacks, Hispanics and other races. This is so in part because the bone structure of Blacks, Hispanics and other races is stronger. The bony structures most often fractures in individuals with osteoporosis are the wrist, the hip and the spine.

The fragile bone fractures associated with osteoporosis amount to about 1.5 million per year in the USA. Between the ages of 40 and 50 years, cortical bone loss is somewhere in the range of 0.2% to 0.5% per year in men. The loss of bone mass per year in some men ranges anywhere from about 40% to 50%. Men tend to lose bone much later than women do. The difference in the incidence of osteoporosis in men of color versus White men and Asian seems to be due to the fact that men of color have higher bone minerals than white men, hence the lesser incidence of osteoporosis seen in men of color.

The annual costs to treat the fractures and other complications of osteoporosis are 18 billion dollars.

There are different causes of osteoporosis:

1. Men who smoke have a higher incidence of osteoporosis as opposed to men who do not smoke.
2. Decrease bone formation due to alcohol abuse can cause osteoporosis.
3. Low dietary calcium consumption can cause osteoporosis.
4. Vitamin D deficiency causes osteoporosis.
5. Lack of exercise can cause osteoporosis.
6. There are certain genetic factors that can interfere with proper Vitamin D absorption, which can cause osteoporosis to develop.
7. If heparin is used for a long period, it can cause osteoporosis.
8. Chronic use of steroids can cause osteoporosis

Many medical conditions are associated with the development of osteoporosis:

1. Osteogenesis imperfecta
2. Cushing syndrome
3. Thyrotoxicosis
4. Calcium deficiency
5. Systemic mastocytosis
6. Rheumatoid arthritis
7. Scurvy
8. Malabsorption
9. Primary hyperparathyroidism

There is a form of osteoporosis called idiopathic, which occurs in children and adolescents of both sexes. The two most common forms of osteoporosis are Type I Osteoporosis, which occurs in a group of postmenopausal women between the ages of 51 and 75. It causes loss of trabecular bones, and fractures of vertebral body and distal forearm are quite common. Type II osteoporosis is seen in men over the age of 70 and these men suffer frequently from fractures of the femoral neck, proximal humeral, proximal tibia and pelvis. Collapse of vertebral bodies frequently occurs, resulting in kyphosis, scoliosis and other deformities as these men get older, and fractures of the hips are quite common, as well.

Many cancers may be associated with osteoporosis, bone pain and vertebrae fractures. Among these cancers are the following:

1. Multiple myeloma
2. Leukemia

3. Lymphoma
4. Metastatic cancer to bones

Multiple myeloma is the most common cancer that is associated with osteopenia/osteoporosis. To diagnose multiple myeloma using x-rays, skeletal survey is the most accurate. Bone scan is the most sensitive test to diagnose metastatic cancer to the bones. Plain x-ray study is the best test to diagnose multiple myeloma, because multiple myeloma causes an osteolytic process. Bone scan is the best test for metastatic cancer to the bones because metastatic cancer to bone is an osteoblastic process. MRI of bones will show cancer in bones, in both osteolytic and osteoblastic processes. However, MRI is an expensive test and is not routinely done to diagnose cancer to the bones, but is done when either the bone scan or the plain x-rays are not definitive.

Another common disease that causes osteoporosis is primary hyperparathyroidism. The reason why primary hyperparathyroidism is associated with osteoporosis is bone resorption.

The bleaching of calcium from the bone causes the bone to become soft and painful, and because the bones are soft, they break easily, resulting in even more pain.

Still, another more common cause of osteoporosis is steroid treatment. Steroid treatment has many major and minor side effects, and prominent among these side effects is osteoporosis. Among the reasons why steroid treatment causes osteoporosis is the fact that it reduces calcium absorption from gastrointestinal tract and increases calcium loss in the urine. As calcium is lost in the urine, the bones become calcium deficient, which ultimately causes soft bones (osteoporosis).

Non-men of color weighing in the 127-pound range are roughly two times more likely to have fractures of the hip, pelvis and ribs, as compared to non-men of color whose weight is in the 161-pound range.

Bone density measurement is the best test to diagnose osteoporosis. That is a painless test, which is quite accurate in diagnosing bone loss of different degrees.

In addition to the bone density study, regular bone x-ray is capable of showing osteopenia/osteoporosis and different degrees of fractures that occur because of osteoporosis.

The following are two examples of osteoporosis as seen on x-rays:

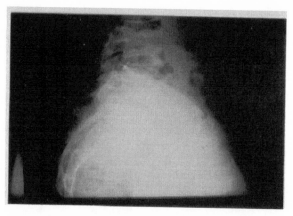

Figure 18.1—Plain x-ray of the lumbar spine of a white person with osteoporosis; multiple wedge compression on osteoporosis with mark osteopenia at L1, L2, L3 and L4.

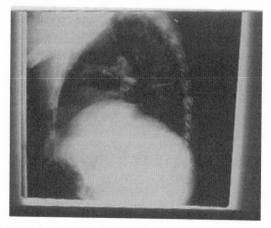

Figure 18.2—Plain x-ray of the thoracic spine of a white individual with osteoporosis; multiple wedge compression on osteoporosis with mark osteopenia at T9, T10, T11 and T12.

An adult needs to take in 1200 mg of calcium daily in a diet, in order to be in calcium balance and 600 IU of vitamin D per day to be in vitamin D balance.

Prevention of osteoporosis is extremely important to avoid the complications of osteoporosis and its associated morbidities and mortality.

Diet plays a major role in the prevention of osteoporosis. Milk and other dairy products such as cheese, yogurt is very good to eat to prevent osteoporosis because they contain calcium. Other foods that contain calcium include beans, egg yolk, kale, cauliflower, chard, molasses, rhubarb, beets, almonds, cabbage, bran, carrots, celery, dates, chocolate, figs, lettuce, lemons, oranges, oysters, pineapples, raspberries, hell fish, spinach, walnuts, watercress and parsnips, among others. While several of the aforementioned do have good calcium source, it must be kept in mind that because some of them are very rich in cholesterol, they must be consumed in moderation. Some of these cholesterol-rich foods are milk, cheese, egg yolk, oysters, shellfish etc. It is a good idea to consume skim milk, as well as cheese made with skim milk, to decrease the amount of cholesterol intake.

Vitamin D is the most important vitamin needed for the absorption of calcium in the human body. Some of the food products that contain Vitamin D are milk, salmon, egg yolk, butterfat and cod liver oil. The human skin contains a substance called ergo sterol, and sunlight, as well as ultraviolet radiation, activates that substance, which leads to the production of Vitamin D, hence, the importance of sunlight exposure. Vitamin D deficiency causes osteoporosis, rickets, caries and a multitude of possible other skeletal malformations. Exercise plays a major role in the prevention of osteoporosis.

Treatments of osteoporosis

Medications that are available in the USA to treat osteoporosis include:
1. Fosamax
2. Actonel
3. Evista
4. Boniva
5. Miacalcin
6. Oscal with Vitamin D 500 IU
7. Vitamin D 600 IU daily.

The National Academy of Sciences, in 2002, recommended the daily intake of Vitamin D to be:

0–50 years 200 IU/day (International Unit)

51–70 years 400–600 IU/day

71 years and older 600–800 IU/day

and the National Academy of Sciences in 2002 also recommended the following daily intake of calcium:

0–6months	200 mg/day
7–12 months	270 mg/day
1–3years	500 mg/day
4–8 years	800 mg/day

9–18 years	1,300 mg/day
19–50 years	1000 mg/day
51 years and older	1,200 mg/day
72 years and older	1,200mg/day

Exercise is important in both the prevention and treatment of osteoporosis. Among the most effective exercises that good for osteoporosis are:

Jumping rope

Stair climbing

Dancing

Walking

Jugging

Running

Hiking

Soccer

Weight lifting

Tennis

Racquetball

Swimming etc;

It is important to understand the different causes of osteoporosis and knowing.

It is also important to know the different subgroup of individuals who have a predisposition and a higher propensity to the development of osteoporosis. Regular exercise and eating a vitamin D and calcium rich diet is highly recommended to prevent osteoporosis. For those men who have osteoporosis medications are available to treat this problem and prevent fractures and the many debilitating side effects of osteoporosis.

CHAPTER 19

LUNG DISEASES IN MEN

THE MOST FREQUENT LUNG DISEASES that men suffer from are as follows:

1. Asthma
2. Chronic Obstructive Pulmonary Disease (COPD)
3. Emphysema
4. Pneumonia
5. Acute bronchitis
6. Pulmonary embolism
7. Lung cancer
8. Primary pulmonary hypertension

About 17.7 million people in the U.S. suffer from asthma and 4,487 individuals died in the years 2000–2001 of asthma in the U.S. There are 10.5 million men with asthma in the U.S. In the year 2000, a total of 2,855 men died of asthma. About half of asthma cases develop before age 10 and about one-third of asthma cases develop before age 40. Most cases of allergic asthma begin in early childhood and frequently are associated with family history of asthma, rhinitis, eczema, hay fever, bronchitis and emphysema. The other common form of asthma is called idiosyncratic asthma, meaning that the individuals who suffer with that type of asthma have no family history of asthma and no history of hay fever, negative skin types were tested, and there is normal IgE level in their blood.

There is still another group of men with a mixed picture, with features of both allergic asthma and idiosyncratic asthma.

What happens in asthma that causes the asthmatic patient to have trouble in breathing is that the bronchioles inside the lungs become obstructed to different degrees, because of being exposed to either one of several irritants. Bronchioles are tube-like structures that are located inside the lungs through which air is channeled in and out the lungs. The irritants that affect the inside of the bronchioles cause swelling, inflammation and secretion of mucoid-like materials to develop. The result is that air gets trapped inside the bronchioles, resulting in shortness of breath, wheezing, marked difficulty in breathing and a feeling of an impending doom.

The wheezing sound that is heard when an asthmatic breathes is due to air fighting to get through the narrow passages that have been created by mucous plug, edema, and swelling inside the bronchioles. The inflammation that occurs at the cellular level is mediated by T lymphocytes that secrete type 2 T-helper cytokines like interleukins 4, 5, and 13. Interleukin 4 and 13 regulate the production of IgE. High-affinity IgE receptor on mast cells mediates the release of histamine, prostaglandins, leukotrienes and inflammatory cytokines, along with interleukins 5 mediation of eosinophils, result in an overall inflammatory process that starts off the asthmatic attack.

Acute asthma attacks can be brought on by a multitude of factors; some are allergenic, environmental, infectious, occupational, and pharmacological and some are emotional.

The most frequent form of allergic asthma is seasonal and is associated with hay fever and pollens. Other allergens that can precipitate acute asthma attacks are such things as animal dander, feathers, dust, mites, molds, paints, roaches, mice, rats and exposure to cats and dogs. Exercise and, in particular, breathing cold air can precipitate an acute asthmatic attack. It is believed that the high incidence of asthma seen in poor communities is the result of the poor living conditions associated with poverty. Many of these individuals live in poorly ventilated, roach-and rat-infested apartments. The high level of crime seen in these communities' forces those who live there to stay behind closed doors to shield themselves from the daily problems associated with living in these communities and under these conditions.

Roaches carry over their body's irritants and materials that get carried by the air which when breathed by the asthmatics, precipitate asthmatic attacks. Rats and mice which live in these apartments, no doubt, leave droppings that, when they get airborne, they also can be inhaled and participate in bringing about most asthmatic attacks. All the things outlined allergens, when inhaled, can precipitate asthmatic attacks.

Environmental factors associated with high incidence of asthma are seen in industrial areas where factories and industrial machines emit sulfur dioxide and nitrogen oxide combining with air, which, when breathed, causes pulmonary diseases of different types, including asthma. Upper airway infection is the most commonly associated precipitating factor triggering asthma attacks. The common infections that frequently precipitate asthmatic attacks are the common cold, which is brought on by rhinoviruses and parainfluenza viruses in adolescents, adults and in young children.

Other infections that can trigger acute asthmatic attacks are respiratory syncytial virus, bacterial infections, such as bacterial bronchitis, bacterial pneumonia, and bacterial sinusitis are all associated with the precipitation of asthmatic attacks. Different types of viral sinusitis, viral bronchitis, and viral pneumonias are also frequently associated with the precipitation of asthmatic attacks.

Occupational exposure plays a major role in both the causation and in the precipitation of asthma. The lists of precipitating materials that men can be exposed to that can cause asthmatic attacks are almost endless. Some of the known industrial materials that are associated with the causation and precipitation of asthma attacks are laundry detergents, different types of fumes, coffee beans, nickel, and platinum dust, etc.

A multitude of pharmacology product drugs, when used by asthmatic men, can bring on an asthmatic attack. Some of the most common drugs that can set off an asthmatic attack are aspirin, beta-blockers, and some coloring medications, such as red dye number 3, and sulfur medications. There is a syndrome of asthma, nasal polyps and aspirin allergy. Some of these men can also have a similar reaction when they ingest NSAIDs.

It is, therefore, always prudent to ask these folks the question, "Are you allergic to aspirin or NSAIDs or have ever taken those medications before with no problem?" before prescribing them for any man who suffers with asthma.

Another common precipitant of asthmatic attacks is exercise. Exercise-induced asthmatic attack seems to be associated with the coldness of the air being breathed in. It is, therefore, not a good idea for asthmatics to participate in sports such as skiing, ice-skating and ice hockey. Sports activity where the air is warm is fine. If an asthmatic man wishes to participate in these activities, he would be wise to get advice from his physician as to what to do to prepare his to partake in them.

Another frequent trigger of asthmatics is emotional stress. The mechanism for that form of asthmatic attack precipitant is not altogether clear, but the overall mental turmoil associated with stress is capable of triggering an asthma attack.

Symptoms of asthma

The most frequent symptoms of asthma are as follows:
1. Shortness of breath
2. Wheezing
3. Coughing spells, and
4. A feeling of impending doom
5. Rapid heart rate

Before starting the evaluation, quickly listen to the lungs for air movement and the heart to check the rate and the rhythm of the heart, and give his nasal oxygen and an injection of epinephrine subcutaneously. Now proceed with the evaluation.

How to evaluate a person presenting with an asthma attack:
1. First the physician must take a history from the patient to find out several things.
2. It is important to watch how the patient is breathing.
3. Does he have labored breathing?
4. It is important to watch how the patient is speaking.
5. Can he hold a sentence and for how long?
6. How does he look?
7. Does he look tired?
8. Ask the question how many hours ago did the attack start?
9. What medication did he take before presenting?
10. Are the nasal passages stuffed up?
11. Is he coughing up sputum?
12. If yes, what color is the sputum—whitish, yellowish, or greenish or bloody?
13. Does he have a fever, chills or body aches?
14. Ask whether he has just been exposed to any of the possible irritants outlined in the preceding paragraphs.

Then quickly do a peak flow, using the breathing meter. Try to ascertain the patient's previous known base peak flow. Do an arterial blood gas to determine whether he is retaining carbon dioxide or not. If so, quickly prepare for possible intubation of the patient to secure the airway, to prevent sudden respiratory arrest. Get a good IV line started to provide medications such as fluid and steroid. Start Alupent nebulizer treatment immediately and continue these treatments every 4–6 hours until the patient is better. Steroid is the backbone and most effective treatment in asthma, but it takes about 6 hours before it starts to work. Get a chest x-ray; look for pneumonia, bronchitis, congestive heart failure and pneumothorax which, if present, will complicate the patient's management. As part of the ER evaluation of the asthmatic patient, a CBC and SMA20 chemistry profile ought to be done. The decision as to whether to admit the patient who presents with an asthmatic attack depends on how the patient looks clinically, how good the peak flow is, and how improved is the examination of the lungs.

If after several hours in the ER with significant and appropriate treatments having been provided without significant improvement in the overall clinical state of the patient, then the patient ought to be admitted for treatments that are more prolonged. An improved peak flow is good objective evidence that the asthmatic patient has gotten better. One of the controversial issues of the treatment of acute asthma associated with upper airway infection is whether to add antibiotics, either by mouth or intravenously. Some respected experts in infectious diseases say, "Don't use antibiotics because the organisms responsible for the infection are viruses," yet there are some who say, "Yes, antibiotics ought to be used." The reason given is that the inflammation that the viral infection causes breaks down the protective membranes within the lining of the upper airway. Once the protective membranes are broken down, local bacteria proliferate, resulting in a superimposed mixed bacterial-viral upper airway infection, precipitating and complicating the asthmatic attack. Even when the upper airway of the asthmatic is irritated with a noxious material, the resulting inflammation can cause the protective membranes to lose their integrity, allowing the bacteria that live in the upper airway to set up an acute asthmatic attack, requiring antibiotic treatment.

The way to diagnose asthma is by:

1. The history
2. Physical examination
3. The chest x-ray and
4. The FEV (forced expiratory volume in 1 second), after administration of 2 puffs of a beta-adrenergic medication and showing that the airway obstruction has been reversed by 15% or greater increase in the FEV. Examination of the chest of the asthmatic patient usually demonstrates different types of wheezes, both inspiratory and expiratory wheezes. Shortness of breath with a fast respiratory rate (normal respiratory 15–20 per minute), the heart rate/pulse rate is fast, 100 or greater per minute. Frequently, the patient uses his abdominal muscles to help to breathe. The chest x-ray shows hyperinflated lungs in asthmatic patients.

Treatment of asthma

Some of the medications used to treat asthma:

1. Alupent inhaler
2. Epinephrine 0.3–0.5 ml. of 1:1000 solution subcutaneously
3. Proventil inhaler
4. Bronchodilators in aerosol solution 0.4%-0.6%
5. Xopenex
6. Salmeterol inhaler
7. Advair Diskus
8. Asmanex
9. Atrovent inhaler
10. Ventolin inhaler
11. Maxair inhaler,
12. Theo-Dur
13. Singulair etc;

    Anti-inflammatory medications in use to treat asthma include:

a. Beclomethasone inhaler
b. Intravenous steroid
c. Azmacort-2 puffs, 3x per day
d. Cromolyn sodium inhaler (non-steroid)
e. Vanceril inhaler
f. Flovent inhaler, etc.
g. Zileuton tablets
h. Montelukast tablets
i. Zafirlukast tablets

Asthma is a chronic inflammatory lung disease and, as such, requires different types of medications working via different mechanisms to treat it both acutely and chronically. One of the most common medications used to treat asthma are steroids. Different types of steroid preparations are used to treat asthma—intravenously, by mouth, or via inhalation technique. Frequently used intravenous steroids in the treatment of acute asthmatic attacks are Solu-Medrol, Decadron and Solu-Cortef. Different irritants, when inhaled, cause an acute inflammatory reaction to occur within the bronchioles (tubes that carry air through the lungs).

Steroid works to decrease that inflammatory reaction, thereby preventing the swelling, mucus production, and spasm within the bronchioles, tissues and other tubes inside the lungs. The spasm and the mucus plugs that occur within the bronchioles prevent air flow from getting in and getting out of the lungs.

The different medications used to treat asthma decrease the spasm, the inflammation and the production of mucus, allowing air to move easier within the lungs, relieving the acute symptoms. In 1996, 10.2 million adults in the U.S. were affected by asthma, according to *the Self-Reported Asthma Prevalence among Adults, U.S. 2000.*

In 1998, the direct and indirect cost of asthma in the U.S. was 12.7 billion dollars. The incidence of asthma is higher in Blacks and Hispanics than Whites: 8.5%. in Blacks vs. 7.1% in Whites. The incidence among other races is 5.6%, and more women suffer from asthma than men: 9.1% vs. 5.1% (Source: CDC, MMWR, 2001; 50: 62.2.686). In addition to medications, removing asthmatic males from high-risk environments to pollutant-free environments will decrease the overall incidence of asthma in men.

COPD is a combination of chronic bronchitis and emphysema or a combination of chronic bronchitis with asthma or emphysema with bronchiolitis.

COPD is fourth leading cause of death in the US after heart disease, stroke and cancer.

There are more than 10 million individuals with COPD in the US and roughly 14 million others with symptoms of COPD.

The direct annual cost of COPD is 14.7 billion dollars and the indirect cost is 15.7 billion dollars annually.

The most common symptoms of COPD are dyspnea, fatigue, cough, anxiety, and depression and sleep disorder.

The tests available to diagnose COPD are Chest X-ray and Pulmonary Function Test.

Emphysema and Chronic Obstructive Pulmonary Disease in Men in The US: Adult men in the U.S. who smoke by age and level of education are as follows:

Age 18 to 24	31.5 percent
25 to 44	30.3 percent
45 to 64	27.7 percent
65 and older	14.6 percent
White men who smoke	26.8 percent
Black men who smoke	30.4 percent
Hispanic men who smoke	26.8 percent
American Indian/Alaskan Native men who smoke	38. 1percent
Asian/Pacific/Islander men who smoke	17.9 percent

38.4% of men with less than high education smoke cigarettes.
48.4% of men with GED diploma smoke cigarettes.

30.9% of men with high school diploma smoke cigarettes.

13.9% of men with college education smoke cigarettes.

9.1% of men with master degree, doctorate and medical degree1 smoke cigarettes.

Source: National Center For health Statistics February 7, 2003, Center for Disease Control& Prevention.

Cigarette smoking is the number-one cause of lung disease and emphysema in men. There are two general forms of emphysema: one form is the pink puffer and the other form is the blue blotter. The pink puffer type is the so-called dried emphysema. It is called dried emphysema because men with pink puffer cough a lot but no sputum comes up. These individuals are called pink puffers because they breathe with a pursed lip to force the air into their lungs and their lips look puffed. In addition, they have barreled chests and they are usually thin in stature. Another distinct feature that differentiates pink puffers from blue blotters is that pink puffers usually do not retain carbon dioxide because they are continuously puffing it out. On the other hand, blue blotter emphysema patients are usually obese; they cough up copious amount of sputum, their lips are blue and retain carbon dioxide. The toxic effects of the tobacco that the smokers inhale, damage the substance of the lungs, resulting in a multitude of anatomical abnormalities, causing trapping of air. It is the trapping of air and the stiffness of the lung that cause the patients with emphysema so much difficulty in breathing. Frequently, men with emphysema develop right-sided heart disease, complicating their overall cardiopulmonary state. The incidence of tobacco use increased significantly in men in the last 40 years, and the result is that lung diseases of different types and severity have increased accordingly. Prominent among these lung diseases are chronic bronchitis, asthma, lung cancer and frequent pneumonia. Because the inner lining of the lungs are damaged by the effects of tobacco, bacterial growth is favored and frequent lung infections develop which can lead to different degrees of respiratory decompositions. Very often, when men with emphysema develop pneumonia, the respiratory system becomes decomposed, resulting in the need for the individuals to be placed on the respirator. The incidence of adult respiratory distress syndrome (ARDS) increases in men who smoke.

In the year 2007, 114,760 men will be diagnosed with lung cancer and 89,510 men will die of lung cancer during that same year. Lung diseases in men are associated with air pollution, exposure to industrial pollutants, tobacco smoking, exposure to asbestos, etc. Exposure to asbestos can lead to the development of a type of cancer called mesothelioma. Characteristic of asbestosis of the lungs is calcification of the lining of the lungs. Emphysema frequently results in end-stage lung disease. End-stage lung disease causes right ventricular heart failure, distended neck veins, swollen abdomen, swollen lower legs, large liver and cardiac arrhythmias of different types, which contributes, often times, to the death of affected men.

Exposure to several other noxious materials is also known to cause damage to the lungs that can lead to chronic pulmonary disease (COPD) in men. One well-known example is coal miner's lung disease. Other examples include exposure to inhalation of cotton fibers by men who work in cotton mills; a similar lung disease can develop in men who work in sugar cane fields/factories.

There is a genetically transmitted disease called alpha-1-antitrypsin deficiency, which can also cause emphysema in men who carry the abnormal gene.

How to evaluate men with emphysema/COPD

The first thing to do is to take a good history from the man to ascertain his symptoms and what kind of noxious materials or environment to which he may have been exposed. It is important to find if he smokes tobacco, if it is via cigarettes, cigars or pipe. What type of work he does? If he does not smoke, it is important to find out whether his husband, boyfriend or significant other, with whom he is frequently in close contact, smokes tobacco. It is also important to find out if he is exposed to tobacco smoke from his co.-workers on the job. The next thing to do is to carry out a complete physical examination, paying close attention to the following:

1. Is he very thin?
2. Is he fat?
3. Is he short of breath?
4. Is he constantly coughing?
5. Is the cough dry or productive of sputum?
6. Is his lips blue or pink?
7. Does he purse his lips when he breathes or not?
8. How hard is his breathing?
9. Can he carry a sentence through without stopping to catch his breath?
10. Is he using accessory abdominal muscles to help to breathe?
11. Does he have clubbed fingers?
12. On listening to his lungs, how well is he moving air? Are there rales or

13. Are wheezes heard in his lungs?
14. On listening to the heart, are the heart sounds distant? Are the heart sounds heard best below the breastbone? Is the heart rhythm regular or irregular?

In men who have the dried type emphysema (pink puffer), the heart sounds are distant and very difficult to hear and the air movement is difficult to hear, as well. The best way to hear the heartbeats in these men is below the breastbone area. That is so because in that type of emphysema, the position of the heart is shifted to that area.

The heart frequently beats irregularly in emphysema patients because of an abnormal rhythm called atrial fibrillation. Another abnormal rhythm such as premature atrial and ventricular contraction is also quite common in patients with emphysema/COPD.

These cardiac abnormalities occur because of a combination of lung and heart malfunctions that emphysema causes. Rales are heard in listening to lungs because of heart failure, which causes fluid to accumulate within the lungs. The most common chamber of the heart that fails in men who have emphysema/COPD is the right ventricle. When the right ventricle fails, the bulk of the work is left to the left ventricle, which ultimately fails as well, resulting in biventricular failure.

After the history and physical examinations are completed, several tests have to be done to document the fact the patient does have emphysema. The first test to do is a chest x-ray, followed by an arterial blood gas and pulmonary function test.

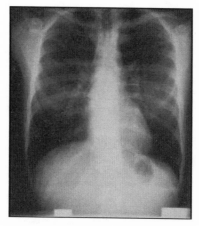

Figure 19.1—Normal chest X-ray in non-smoking female

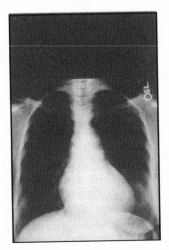

Figure 19.2—Abnormal chest X-ray in male smoker with emphysema

Frequently both arterial blood gas and the pulmonary function tests are abnormal in COPD patients.

The Medications available to treat COPD/Emphysema are in many instances similar to that of asthma.
The most frequently used medications in COPD/Emphysem
Advair Diskus
Ventolin
Atrovent
Spiriva
Nebulizer treatment
Steroid
Antibiotics
Oxygen etc,
When emphysema is discovered in a non-smoker with no exposure to secondary tobacco smoke and no exposure to industrial air pollution, etc., it is likely to be due to a hereditary condition known as alpha-1-antitrypsin deficiency.

There is a commercial blood test available to test for alpha-1-antitrypsin level in the blood.

Men with chronic bronchitis/emphysema/COPD develop infection in the lungs very frequently, as well as infection of the upper airway. The very nature of that disease predisposes these men to those infections.

Frequently, these infections are mixed infections, associated with more than one bacterial organism causing the infection. Frequently, these upper airway infections start out with viral URI and become complicated with a secondary bacterial infection. Any infection affecting the airway of men with chronic bronchitis/emphysema/COPD usually causes their pulmonary status to become decompensated, resulting in difficulty of breathing and anoxia. If the infection in the upper airway is not treated early and aggressively with antibiotic, the result oftentimes is the development of pneumonia.

Pneumonia and its complications are frequently the cause of death of individuals who suffer from chronic bronchitis/emphysema/COPD. The effects of tobacco smoking and other inhaled toxins damage the tissues of the lungs, and the chronic nature of these diseases places these individuals in an immuno-suppressed state, which predisposes them to the development of pulmonary infections of different types and severity.

The organisms that most frequently cause pneumonia in men with emphysema/COPD are the following:
> Haemophilus influenzae
> Haemophilus parainfluenzae
> Streptococcus pneumonia
> Moraxella catarrhalis
> Klebsiella pneumoniae
> Serratia marcescens
> Pseudomonas
> Staphylococcus aureus etc;

Different viruses and different fungi also can cause pneumonia in these individuals.

How to evaluate a patient with emphysema for pneumonia

The first thing to do is to take a good history from the patient. Ask him: Are you coughing and for how many days? Is the cough productive? What is the color of the sputum? Is the sputum yellow, green, dark green, bloody, or whitish? Do you have a fever? Are you having chills? Does your chest hurt when you cough? Are you having headaches? Is your nose stuffed? Do you have a runny nose? Do you have generalized body aches and pain? Who else is sick in your household? Do you have birds in the house? Have you traveled recently out of the country or to other states in the USA? Do you have night sweats? Have you lost weight? Do you have poor appetite? The next thing to do is a physical examination.

When a physician suspects pneumonia in a patient, the most important parts of the physical examination are as follows:

1. The respiratory rate: Is it greater than 20?
2. The pulse rate: Is it 100 or greater?
3. Is the blood pressure normal or is it abnormally low?
4. Is the patient using abdominal muscle to help in breathing?
5. Does the patient look pale? Is the skin warm and moist?
6. How sick does the patient look?
7. Is the temperature below 98.6°F or 100.4°F or greater?
8. How fast is the heart rate?
9. How do the lungs sound?
10. Is the patient moving air well?
11. Are there pneumonia sounds (rales) in the lungs? If so, where are they located in the lungs?
12. Is the patient wheezing?

Once the physical examination is completed, the next step is look at the chest x-ray. Are there infiltrates in the lung fields? What do those infiltrates look like? What does the arterial blood gas look like? Is the patient hypoxic (low oxygen)? In the case of the patient with emphysema, is he retaining carbon dioxide? If so how much? Is the patient producing sputum? What is the color of the sputum? Is it yellow? Is it green? Is it bloody? Alternatively, is it whitish? Alternatively, is it a mixture of all these colors?

Once the physical examination has been completed, the next thing to do is to order some tests. The most appropriate tests to order are the following:

1. Chest x-ray
2. ABG
3. Pulmonary Function Test
4. EKG
5. CBC
6. Chemistry profile (SMA 20)
7. 2 sets of blood cultures
8. Sputum gram stain
9. Sputum culture and sensitivity

Once these tests have been ordered, treatment for pneumonia in Emphysema/COPD can be started.

1. The type of IV fluid that is given to these patients depends on the level of dehydration that the patient presents with. Usually Dextrose

with normal saline or health normal saline, either alone or with dextrose at a reasonable rate of 125 cc per hour can be started. If the patient is a diabetic, ½ normal saline or normal saline can be given at the same rate.

2.   Oxygen can be given via nasal canals of 2–3 liters per minute in patients who have pneumonia and no emphysema. If the patient has emphysema/COPD and pneumonia, it is best to give oxygen via venti-mask, to prevent too much oxygen from being administered, since, in a patient who is suffering from emphysema, such as a blue blotter who retains carbon dioxide, too much oxygen can cause more carbon dioxide to be retained. The higher the level of carbon dioxide in the body, the sicker he becomes. If that high concentration of carbon dioxide is allowed to persist, several major complications, including inability of the heart and brain to function properly, can develop. Frequently, patients with emphysema who have pneumonia develop respiratory failure, necessitating placement on the respirator for breathing assistance. The next step is to administrate antibiotics intravenously. If the patient comes from home, then a protocol that provides antibiotic coverage for community-acquired pneumonia is put into place. Examples of the intravenous antibiotics that can be used are the following:

    a.   Ceftriaxone, 1 or 2 grams every 24 hours, or
    b.   Levaquin, 500 mg. IV every 24 hours, or
    c.   Penicillin G, 10 to 20 million units daily in divided doses of IV, or
    d.   Ampicillin, 2–4 grams every 6 hours IV or,
    e.   In penicillin-allergic patients, Cipro, 400 mg. IV daily, or
    f.   Erythromycin, 500 mg. IV every 6 hours or
    g.   Tequin, 400 mg IV

Even though the patient is coming from the community, the health profile of the patient determines whether the patient gets started on one or more antibiotics. The types of work the patient does for a living, as well, where the patient may have been prior to getting sick, also determines whether he gets started on one or more antibiotics and what type of antibiotics are used to start treatment. Erythromycin is an excellent antibiotic to use, especially in the setting where atypical pneumonia and organisms such as legionella is suspected. Once the result of sputum gram stain/culture is back, antibiotic treatment is adjusted according to the results of these two tests.

Men who are coming from a nursing home or who are in the hospital, and who develop pneumonia, are treated with different antibiotics, because bacterial organisms such as pseudomonas and staphylococcus for which specific antibiotics are required for treatment, frequently colonize these men. The best antibiotic to use to treat pseudomonas is Ceftazidime and the best antibiotic to use to treat staphylococcus is Vancomycin. Examples of IV antibiotics that can be used to treat hospitalized patients with pneumonia and their usual doses are as follows:

1. Ceftriaxone, 1–2 grams IV every 12 to 24 hours
2. Cefotaxime, 1–2 grams IV every 8–12 hours
3. Cefuroxime, 750 mg IV every 8 hours
4. Cipro, 400 mg IV every 24 hours
5. Erythromycin, 500 mg IV or by mouth every 6 hours
6. Imipenem, 500 ml IV every 6 hours
7. Nafcillin, 2 grams IV every 4–6 hours
8. Penicillin G, 2 million units every 6 hours IV
9. Vancomycin, 1 gram IV every 12 hours
10. Flagyl, 500 ml IV every 6 hours
11. Clindamycin, 600 ml IV every 8 hours
12. Levaquin, 500 ml IV once per day
13. Ceftazidime, 1gram IV every 8 hours
14. Tequin, 400mg IV every 24 hours
15. Bactrim DS, one tablet 2 times per day or IV Bactrim when the situation calls for it.

In the office setting, Levaquin, Tequin, Zithromax, Cipro, and Bactrim DS can be a single antibiotic, to treat appropriate men for pulmonary infection.

Other medications that are used to treat patients with pneumonia and emphysema include: steroid IV or by mouth; Ventolin inhaler; Albuterol inhaler Alupent treatment; Maxair inhaler; Serevent; Flovent; and Singulair by mouth, etc. together with oxygen, IV fluid, cough syrup and pulmonary toilet.

Viral pneumonia is treated with IV steroid, Alupent treatment, IV fluid, oxygen; cough syrup, and pulmonary toilet. In patients with chronic lung disease and viral pneumonia, broad-spectrum antibiotics must be added to their treatments to cover for the possibility of secondary bacterial infection which inevitably always becomes part of the pulmonary infection. If it is determined that the clinical picture is that of pure viral pneumonia, then the antibiotics can be stopped.

That determination can sometime be made through viral titers.

As for fungal infection of the lung, that diagnosis is more appropriately established with specimen taken during bronchoscopic examination with biopsy/brushing, then treatment can be started with Amphotericin B or Fluconazole. Pneumocystis carinii pneumonia (PCP) is more commonly seen in patients with AIDS. The diagnosis is usually made by the history, the clinical picture with breathing difficulty, hypoxemia, fever, chills, night sweat, weight loss, the chest x-ray characteristics, the propensity for oxygen desaturation on exercising, O concentration under 70, alveolar-arterial oxygen gradient over 35, elevated LDL and the recovering of the PCP organism on pulmonary washing or on lung biopsy.

Acute PCP is treated with IV Bactrim and IV steroid or steroid by mouth for 21 days.

Pentamidine IV can also be used in patients who are allergic to Bactrim. Pentamidine has serious cardiac, kidney, and pancreatic complications, including severe hypoglycemia (low blood sugar).

Other common lung diseases that afflict men include:
1. Sarcoidosis
2. Pulmonary hypertension
3. Pulmonary embolism
4. Hypersensitivity pneumonitis
5. Eosinophilic pneumonitis
6. Cystic fibrosis
7. Interstitial lung diseases, etc.,

Sarcoidosis is a very common disease of unknown etiology that frequently affects the lungs of men. The lungs are the most frequently affected organs with sarcoidosis and most definitely the most important organ to be affected by that disease.

The most frequent symptoms of pulmonary sarcoidosis are the following:
1. Shortness of breath
2. Coughing
3. Wheezing
4. Fever
5. Night sweats
6. Weight loss

Infiltrates and nodules of different sizes can be seen on chest x-ray. The pulmonary function test is abnormal in pulmonary sarcoidosis. In time, there will be the development of pulmonary fibrosis. The diagnosis of sarcoidosis is usually established by taking a biopsy of a pulmonary nodule during a bronchoscopic examination or by biopsying a palpable lymph node. The characteristic histopathological finding on tissues taken from a man with sarcoidosis is non-caseating granuloma. The angiotensin-1-converting enzyme blood test is usually elevated in men suffering from sarcoidosis. Sarcoidosis is a multi-system disease that affects many organs in the human body

Clinical manifestations of sarcoidosis

Sarcoidosis has the potential to affect all organs in the body and its manifestations may be felt throughout the body. The organs most frequently affected are the following:

1. The lungs
2. The lymph nodes
3. The eyes
4. The skin
5. The upper respiratory tract
6. The liver
7. The spleen
8. The bone marrow
9. The kidney
10. The heart
11. The nervous system
12. The endocrine system
13. The gastrointestinal tract
14. The exocrine glands and
15. The musculoskeletal system

The most frequent symptoms of sarcoidosis include:

1. Shortness of breath and wheezing
2. Cough
3. Fever
4. Night sweats
5. Weight loss
6. General weakness
7. Difficulty seeing
8. Kidney stones
9. Swollen joints
10. Hoarseness
11. Irregular pulse
12. Palpitations
13. Facial paralysis

14. Seizures

15. Excessive urination

About 90% of people with sarcoidosis have their lungs involved with the disease process. Approximately, 50% of these individuals develop permanent lung abnormalities and about 15% develop pulmonary fibrosis, and a significant percentage of these people go on to die of respiratory failure.

Fever of unknown origin is frequently due to sarcoidosis. Weight loss, night sweats, general weakness, and poor appetite can be seen in sarcoidosis. Blurry vision and bleeding into the eyes can also be seen in sarcoidosis, 25% of the time. The usual types of the eye problems that are frequently seen in sarcoidosis are uveitis, detached retina, etc. When the eyes are affected, soreness, redness and pain in the eyes with dryness can develop and if left untreated, blindness is the usual result.

Kidney stones with acute back pain and kidney stones in the urine can occur in sarcoidosis because of high serum calcium. Sarcoidosis is frequently associated with hypercalcemia (high serum calcium), and when the calcium is high in the blood, it can precipitate in the kidneys, resulting in calcium kidney stones.

Multiple and different joints and muscles can get involved in sarcoidosis, resulting in severe pain, arthralgias, arthritis, and different bone abnormalities. Carpal tunnel syndrome can also be seen in sarcoidosis. Muscle weakness, such as polymyositis, has also been described in sarcoidosis.

Sarcoidosis can involve the heart 5% of the time. The parts of the heart most frequently affected by sarcoidosis are the left ventricle, the conductive system causing complete heart block, etc. Both congestive heart failure and different types of cardiac arrhythmias can also occur in sarcoidosis.

The neurological system is commonly affected by sarcoidosis and in about 5% of the time a neurological finding is documented. Damage to the nerve, resulting in Bell's palsy (paralysis of one side of the face), can be seen in sarcoidosis. Damage to the liver and spleen can be seen in sarcoidosis, resulting in enlargement of both the liver and spleen, causing significant abnormalities in liver functions and white blood cells, red blood cells, as well as platelets.

The bone marrow is involved in about 40% of cases of sarcoidosis.

The manifestation of the bone marrow involvement with sarcoidosis is reflected by anemia, leukopenia, and thrombocytopenia.

The skin is commonly involved in sarcoidosis in up to 20%-25% of the cases.

Among the most commonly, seen skin lesions in cases of sarcoidosis are erythema nodosum and alopecia.

Enlargement of the lymph nodes is quite frequently seen in sarcoidosis.

Mediastinal nodes are enlarged in about 90% of patients with sarcoidosis. Other nodes that are frequently enlarged in sarcoidosis are axillary notes, cervical nodes, inguinal nodes, etc.

Several laboratory tests can be abnormal in sarcoidosis; examples are low white blood cells, low red blood cells, low platelets, high serum calcium, and high sedimentation rate. Steroid is the treatment of choice for all forms of sarcoidosis. Cytoxan can also be used in cases where the side effects of steroid are too bothersome.

Pulmonary failure leading to death can be the result of pulmonary sarcoidosis in many men who suffer from sarcoidosis.

Tuberculosis is one of the world's most common infections that affect the lungs.

Worldwide there are 2 billion people who are infected with tuberculosis.

Men are affected frequently by tuberculosis. In 1995, the World Health Organization reported that 8.8 million cases of tuberculosis occurred annualy worldwide and that 3 million people died in the world from tuberculosis during that same period. About 98% of these cases of tuberculosis occurred in the underdeveloped countries of the world.

About 10% of new tuberculosis cases that occur in the U.S. occur in individuals who were skin-test positive for TB, therefore that group of individuals serves as a reservoir for new TB cases.

The organism that causes tuberculosis is mycobacterium tuberculosis. Infected individuals with whom they come in contact infected men with tuberculosis through droplets that came from the lungs through sputum that is coughed up.

Once the TB organism enters into the lungs of the man being infected, it locates itself in the upper/posterior part of the lung, where the oxygenation of that area of the lung favors its growth.

Symptoms of pulmonary tuberculosis include:

1. Fever
2. Chills
3. Weight loss
4. Loss of appetite
5. Night sweats
6. Cough

7. Hemoptysis (coughing blood)
8. Shortness of breath

Findings on physical examinations may be positive for enlarged lymph nodes, large spleen, large liver, fever, and evidence of weight loss. Evidence of fluid in the lungs may show evidence of fluid around the heart (cardiac tamponade pericardial effusion). X-ray findings frequently seen in tuberculosis include:

1. Infiltrate seen on chest x-ray
2. Cavity seen on chest x-ray

Non-specific laboratory tests that may be abnormal in pulmonary tuberculosis:

1. Low white blood cells
2. High white blood cells
3. Low red blood cells (anemia)
4. Low platelet count
5. High platelet count
6. High serum calcium
7. High alkaline phosphatase
8. High serum protein
9. Low serum albumin
10. High LDH (lactic dehydrogenase)
11. Low serum sodium, etc.

Specific laboratory tests that are positive in pulmonary tuberculosis are as follows:

1. Acid fast bacteria (AFB) seen on stain of sputum coughed up by the patient.
2. Acid fast bacteria (AFB) seen on stain of washing/tissues taken during bronchial examination of the lungs/pleural biopsy of pleural fluid.
3. M. tuberculosis organism grown on AFB culture six weeks after it is plated on appropriate culture medium.
4. AFB organism seen on lymph node biopsy from patients suspected of suffering with tuberculosis

The pathological finding seen on tissue specimens taken from an individual suspected of suffering from tuberculosis is caseating granuloma.

Positive sputum for AFB does not necessarily mean that the person has M. tuberculosis because mycobacterium avium intracellulare (MAI) also stains positive for AFB. However, using DNA probe test, MAI can be differentiated from M. tuberculosis quickly.

How to test the skin for TB

When an individual has been exposed to a person infected with tuberculosis, the first thing to do is to plant a PPD 5TU on the person's arm. If the PPD is positive and the person being tested has not been vaccinated with BCG that then raises the possibility that the individual may in fact have been exposed to TB. That finding has an even stronger meaning if the person being tested is known to have had a negative PPD in the past. The PPD test must be read within 48 hours to 72 hours from the time it was planted.

The next thing to do is a chest x-ray. If the chest is positive for TB, then the man is treated for TB. If on the other hand, the chest x-ray is negative, the man then is to be given prophylaxis with Isoniazid (INH) 300mg daily for 6 months together with Vitamin B6 one tablet per day.

Treatment for tuberculosis

The medications that are used to treat M. tuberculosis are Rifampin, Isoniazid, Pyrazinamide, Ethambutol and Streptomycin. The usual period of time that individuals are treated for TB is 9–12 months. The usual adult doses of these medications are: 1) Isoniazid—150 mg by mouth twice a day; 2) Rifampin—300 mg by mouth twice per day; and 3) Pyrazinamide—2 grams per day by mouth and Ethambutol 15 mg/kg body weight per day by mouth and Streptomycin 10–15 mg/kg body weight per day. Usually after the first month of treatment, the sputum becomes negative for AFB.

During treatment for TB, complete blood count and liver function tests must be done every 6–8 weeks to monitor for possible low platelets, low white blood cells, low red cells count and medication-induced hepatitis with elevated liver function tests.

Another common disease of the lung that affects men is pulmonary embolism (clot in the lung).

Deep vein thrombophlebitis (DVT) is the condition that causes pulmonary embolism to develop in most instances. Every year 2.5 million individuals develop DVT in the US. The clot breaks off from the DVT and migrates into the lung resulting in pulmonary embolism.

Every year 600,000 individuals in the U.S. develop pulmonary embolism, resulting in 300,000 deaths, and many of these individuals are men. About 60,000 individuals die yearly in the U.S. because of undiagnosed pulmonary embolism.

Conditions that predispose men to pulmonary embolism include:

1. Obesity
2. Birth control
3. Hormone replacement therapy
4. Post-surgery immobilization
5. Multiple traumas
6. Immobilization after a stroke
7. Hypercoagulable state due to cancer of different types (secondary to thrombophylias)
8. Deep vein thrombophlebitis (DVT)
9. Polycythemia vera
10. Post-partum state
11. Elevated homocysteine level
12. Anti-thrombin III deficiency
13. Protein C deficiency
14. Protein S deficiency
15. Elevated lipoprotein—a
16. Factor V Leiden abnormality
17. Antiphospholipid antibody
18. Lupus anticoagulant ect,

The most frequent symptoms of pulmonary embolism consist of:

1. Shortness of breath
2. Tachycardia (rapid pulse rate)
3. Pleuritic chest pain
4. Sweating
5. Paleness
6. Restlessness
7. Coughing
8. Coughing up blood
9. Pain in calf muscle
10. Syncopal episode
11. In massive pulmonary embolism, sudden death can occur

Following the history and physical examination, the most sensitive tests to do to confirm the presence of pulmonary embolism consist of:

1. Arterial blood gas (ABG) 2. d-Dimer
3. Chest x-ray
4. Ultrasound of the liver extremities
5. Lung scan

The most definitive test to do to establish the diagnosis of pulmonary embolism is the pulmonary angiogram, but that test is hardly ever necessary nowadays because D-dimer; ultrasound of the lower extremities and the high probability lung scan are sufficient to arrive at the diagnosis of pulmonary embolism. The D-dimer blood test is extremely important because when pulmonary embolism is present, that test is positive. Whenever a clot is formed anywhere in the body, the D-dimer is elevated greater than 500 mg/ml. So if the lung scan is read as high probability for pulmonary embolism, the D-dimer is elevated, and if the ultrasound of the extremity shows a DVT, the possibility that the patient has pulmonary embolism is greater than 90%.

Treatment for pulmonary embolism

The treatment choice for pulmonary embolism is intravenous heparin. However, before starting heparin, several blood tests must be done:
1. Prothrombin time (PT)
2. Partial thromboplastin time (PTT)
3. Hematocrit
4. Platelet count
5. Stool hemoccult
6. Protein C
7. Proein S
8. Anti-thrombin III
9. Factor V Lieden
10. Prothrombin 2 gene mutation
11. Lupus anticoagulant
12. Anti-phospholipin antibody
13. Lipoprotein—a

Any abnormality from # 6 above to # 13 may be the reason why the DTV develops which then can lead to pulmonary embolism.

The importance of the PT and PTT is to ensure that the patient's coagulation system is working normally, so as not to precipitate bleeding. The importance of the platelet count is 1) to make sure the platelet count is not too low prior to starting heparin. 2) Do a baseline platelet count. 3) The rationale for establishing that the baseline platelet count is normal is that in the event that if the platelet count drops to 50% of the baseline platelet count that means that the patient is developing platelet-induced thrombocytopenia. Therefore, the heparin administration must be stopped immediately. The reason to check the hematocrit every day in a patient receiving heparin is that the heparin can cause bleeding to occur and a drop in hematocrit would document that. Checking the stool for blood every day is important, because if the stool is positive for blood, it means that the patient is bleeding and the heparin must be stopped.

Once these tests are done, then heparin can be infused as a 5000 unit's bolus IV, followed by 1000 units per hour intravenously. While on heparin, the patient must be monitored with daily PTT and CBC.

It is a good idea to keep the patient with pulmonary embolism on heparin for 7 to 10 days. Then Coumadin ought to be started while the patient is still on heparin. After 5 days of being on Coumadin the heparin can be stopped if the prothrombin time and the INR (international normalized ratio) are in therapeutic range. The Coumadin can be continued for 6 months to 1 year. Anticoagulation may need to be continued for life, if the pulmonary embolism is associated with a hereditary thrombophylia.

Another lung disease that afflicts men is primary pulmonary hypertension. The root cause of primary pulmonary hypertension is not known. The basic cause of that disease seems to be due to failure of the smooth muscles within some of the small vessels in the circulation of the lungs to relax, resulting in constriction and narrowing of these vessels, thereby impeding blood flow and oxygen flow. The most common symptoms of primary pulmonary hypertension are shortness of breath on exertion, fatigue, weakness, chest pain, syncope, etc. Physical findings include distended jugular veins, rales in the lungs, different abnormal heart sounds, swelling of lower legs and ankles, representing evidence of right failure, causing right lung symptoms.

Treatments of primary pulmonary hypertension include diuretics such as Lasix or Bumex by mouth or IV, digitalis by mouth, nasal oxygen, and anticoagulation to prevent pulmonary embolism. In certain cases lung transplantation can be tried.

Secondary pulmonary hypertension is associated with many cardio/pulmonary conditions and their treatments depend on the particular underlying disease.

There are many other diseases of the lungs that some men are afflicted which are not mentioned in this chapter.

The most preventable lung diseases that men suffer from are COPD/Emphysema and lung cancers; both of them are, in most part, due to tobacco smoking. About 47 million individuals in the U.S. smoke tobacco and a significant percentage of these individuals are men. Smoking tobacco is a deadly habit, which accounts for roughly 430,000 deaths per year in the United States, all of which are preventable. The way to put a stop to this trend is for men to stop smoking.

CHAPTER 20

THYROID DISEASES
IN MEN

THYROID DISEASES ARE QUITE COMMON in men. The thyroid gland is located in the neck and its normal functions are under the control of the pituitary gland, which produces the thyroid-stimulating hormone, which is located at the base of the brain. The hormones, which the thyroid secretes, are necessary for proper body functions. The most common diseases of the thyroid found in men are as follows:

1. Thyroid goiter
2. Hypothyroidism
3. Hyperthyroidism
4. Goiter disease
5. Acute thyroiditis
6. Chronic thyroiditis
7. Hashisoto's thyroiditis
8. Thyroid nodules
9. Thyroid cancer

There are two different types of goiters: simple goiter and nontoxic goiter. Simple goiter is quite common in men and is due to lack of iodine in the water and diet of those who are affected. Simple goiter causes enlargement of the thyroid gland. Toxic goiter occurs when the thyroid gland is enlarged because of either an acute inflammation of the thyroid gland or thyroid cancer.

Hypothyroidism

Hypothyroidism occurs because of failure of the thyroid gland to produce enough thyroid hormone. The most frequent causes of hypothyroidism consist of: 1) Surgical removal of the thyroid gland, due to disease, 2) Destruction of the thyroid gland with radioactive iodine as treatment for hyperthyroidism, 3) Hashisoto's thyroiditis with resulting hypothyroidism.

Hyperthyroidism is sometimes seen in association with lupus, vitiligo, rheumatoid arthritis and pernicious anemia.

Sometimes the neck becomes painful and a man may think he has an ordinary sore throat, and sometimes it occurs with no symptoms at all. Both acute and sub-acute thyroiditis can lead to either transient or permanent hypothyroidism.

Hyperthyroidism is divided in two major parts:
1. Hyperthyroidism due to excessive production of thyroid hormones, resulting in the clinical hyperthyroid state
2. Grave diseases with its three parts:
    a. A large goiter
    b. Large protruding eyes (exophthalmus)
    c. Skin abnormalities (dermatopathy)

Cancer of the thyroid

About 6.4% of men have thyroid nodules. Most of those nodules are not malignant. There are two types of thyroid nodules: hot nodule and cold nodule. Hot nodules are usually benign and are not cancerous. Most cold nodules are not associated with cancer, but when local thyroid cancers develop, frequently, they arise from a cold nodule. Because the thyroid gland is extremely vascular, a lot of blood passes through it, and consequently metastatic cancer of the thyroid from lung, breast, melanoma and esophagus occur frequently. Lymphoma of the thyroid also occurs and represents about 5% of all thyroid cancers.

The most common form of thyroid cancer is papillary carcinoma, which is 70% of thyroid cancers. Follicular carcinoma represents 15% of thyroid cancer, and anaplastic cancer of the thyroid occurs 5% of the time. The most malignant and aggressive type of thyroid cancer is the follicular type.

Among the risks for the development of thyroid cancer are being female and exposure to radiation. Men who have had radiation treatment to their tonsils as a child have high incidence of thyroid cancer when they become adults.

To diagnose thyroid cancer, the first thing to do is to:

1. Take history from the patient.
2. Palpate the thyroid gland, looking for a nodule.
3. Examine carefully the anterior and posterior cervical areas of the neck, looking for enlargement of nodes.
4. Do a thyroid scan.
5. Do a thyroid ultrasound.
6. Do thyroid function tests (T4 and TSH).
7. Do a fine-needle aspiration biopsy of the thyroid nodule (that is done usually by an endocrinologist) or by a surgeon.

Once biopsy documents that thyroid cancer is present, surgical removal of the thyroid gland must be carried out. The extent of the surgical incision depends on the cell type of the cancer. Following resection of the thyroid cancer, radioactive iodine must be administered to destroy all remaining thyroid tissues. The other necessary treatment is Synthroid by mouth both for suppression and treatment for life. There is no effective chemotherapy available for thyroid cancer except for VP16 which has shown some response. Men with thyroid cancer must remain under the care of an endocrinologist for many years.

Symptoms, physical findings, evaluation and treatment of thyroid goiter

The first sign of goiter is a swelling in the neck, either on both sides or on one side. On palpitation of the neck, the goiter can be felt.

On auscultation with a stethoscope, a bruit sometimes can be heard. Sometimes the goiter may be located under the collarbone and is seen only during x-ray test of the upper chest. Sometimes the first indication that a person has goiter is difficulty swallowing or breathing, due to pressure on the trachea and upper esophagus, and at times hoarseness can occur due to pressure on the vocal cords.

To evaluate a thyroid goiter, the tests that are done are ultrasound of the neck along with a thyroid scan.

Treatment of thyroid goiter consists of surgical removal or suppressive treatment with Synthroid to try to shrink the size of the gland.

Symptoms, evaluations and treatment by hyperthyroidism

The symptoms of hyperthyroidism (overactive thyroid gland) are as follows: weight loss, diarrhea, agitation, insomnia, palpitations, cardiac arrhythmia, chest pain, shortness of breath, poor appetite, weakness, depression, nervousness, sweatiness, warm feeling, psychosis, mental confusion, poor memory and possible thyroid storm, etc. The usual findings on physical examination of men who are suffering from hyperthyroidism/Graves' disease includes:

1. Large thyroid gland, tender or non-tender
2. Protruding eyes
3. Fine, smooth skin
4. Sweaty palms
5. Fast pulse rate
6. Irregular heartbeat
7. Fluid in the lungs
8. Heart murmur.

Laboratory evaluations in hyperthyroidism consist of:

1. Serum T4, TSH, free T4 and T3
2. ANA, serum B12
3. CBC
4. Reticulocytes count
5. Liver Function Tests
6. Anti-thyroid antibody and anti-microsomal antibodies
7. Thyroid scan
8. Thyroid ultrasound

In hyperthyroidism, serum T4, T3 and free T4 are high and serum TSH (thyroid-stimulating hormone) is low.

There is a subgroup of hyperthyroidism called apathetic hyperthyroidism (or T3 thyrotoxicosis) with high serum T3 and low serum TSH, seen often in elderly men.

These men usually become bed-bound and show no obvious signs of overactive thyroid, except for a fast heart rate, weakness, poor appetite and poor memory. The fast heart rate and the apathetic look in the patient's face are the red flags that overactive thyroid is responsible for the patient's total body weakness which, if left untreated, can lead to the death of the affected man.

Graves' disease is a form of hyperthyroidism (overactive thyroid) state, during which the thyroid gland is enlarged and tender. The eyes are markedly enlarged (exophthalmus), the skin areas that are affected are thickened and edematous. The swelling around the eyes is due to infiltration by lymphocytes and mononuclear cells. Graves' disease occurs commonly in men. Graves' disease may be an autoimmune disease. There exists a link between Graves' disease, Hashisoto's disease, hypothyroidism, pernicious anemia and vitiligo, etc.

The evaluations of Graves' disease (hyperthyroidism) are as described earlier. The treatments of Graves' disease are the same as that of hyperthyroidism.

The different types of treatments used to treat hyperthyroidism are as follows: high

1. Surgical removal of part of the thyroid
2. Medication to suppress the thyroid glands' ability to produce thyroid hormone
3. Steroid IV or PO
4. Radioactive iodine to destroy the thyroid glands

Treatments that are preferable to treat hyperthyroidism in men who are pregnant are surgical removal of the thyroid gland or administering Propylthiouracil by mouth. In men who are not in childbearing age or who are elderly, radioactive iodine is preferable. For men who present with hyperthyroidism and a fast heart rate, Inderal by mouth is given to slow the rate of the heart down to prevent cardiac decompensation and possible cardiac arrhythmia that can develop if the heart rate is allowed to remain fast. Whether or not the treatment is given inside the hospital or in the office setup depends on the judgment of the treating physician or how sick the patient looks.

The next thing to do is to give medication to shut down the production of thyroid hormones. The most frequently used anti-thyroid medications are Propylthiouracil and Tapazole. The usual dose of Propylthiouracil is 100 to 150 mg every 6 or 8 hours, by mouth. Propylthiouracil works to decrease the symptoms of hyperthyroidism by preventing the conversion of T4 to T3 in the bloodstream. Tapazole works to decrease the symptoms of hyperthyroidism by inhibiting the production of thyroid hormone by the thyroid gland. The usual dose of Tapazole is 30–40mg in divided doses 2–3 times per day by mouth.

In the acute hyperthyroidism state to prevent the so-called thyroid storm, large doses of Dexamethasone 2 grams every 6 hours can be given in addition, to reduce the level of T4 in the body, thereby improving the overall condition of the affected man. Either Propylthiouracil or Tapazole can be used for up to 2 years, while a decision is being made regarding a long-term modality of treatment. During the administration of these medications, a complete blood count must be done every month or so, because leukopenia and low platelet count can develop.

When it is decided based on clinical facts and the appropriate patients that radioactive iodine is the treatment modality, an endocrinologist will administer the proper dose of radioactive iodine to the patient to destroy the thyroid gland. Following the administration of the radioactive iodine, the patient will be monitored for many years, waiting for the development of the hypothyroidism state, which is guaranteed to develop in time. When the T4 and TSH evaluation indicates that the patient has developed hypothyroidism, then Synthroid by mouth for life will be given to him.

Hypothyroidism is much more common in women than men. Some of the conditions that can cause hypothyroidism include:

1. Surgical removal of the thyroid gland
2. Treatment with radioactive iodine to treat overactive-state thyroid gland
3. Hashisoto's thyroiditis

Hashisoto's thyroiditis is a chronic inflammatory/autoimmune disease that, when present, causes the thyroid gland to hypo-function, resulting in the state of hypothyroidism. Hashisoto's thyroiditis is frequently seen associated with pernicious anemia, rheumatoid arthritis, systemic lupus erythematosus, diabetes mellitus, and adrenal deficiency.

Sometime Hashisoto's thyroiditis can present with a goiter, but frequently there are no obvious physical findings in the thyroid gland.

Symptoms of Hypothyroidism:

1. Weight gain
2. Tiredness
3. Sleepiness
4. Hair loss
5. Depression
6. Slow heart rate
7. Anemia
8. Dry skin
9. Swollen legs
10. Irregular menstrual periods
11. Bleeding between menstrual periods
12. Loss of eyebrows, etc.

The diagnosis is usually made when a patient presents to the doctor with complaints of not feeling well, feeling tired, and other vague complaints, and an evaluation is carried out which includes T4 and TSH blood tests. If the T4 is low and the TSH is high that establishes a diagnosis of hypothyroidism. If the T4 is normal and the TSH is high that also establishes the diagnosis of normal T4 hypothyroidism. Other tests to order are anti-thyroid antibody and anti microsomal antibody, ANA, B12, rheumatoid factor, ESR, and fasting blood sugar. If the anti-thyroid is positive, the diagnosis of Hashisoto's thyroiditis is established.

The next thing to do is a thyroid scan, to look at the anatomy of the thyroid gland. Once these tests have been done, then treatment with Synthroid can be started. Hashisoto's thyroiditis may be responsible for 90% of the cases of the cases of hypothyroidism. It does not matter what causes the state of hypothyroidism; once it occurs, the treatment choice is thyroid hormone replacement, and most of the time for life.

The dose of Synthroid that is used to treat hypothyroidism in mcg must be individualized from patients to patients, while monitoring the serum T4 and TSH to adjust the dose.

About the author

VALIERE ALCENA, M.D., F.A.C.P.,

Dr. Alcena is a clinician and a medical educator. He is in private practice of internal medicine hematology and medical oncology in White Plains N.Y.

He is clinical professor of medicine at Albert Einstein College of Medicine Bronx New York and Adjunct professor of medicine at New York Medical College Valhalla N.Y.

Dr Alcena is the 2007 winner of the ICM teacher of the year Award from the Albert Einstein College of Medicine of Yeshiva University Bronx N.Y.

Dr Alcena has beeen elected to the American College of Physicians as MASTER (MACP).

He is founder and Chairman of the Minority Affairs Committee at Albert Einstein College of Medicine Bronx N.Y.

He is Chief Emeritus of the Department of Medicine at St Agnes Hospital White Plains N.Y.

He is former co-Director of the Department of Medicine at St Agnes Hospital White Plains N.Y.

He is founder of the Annual Sam Seifter Lecture at Albert Einstein College of Medicine Bronx N.Y.

He is a TV Journalist, TV producer and host of two Award winning TV shows

He is President, Publisher and Editor of LeNegre Publishing of White Plains N.Y.

He is Editor in Chief of Prestige Medical News

He is President and CEO of Alcena Medical Communications INC.

He is Chairman of White Plains Cable Access Commission-City of White Plains N.Y.

He is founder and Chairman of the Board of Alcena Africa Hunger Relief Fund

He is founder, President and Chairman of the Board of White Plains Community Health Fair INC

His previous books are:

1. Women's Health and Wellness for the Millennium, Published by LeNegre Publishing (Hard Cover) June, 2005
2. Women's Health and Wellness for the Millennium, Published by LeNegre Publishing (Paper Back) Feb, 2006
3. *African American Women's Health Book*, published by Barricade Books. 2001.
4. *AIDS, The Expanding Epidemic: What the Public Needs to Know, A Multi-Cultural Overview*, published by Alcena Medical Communications, Inc., 1994.
5. *The African American Health Book*, New York Citadel Press. Carol Publishing Group (paperback edition), 1994.
6. *The African American Health Book*, New York Birch Lane Press. Carol Publishing Group, 1994.(Hard Cover)
7. *Third World Tropical Diet, Health, Maintenance and Medical Management-Program*. Published by Alcena Medical Communications, Inc., 1992.
8. *The Status of Health of Blacks in the United States of America: A Prescription for Improvement*, published by Kendall/Hunt Publishing Company, 1992.
9. He has published numerous articles in many prestigious medical Journals About health issues
10. Dr Alcena is the physician who first proposed the idea that male circumcision would decrease the incidence of HIV/AIDS in August of 1986 in the NY State Journal of Med. He has been fully credited in the medical literature for this extraordinary contribution to the scientific world and humankind which is helping to solve some of the problems in HIV/AIDS epidemic.
11. He has lectured all over the US and Internationally.
12 He is a well-respected Book reviewer and reviews scientific articles for prestigious medical Journals.

978-0-595-45782-3
0-595-45782-7

Made in the USA